Disorders of Human Learning, Behavior, and Communication

Ronald L. Taylor and Les Sternberg
Series Editors

James K. Luiselli

Editor

Behavioral Medicine and Developmental Disabilities

Springer-Verlag
New York Berlin Heidelberg
London Paris Tokyo

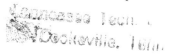

James K. Luiselli, Behavioral and Educational Resource Associates, Concord, Massachusetts 01742, USA

Series Editors: Ronald L. Taylor and Les Sternberg, Exceptional Student Education, Florida Atlantic University, Boca Raton, Florida 33431-0991, USA

Library of Congress Cataloging-in-Publication Data
Behavioral medicine and developmental disabilities.
   (Disorders of human learning, behavior, and
communication)
   Includes bibliographies.
   1. Medicine and psychology.   I. Luiselli, James K.
II. Series. [DNLM: 1. Behavior Therapy.   2. Child
Development Disorders.   WS 350.6 B4184]
R726.5.B4252 1989   616.89′142   88-29475
ISBN 0-387-96875-X (alk. paper)

Printed on acid-free paper

Typeset by Publishers Service, Bozeman, Montana.
Printed and bound by Edwards Brothers, Ann Arbor, Michigan.
Printed in the United States of America.

9 8 7 6 5 4 3 2 1

ISBN 0-387-96875-X Springer-Verlag New York Berlin Heidelberg
ISBN 3-540-96875-X Springer-Verlag Berlin Heidelberg New York

Preface

As a graduate student a decade ago, I recall vividly reading the inaugural issue of the *Journal of Behavioral Medicine* when it appeared in 1978. Its purpose was described as "a broadly conceived interdisciplinary publication devoted to furthering our understanding of physical health and illness through knowledge and techniques of behavioral science." The articles in that first issue addressed such topics as the biofeedback treatment of neuromuscular disorders, anxiety management of Type A behavior, and premorbid psychological factors related to cancer incidence. At that time, coursework in behavioral medicine was in its infancy at my university, and I, along with many classmates, was eager to learn more of this "new and emerging field."

Thinking back to those times, it is astonishing for one to reflect on the rapid evolution of behavioral medicine and its current status as a clinical and scientific discipline. Organizations such as the Society of Behavioral Medicine now include a broad-based membership that is convened yearly at a major convention. In addition to the *Journal of Behavioral Medicine*, professionals can avail themselves of several other specialty journals (*Annals of Behavioral Medicine*, *Behavioral Medicine Abstracts*, *Journal of Developmental and Behavioral Pediatrics*) as well as the numerous articles on behavioral medicine that appear regularly in the clinical psychology, psychiatry, rehabilitation, and behavior therapy literature. And behavioral medicine services and training programs are encountered with increasing frequency within clinic, hospital, and academic settings.

Keeping pace with the latest developments in behavioral medicine can be an arduous task for even the most fastidious reader. For this reason, edited volumes provide a useful function by presenting timely reviews of topical areas, synthesizing research findings, and critically evaluating our current knowledge base. In recent years, several such volumes have been prepared on both general issues in behavioral medicine and more narrowly defined clinical categories (e.g., behavioral pediatrics). This book also represents an attempt to consolidate our recent clinical and research advances, but differs from previous volumes in two primary ways. First, whereas the majority of prior books have concentrated on the population of nonhandicapped persons, the present edition addresses the topic of behavioral medicine treatment and research with developmentally disabled individuals. The involvement of behavioral medicine specialists with handicapped persons has been expanding over the years, given advances in biomedical research, refinements in treatment technology, and the growing alliance among psychologists and physicians. Second, this book focuses on the contributions of applied behavior analysis to assessment, intervention, and evaluation. Behavior analysts have been instrumental in the design of habilitation programs for developmentally disabled persons and, from the beginning, have helped shape and define the field of behavioral medicine as a whole. Although several journal articles and book chapters have described behavioral medicine applications with handicapped persons, this book is one of the first efforts to present this information in the context of a single edited volume.

The book is geared toward clinicians, physicians, practitioners, researchers, and advanced graduate students in the areas of psychology, rehabilitation, special education, and medicine. Psychologists and physicians should find the book useful in identifying effective therapeutic strategies and methods to design comprehensive therapy programs. Because of the integrated review of experimental findings contained in the book, academic and applied researchers will be able to locate timely data from varied perspectives. The critical appraisal of research provided by the authors should also aid in the design and implementation of future studies. The student population can utilize the book as a reference source that provides an overview of specialized areas of treatment and research. As always, it will be left to the reader to decide whether these objectives have been fulfilled.

I am indebted to the people at Springer-Verlag for their support and assistance throughout the conception and completion of this work. Special thanks are also extended to Dr. Ronald L. Taylor and Dr. Les Sternberg for providing much help along the way. I am grateful to many colleagues, too numerous to mention, who have helped shape my thinking over the years, given encouragement, and lent an ear. Finally, this book is dedicated to my parents, who have always been my finest teachers and a constant source of love and inspiration.

James K. Luiselli

Contents

Contributors

Kathryn Larsen Burgio, PHD, Section on Geriatric Medicine, University of Pittsburgh School of Medicine, Pittsburgh, PA 15213, USA.

Louis D. Burgio, PHD, University of Pittsburgh School of Medicine, Pittsburgh, PA 15213, USA.

Ronald S. Drabman, PHD, Department of Psychiatry and Human Behavior, University of Mississippi Medical Center, Jackson, MS 39216, USA.

Robert A. Fox, PHD, School of Education, Marquette University, Milwaukee, WI 53233, USA.

Carol Lewis, PHD, Private practice, Gainesville, FL 32601, USA.

Thomas R. Linscheid, PHD, Department of Pediatrics, Children's Hospital, Columbus, OH 43205, USA.

James K. Luiselli, EDD, Behavioral and Educational Resource Associates, Concord, MA 01742, USA.

Donald J. Meyer, PHD, School of Education, Marquette University, Milwaukee, WI 53233, USA.

James A. Mulick, PHD, Department of Psychology, Ohio State University, Columbus, OH 43205, USA.

L. Kaye Rasnake, PHD, Department of Pediatrics, Children's Hospital, Columbus, OH 43205, USA.

Anthony F. Rotatori, PHD, School of Education and Allied Professions, Fairfield University, Fairfield, CT 06430, USA.

Nirbhay N. Singh, PHD, Educational and Research Service Center, Northern Illinois University, DeKalb, IL 60115, USA.

Lori A. Sisson, PHD, Department of Psychiatry, Western Psychiatric Institute and Clinic, Pittsburgh, PA 15261, USA.

Don P. Sugai, PhD, Department of Behavioral Medicine and Psychiatry, Lahey Clinic Medical Center, Burlington, MA 01803, USA.

Kenneth J. Tarnowski, PhD, Department of Pediatrics, Children's Hospital, Columbus, OH 43205, USA.

Vincent B. Van Hasselt, PhD, Department of Psychiatry and Human Behavior, Irvine Medical Center, Orange, CA 92668, USA.

Alan S.W. Winton, PhD, Department of Psychology, Massey University, Christchurch, New Zealand.

1
Behavioral Medicine, Behavior Therapy, and Developmental Disabilities: An Overview

JAMES K. LUISELLI

In its broadest terms, behavioral medicine represents, "the integration of behavioral and biomedical expertise in the search for solutions to problems of health and illness" (Schwartz & Weiss, 1978, p. 4). Although scientific inquiry in the behavioral sciences and medicine has a long history, the confluence of these disciplines is a relatively new area of investigation. Some authors have suggested that the term *behavioral medicine* first appeared in 1973 with the publication of Birk's volume, *Behavioral Medicine: Biofeedback* (Blanchard, 1982; Russo & Varni, 1982). Beginning in 1977, significant organizing events occurred, such as the Yale Conference on Behavioral Medicine and the formation of special-interest groups such as the Society of Behavioral Medicine and the Academy of Behavioral Medicine Research. Another area of development originating in the late 1970s was the establishment of several university-affiliated centers specializing in behavioral medicine treatment and research. As an outflow of this increased clinical and experimental activity, scholarly publications in behavioral medicine proliferated during the decade of 1977 to 1987. These include the appearance of peer-refereed journals (*Journal of Behavioral Medicine, Annals of Behavioral Medicine*) and numerous texts addressing general issues in behavioral medicine (Ferguson & Taylor, 1980; Pomerleau & Brady, 1979; Williams & Gentry, 1977), as well as more circumscribed target areas such as cardiology (Surwit, Williams, & Shapiro, 1982), rehabilitation (Ince, 1976), and pediatrics (Russo & Varni, 1982; Varni, 1983).

Although behavioral medicine clearly appears to be a discipline "whose time has come," there is still no uniformly accepted definition of the field. In fact, as discussed subsequently, considerable disagreement prevails concerning focus, scope, and methodology. As with any emerging, investigative area, definitive boundary conditions have yet to be established. It is, perhaps, more useful to view behavioral medicine as a *general orientation* towards the psychological and environmental treatment of illness and disease rather than a fixed set of principles and procedures.

The intent of this chapter is to provide an overview of behavioral medicine, its relevance to the treatment of developmentally disabled persons, and the components comprising a behavior therapeutic approach.[1] The chapter begins with a discussion of several trends that influenced the emergence of behavioral medicine as a specialty discipline. Next, various definitions of the field are compared and contrasted in an effort to identify commonalities and divergent interpretations. This is followed with a presentation of behavior analysis assessment, treatment, and evaluation methodologies. The chapter concludes by discussing the importance of behavioral medicine treatment and research with developmentally disabled persons.

Trends and Influences

The establishment of behavioral medicine as an area of clinical practice and scientific inquiry cannot be linked to a single point of origin. Rather, its development appears to be the result of several trends related to health care service delivery, conceptualizations of illness, advances in treatment methodologies, and cross-fertilization among disciplines. Blanchard (1982), for example, traces the evolution of behavioral medicine to three patterns initiating in the late 1960s and early 1970s. One development was the growing alliance between behaviorally oriented psychologists and physicians. As a function of their involvement in university-affiliated hospitals and clinics, behavioral psychologists began applying treatment strategies demonstrated to be effective with psychiatric patients to clients referred from such departments as neurology, gastroenterology, and internal medicine. To illustrate, clinical studies by Hersen and associates out of the University of Mississippi Medical Center revealed positive therapeutic effects from behavioral intervention programs for spasmodic torticollis (Bernhardt, Hersen, & Barlow, 1972), anorexia nervosa (Elkin, Hersen, Eisler, & Williams, 1972), and conversion reaction (Kallman, Hersen, & O'Toole, 1975). Other examples of this increasing psychological-medical affiliation include interventions for smoking (Lichtenstein, 1982), insomnia (Borkovec, 1982), and chronic pain (Keefe, 1982).

The second influence suggested by Blanchard (1982) was biofeedback. The process of biofeedback consists of detecting and amplifying the body's bioelectrical potentials, transforming this information into comprehensible stimuli, and making it available (feeding it back) to the individual. In this manner, one learns to control physiological responses that are usually considered to be involuntary or responses that are normally controllable but are no longer so due to disease or trauma (Blanchard & Epstein, 1978). At about the time of the late 1960s, most biofeedback research concerned the self-regulation of bodily processes such as heart rate, galvanic skin response (GSR), and electroencephalographic activity (EEG). The demonstration of learned control over these and other responses led to applications of biofeedback for the treatment of

---

[1]The terms *behavior therapy, behavior modification*, and *applied behavior analysis* are used synonymously throughout the text of this chapter (cf. Kazdin, 1982a; Rimm & Masters, 1979).

medical disorders. For instance, cardiovascular biofeedback methods were utilized for the regulation of blood pressure in patients with hypertension; vascular conditioning approaches were applied to treat migraine headache and Raynaud's disease. Similarly, the results of earlier studies on motor control were translated into therapy programs for muscular reeducation in cerebral palsy and poststroke rehabilitation (Epstein, Malone, & Cunningham, 1978). Presently, biofeedback is one of the most frequently employed therapeutic modalities in behavioral medicine.

The final significant influence on behavioral medicine was a change in the epidemiology of disease. As Blanchard (1982) notes, by the decade of the 1960s the threat of acute, infectious disease had largely been overcome. The challenge to medical practice now became the management of chronic illness. This shift in focus brought with it a heightened awareness of the role of psychological, behavioral, and environmental factors in the pathogenesis and maintenance of chronic disease states. Thus, issues such as exposure to stress, Type A behavior pattern, sedentary lifestyle, and diet were implicated in the development of coronary heart disease (Surwit et al., 1982). With recognition of these and similar causal variables, behavioral psychologists became involved in the area of "lifestyle management," in effect, teaching individuals to control those influences contributing to their medical problems. The concern for therapeutic intervention also included training afflicted persons to cope more effectively with the sequelae of their illness as, for example, teaching cancer patients to control the toxic side effects from chemotherapy (Redd & Andresen, 1981). Enhancing adherence to therapeutic regimens and compliance with medication taking represents another target area brought to the forefront with an emerging emphasis on chronic care (Epstein & Cluss, 1982).

Finally, the growth of behavioral medicine over the past decade likely reflects certain limitations of traditional medical practice (Epstein, Katz, & Zlutnick, 1979). For one, "psychological" treatment may lead to fewer side effects when contrasted to invasive physical procedures or pharmacological management. Also, the cost efficiency of health care delivery may be enhanced. This is particularly true since many behavioral medicine approaches stress the self-management of treatment protocols. In some cases, patients may request alternative methods over those offered in typical medical settings. And lastly, the application of behavioral and psychological principles have been utilized in preparing patients for surgery (Varni, 1983), reducing distress during medical evaluations (Melamed, Robbins, & Graves, 1982), and organizing intensive care units (Cataldo, Jacobs, & Rogers, 1982), thereby increasing the proficiency of hospital-administered services.

Definitions

The Yale Conference on Behavioral Medicine was convened in 1976 and was one of the first organizing efforts of this newly emerging and rapidly expanding field. The conference brought together a diverse group of behavioral and biomedical scientists with the goals of defining behavioral medicine, its content areas, and exclusion criteria. The definition emanating from the conference was reported subsequently by Schwartz and Weiss (1978). It reads:

Behavioral medicine is the field concerned with the development of behavioral science knowledge and techniques relevant to the understanding of physical health and illness and the application of this knowledge and those techniques to prevention, diagnosis, treatment, and rehabilitation. Psychosis, neurosis, and substance abuse are included only in so far as they contribute to physical disorders as an end point (p. 7).

In addition to presenting this definition, Schwartz and Weiss (1978) discussed some of the issues stressed by the conference participants and emphasized in the formal description. First, they indicated that the intent of the conference definition was to describe behavioral medicine in terms that were neither "too narrow nor too broad." This qualifier resulted in a definition that clearly focused upon the integration of behavioral and biomedical sciences but was not restricted to a specific orientation within these fields. Thus, psychology, sociology, anthropology, education, epidemiology, biostatistics, and psychiatry were considered to be equally relevant disciplines. Similarly, behavioral medicine was viewed as multidimensional in scope including the areas of etiology, diagnosis, pathogenesis, treatment, rehabilitation, and prevention. Another important characteristic was the attention given to issues of both disease *and* health. It became essential to define behavioral medicine not only as an approach to the therapeutic management of chronic conditions, but also as a methodology to promote physical well-being. As for research orientation, basic, applied, and therapeutic trials were included. Areas of research excluded from the Yale Conference definition were mental illness, substance abuse, mental retardation, and social welfare problems per se.

The description of behavioral medicine offered by Schwartz and Weiss (1978) constitutes a broad-spectrum approach with regard to treatment modality. Clinical and preventive interventions, for example, are derived equally from psychosocial, physiological, sociocultural, and environmental influences. However, not all descriptors of the field are characterized by such a multifaceted perspective. Behavior therapists in particular have attempted to bring the evolution and current status of behavioral medicine more within the domain of learning theory and experimental psychology. Agras (1975) noted that medical professionals tended to underemphasize the relationship between behavior and health until behavior modification procedures were demonstrated to be clinically efficacious. In commenting on the types of activities within the purview of behavioral medicine, Mostofsky (1981) stated: "The behavior therapist, perhaps more than any other, occupies a prominent position in his/her ability to contribute significantly to the formulation of treatment and clinical services" (p. 449). Similar views have been posited by other contemporary theorists (Pomerleau, 1982; Varni, 1983).

Pomerleau (1979) highlights the integration of behavioral psychology and behavioral medicine with this definition:

Behavioral medicine consists of (a) the clinical use of techniques derived from the experimental analysis of behavior – behavior therapy and behavior modification – for the prevention, management, or treatment of physical disease or physiological dysfunction, and (b) the conduct of research contributing to the functional analysis and understanding of behavior associated with medical disorders and problems of health care (p. 656).

This more narrowly focused description equates behavioral medicine with the study and manipulation of respondent, operant, and social learning principles within the framework of an applied behavior analytic methodology. In a similar vein, Surwit, Feinglos, and Scovern (1983) defined behavioral medicine "in terms of inducing changes in both physiology and behavior using behavioral techniques. Intervention is aimed either at direct behavioral manipulation of physiology or at alteration of secondary behaviors related to disease or its therapy" (p. 257).

To underscore further the differences in descriptive terminology, consider Matarazzo's (1980) distinctions between behavioral medicine, behavioral health, and health psychology. His definition of behavioral medicine is the interdisciplinary field concerned with the treatment of disease, illness, and health-threatening conditions. Behavioral health is considered to be a specialty area within behavioral medicine aimed at disease prevention and health maintenance in nonafflicted persons. Health psychology is the field that addresses specifically the role of psychological processes in medicine.

Although divergent opinions regarding the focus, methods, and directions of behavioral medicine are readily apparent, it is also true that commonalities exist among descriptions. In fact, as stated previously, it is, perhaps, more productive to define behavioral medicine as a general orientation and not a discipline-bound approach. The concentration on behavior therapy and analysis in this volume, for example, is not intended to equate behavioral medicine with this particular theoretical and clinical viewpoint. Instead, behavior therapy is viewed as one methodology, perhaps a subspecialty, within the interdisciplinary field that combines behavioral science and medical expertise.

Characteristics of Behavior Therapy and Analysis in Behavioral Medicine

Behavior therapy shares a common ground with many of the goals and objectives stated in the previous descriptions of behavioral medicine. It is also comprised of principles, strategies, and procedures that distinguish it from other "psychological" doctrine. The purpose of this section is to review these similar and unique characteristics.

Interdisciplinary

One area of consensus among descriptions of behavioral medicine is that the field is interdisciplinary in scope. Varni (1983) addresses cogently the distinction between *multi*disciplinary and *inter*disciplinary approaches:

Multidisciplinary refers to activities involving the efforts of professionals from a number of disciplines approaching the patient primarily through an uncoordinated discipline-specific fashion. This approach requires that each professional only know the skills specific to his/her own discipline. In contrast, the interdisciplinary approach requires that physicians, nurses, physical therapists, occupational therapists, medical social workers, psychologists, and other allied health professionals have a working knowledge of the other team members' skills and specialties. Thus, the interdisciplinary approach is synergistic, integrating the knowledge and skills from the various disciplines into a coordinated plan for patient care (pp. 4–5).

An interdisciplinary perspective, then, is formulated on an integrated and inter-dependent team concept. Within the field of behavioral pediatrics as an example, specialists must consider factors such as developmental psychology, children's attitude towards illness, psychosocial impact of hospitalization, and family dynamics as well as the particulars of medical knowledge pertaining to specific disorders (Russo & Varni, 1982). Within developmental disabilities, practitioners should have a working knowledge in the areas of abnormal development, genetics, special education, and pharmacology just to name a few. This interdisciplinary model extends to a familiarity with diagnostic, assessment, evaluation, and therapeutic practices.

   Although the early history of behavior therapy in behavioral medicine suggests a somewhat isolated stance (primarily because behavioral clinicians were typically sought out "when all else fails"), present conditions reflect a growing interdisciplinary flavor. More and more, behavioral psychologists are becoming regular additions to "in-house" hospital and clinic staffs. Both medical school and residency training programs are showing an increasing collaborative relationship with behaviorally oriented professionals (Christophersen & Abernathy, 1982). This integration between disciplines is exemplified in subsequent chapters on professional training and behavioral consultation (Chapters 8 and 9).

Basic and Applied Research

Another common feature of most descriptions of behavioral medicine is the inclusion of both basic and applied research experimentation. As noted by Russo, Bird, and Masek (1980), behavioral medicine researchers should be concerned not only with the evaluation of methods that produce symptomatic relief but also with identifying underlying mechanisms responsible for maladaptive functioning. This attention to basic processes such as biochemistry and electrophysiology contributes to a better understanding of the etiology of certain pathological conditions and how these indices covary with therapeutic intervention.

   Illustrations of the interaction between basic and applied research include the application of behavioral assessment methods to demonstrate how overt seizure activity corresponds to moment-by-moment alterations in electroencephalographic patterns (Cataldo, Russo, & Freeman, 1979) and how electromyography is affected in the operant control of neuromuscular orofacial dysfunction (Parker et al., 1984). Similarly, infrahuman research has identified the influence of specific neurotransmitters (serotonin, dopamine) on agitated/aggressive responding, findings that may provide a biological explanation for some forms of self-injurious behavior (Cataldo & Harris, 1982). As another illustration, Sandman et al. (1983) hypothesized that the presence of self-injury in some disabled clients may stem from increased pain thresholds that, in turn, exist due to elevated levels of endogenous opiates. In a study with two self-injurious, mentally retarded adults, these investigators were able to reduce occurrences of self-injury following injections of naloxone, an opiate antagonist. And Nidiffer, Iwata, Kelly, and Ward-Zimmerman (1983) documented biochemical changes concurrent with a reduction in self-mutilation in a child with Lesch-Nyhan syndrome. These cases highlight how the study of interrelationships between basic biological mechanisms and behavior can lead to advances in the conceptual understanding and clinical management of certain behavioral/medical disorders.

Therapeutic Management and Prevention

Essentially all descriptions of behavioral medicine have emphasized a dual focus on treatment and prevention. Behavior therapy and analysis are concerned with similar efforts. In effect, three preventive, intervention perspectives may be identified (Luiselli, 1987; Masek, Epstein, & Russo, 1981). First, *tertiary prevention* addresses the therapeutic management and care of individuals presenting a dysfunctional condition. Examples in this book include chapters on bladder and bowel disturbances and feeding problems. Programming with such patients is aimed at eliminating or reducing the dysfunction resulting from a particular affliction (e.g., decreasing spasticity in a cerebral-palsied individual), alleviating associated distress, and improving overall life-style functioning. To date, the majority of behavior therapy interventions in behavioral medicine fall within the category of tertiary prevention.

Secondary prevention approaches are aimed at the identification of conditions that place one at risk for subsequent difficulties and the direct modification of these behavioral risk factors. One form of application in this regard has been the establishment of systematic health monitoring programs such as mass-screening projects for hypertension, breast cancer, diabetes, and cardiovascular disorders. Studies in the area of behavioral epidemiology (Epstein & LaPorte, 1978) have been useful in detecting a number of health risks relative to life-style activity. Thus, cigarette smoking, elevated cholesterol levels, and sedentary existence contribute to the development of coronary heart disease (Surwit et al., 1982). Behavior therapy procedures in particular can be utilized to change these deleterious influences through programs aimed at reducing cigarette consumption, changing dietary intake, and increasing physical exercise. As applied to developmentally handicapped populations, many behavioral techniques have been employed successfully to decrease operant responses that are health threatening, a topic reviewed in detail in Chapter 6.

The aim of *primary prevention* is to prevent the occurrence of disease or development of a pathophysiological risk factor. Immunization against infectious disease represents a major primary prevention effort within traditional medical practice. Examples of behavioral treatment strategies include designing instructional programs that teach parents how to prepare nutritionally sound meals (Sarber, Halasz, Messmer, Bickett, & Lutzker, 1983), increasing physical exercise (Martin & Dubbert, 1982), establishing routine dental care (Horner & Keilitz, 1975), and improving hospital and clinic appointment keeping (Parrish, Charlop, & Fenton, 1986). Treatment to prevent accidents and physical injury is another goal of primary prevention. Contrary to popular belief, many childhood accidents are preventable and can benefit from psychological and community-based interventions (Roberts, 1986). In several studies, parents have increased their children's use of automobile safety seats through application of standard reinforcement techniques (Roberts & Turner, 1986). Home safety can also be improved with the implementation of several behaviorally based instructional programs (Peterson, 1984).

Assessment

Assessment is one of the foundations of behavior therapy and applied behavior analysis. The principles of behavioral assessment have been presented in a number of exemplary texts (Hersen & Bellack, 1981; Kazdin, 1984) and are reviewed relevant to the area of behavioral medicine in Chapter 2 of this book. Therefore, this section will serve as a cursory overview of assessment methodology, highlighting primary features and functions.

According to Nelson and Hayes (1981), "Behavioral assessment is the identification and measurement of meaningful response units and their controlling variables (both environmental and organismic) for the purposes of understanding and altering human behavior" (p. 3). In contrast to traditional psychometric measurement whereby a "test score" is presumed to reflect some underlying condition or fixed trait, behavioral assessment focuses upon quantifiable responses that occur within and are influenced by different environmental setting conditions. Put simply, behavioral assessment addresses what a person *does* as opposed to what a person *has* (Nelson & Hayes, 1981).

Quantification within behavioral assessment entails identifying relevant target responses, operationally defining these responses into measurable units, and designing a recording protocol. Responses selected for assessment may fall within three domains: 1) overt motor behaviors, 2) physiological activity, and 3) cognitive processes. Typically, assessment methods consist of on-line, observational recording for motor behaviors, biochemical and electrodiagnostic measurement for physiological recording, and self-report for cognitions. It is important to note that within behavioral medicine, emphasis is placed upon a multimethod assessment approach (Russo et al., 1980; Varni, 1983). For example, in the treatment of chronic pain it is possible to assess the behavioral expression of discomfort (grimacing, posturing, crying), biological parameters (skin temperature, EMG), self-report of distress, and administration of analgesics. In the treatment of seizure disorders assessment can be performed on the frequency of seizures per day, anticipatory anxiety, and electroencephalographic activity (Wells, Turner, Bellack, & Hersen, 1978). The assessment of multiple dependent measures ensures that the practitioner/researcher is provided with a total "clinical picture" of the presenting disorder plus allows for the determination of behavioral covariation among component responses. It is also worth noting that behavioral assessment within behavioral medicine encompasses the measurement of both physical dysfunction and well-being. Thus, citing the example of chronic pain once again, assessment would be directed at indices of discomfort as well as improvements in activities of daily living, functional abilities, emotional adjustment, and so on.

Reliability and validity are significant issues in any discussion of behavioral assessment. Reliability refers to the consistency of a particular assessment device and is determined through the simultaneous and independent recordings of two observers. A standard interobserver agreement score (typically an average of 80% or greater) is utilized as a criterion to judge the acceptability of recorded data. Low reliability estimates indicate that observers are not recording uniformly the same dependent measures. Validity refers to the accuracy of the assessment protocol, namely, does it measure what it purports to measure? Estimates of validity are obtained by the degree of correlation between two or more dependent measures (e.g., self-report and motor responding). In recent years, the construct of *social validation* has received increased attention (Kazdin, 1977; Wolf, 1978). One type of social validity attempts to ascertain the clinical significance of behavior-change interventions. This process may involve comparing persons who received treatment to a normative sample and/or having "expert" judges rate the degree of clinical improvement. Another form of social validity concerns the acceptability of treatment. Assessments of this type request consumers to register their satisfaction with service delivery and therapeutic outcome.

Another primary function of behavioral assessment is to identify the variables that control and maintain responding. Rather than concentrating on purported historical determinants of behavior, the process of conducting a "behavior analysis" stresses identification of presently operative organismic, interpersonal, and environmental influences. Some of the categories of controlling variables emphasized by behavior analysts include: 1) organic dysfunction such as anatomical, biochemical, and neuromuscular deficits; 2) anxiety- or frustration-provoking antecedent stimuli; 3) sensory reinforcing events; and 4) contingent consequences that produce social attention or allow avoidance of or escape from the interpersonal environment. Performing a detailed behavior analysis is a critical step in the assessment process because the information obtained will dictate the selection of relevant intervention methods (see Chapter 6 for an expanded discussion on this topic).

Single-Case Research Design

The development of single-case research methodology, also known as within-subject or $N = 1$ evaluation designs, is one of the most significant contributions of applied behavior analysis (Barlow, Hayes, & Nelson, 1984; Hersen & Barlow, 1976; Kazdin, 1982b). Like traditional between-group research formats, single-case approaches seek to isolate the effects of treatment variables by ruling out influences such as maturation, attention-placebo factors, and other uncontrolled events. The experimental rigor imposed by single-case designs is accomplished by having each research participant serve as his or her own control. In contrast to group research methodology, single-case studies do not require the recruitment of large sample sizes or the uniform matching of subject variables and presenting problems. This is a noteworthy consideration in research with developmentally disabled populations since it is usually difficult to find numerous participants who display the same behavior of interest. In fact, many of the clients referred to behavioral medicine specialists present unique and oftentimes idiosyncratic disorders.

Single-case research is also advantageous for clinical assessment and decision making. Because the results from between-group research are reported as *statistically significant* outcomes, the individual therapeutic responsiveness of subjects is obscured. It is possible, for example, for a statistically significant effect to be obtained even though some subjects fail to demonstrate improvement. Therefore, group designs are not ideal for evaluating the *clinical significance* of treatment outcome or the processes responsible for subject-specific changes. Single-case strategies, on the other hand, assess variability in subject behavior continuously as treatment variables are presented, removed, and altered. This approach enables the investigator to determine the most optimal intervention strategy and decide upon its application in a clinically efficacious manner. Furthermore, the effectiveness of different treatment techniques with a single subject can be compared.

Although it is beyond the scope of this section to discuss the tenets of single-case research in detail, it would be worthwhile to describe several designs briefly since they will be encountered frequently in the chapters that follow. Overall, the format of these designs entails the repeated measurement of dependent variables under varying conditions of baseline and treatment. Changes in measured behaviors under these conditions permit conclusions to be inferred concerning the influence of treatment (independent) variables. One type of single-case evaluation, the *reversal design*, consists of an initial phase of baseline assessment followed by the subsequent introduction, removal, and reinstatement of treatment. Functional control of intervention is revealed by demonstrating that the subject's behavior improves when treatment is present and deteriorates in its absence. The reversal design has been a popular strategy within behavioral research but it is not without problems. One difficulty is that some behaviors are unlikely to change during the reversal phase due to a learning effect. Say, for example, the number of steps taken by a child with motor impairment are recorded during an initial baseline condition. During the application of a training program to establish ambulation, a significant increase in walking is demonstrated. Removing the program during a subsequent reversal-to-baseline phase may not result in a loss of treatment effect since it is likely that natural reinforcers for walking would be operating (e.g., exploration of the environment). Therefore, behaviors that might change in a permanent fashion are not suitable for evaluation using a reversal design. A second limitation is that it is ethically objectionable to discontinue an effective treatment for certain clinical disorders. To illustrate, one would not want to withdraw a successful therapy program for a youngster with lead poisoning stemming from chronic pica behavior.

One way to overcome the problems associated with reversal strategies is to incorporate a *multiple-baseline design*. In a multiple baseline, two or more dependent measures are recorded simultaneously under pretreatment conditions. These measures may consist of several behaviors exhibited by a single person (multiple baseline across behaviors), the same behavior displayed by several individuals (multiple baseline across subjects), or the behavior of one person within different environments (multiple baseline across settings). Treatment is then introduced for one measure while baseline conditions continue for the remaining measures. Over time, treatment is applied successively in a staggered fashion across measures. By showing that therapeutic changes only occur following intervention, valid conclusions may be drawn regarding the controlling effects of treatment. Since a withdrawal of treatment is not required with a multiple-baseline design, the difficulties of irreversibility and ethical restraints are not encountered.

A third type of single-case experimental design is the *changing criterion design*. This approach also begins with a period of baseline assessment. Functional control is assessed by introducing treatment at a predefined standard (criterion), gradually altering the imposed standard, and demonstrating that each criterion change is accompanied by a respective change in the behavior under study. As a clinical demonstration, a treatment program might be designed for a child with diurnal enuresis. During the first treatment phase, reinforcers are presented for appropriate voiding and displaying minimal wettings, say no more than five incidents each week. Following a decrease in wettings, the criterion for reinforcement would be reduced to three wettings per week, one wetting, and ultimately an absence of the behaviors. If this child's frequency of wetting stays at or below the imposed criterion each time it is changed, it would suggest strongly that the treatment program was responsible for the desired outcome. The changing criterion design is particularly well suited to studying the effects of behavioral shaping programs and response acquisition.

Previously it was stated that single-case methodology allows for the comparative analysis of different treatments in one person. However, comparing treatments within single-case research requires the control of sequence or order effects. For example, a study incorporating a reversal design might consist of the following sequential phases: baseline, Treatment A, baseline, Treatment B. If the results of Treatment B are more clinically significant than Treatment A, it is not possible to conclude unequivocally that the latter treatment is superior. The subject's response to Treatment B may have occurred, in part, from his or her prior exposure to Treatment A. To control for potential order effects, the clinician/researcher can implement an *alternating treatments design*. This design consists of an initial baseline phase, an alternating treatments phase during which two or more interventions are compared, and usually a third condition wherein the most beneficial treatment is utilized exclusively. To conduct the comparison during the second evaluation phase, the subject is exposed to the different treatments that are counterbalanced across stimulus conditions (e.g., time of day, therapy settings). In some cases, a no-treatment baseline condition may also be programmed as an additional control. The levels of responding associated with each treatment (or the absence of treatment) indicate comparative differences or similarities. If one form of treatment is clearly superior to the other(s), it can then be introduced uniformly across stimulus conditions.

In concluding this discussion of single-case designs, it is important to stress that the emphasis on this methodology within applied behavior analysis neither overlooks nor excludes the utilization of between-group strategies. Indeed, group approaches provide a means to carry out tightly controlled research, examine theoretical issues, and investigate procedural parameters (Wilson & O'Leary, 1980). The strengths of single-case designs are that they are technique oriented, problem solving in approach, and extremely adaptable to studying clinical phenomena. Ultimately, the choice of experimental design depends upon the particular questions that are posed and the skill of the researcher in tailoring the method of evaluation to these concerns. In the end, advances in behavioral medicine will accrue from the combined use of single-case and between-group analyses and not an exclusive reliance on one experimental format.

Empirically Based Treatment [2]

The field of behavior therapy and analysis is one area of clinical assessment and treatment subsumed under the general category of behavioral psychology. Both the conceptual bases and treatment techniques comprising behavior therapy are formulated largely on principles of learning derived from laboratory research. Although many persons still associate the term behavior therapy with early Watsonian behaviorism, its actual constitution is quite different and diverse. Contemporary behavioral approaches, for example, encompass respondent and operant conditioning, modeling, cognitive learning, and self-regulation (Wilson & O'Leary, 1980). The conceptualizations based on these approaches and respective therapeutic strategies share a common ground that is characterized by systematic empirical validation. Treatment procedures are routinely evaluated within analogue, clinical, and applied contexts. This commitment to empiricism is, perhaps, the primary descriptive feature of a behavioral therapeutic approach (Rimm & Masters, 1979).

This section describes three categories of behavior therapy techniques commonly employed in behavioral medicine. The first category, *Contingency Management*, consists of arranging environmental consequences in a manner that encourages (increases) the display of adaptive behaviors and discourages

---

[2]Portions of this section are adapted from Luiselli (1987).

(decreases) the display of maladaptive behaviors. The goal of increasing desired responses is addressed through utilization of *positive reinforcement* methods that consist of making pleasurable consequences contingent on the occurrence of specified target responses. There are several procedural variations when implementing positive reinforcement. One set of techniques consists of time-based schedules, the two most popular forms being the differential reinforcement of other behavior (DRO) and the differential reinforcement of incompatible behavior (DRI). With DRO, reinforcement is delivered if a target response does not occur after a predetermined interval of time elapses. DRI is similar except that reinforcement is made contingent on behaviors that are physically incompatible with the target problem. Another method of programming positive reinforcement is in the form of a token economy. Tokens are any inanimate object such as stars, poker chips, or marks on a paper that acquire reinforcing properties through their association with pleasurable stimuli. In the typical token economy system, an individual earns tokens for engaging in desired behaviors and/or inhibiting problematic responses and then exchanges accumulated tokens at scheduled times for preferred items or events (termed "backup" reinforcers). The final method of programming positive reinforcement is through *contingency contracting*. This approach entails specified parties (e.g., a child and parents) developing a written contract that designates that particular reinforcing activities will be provided upon performance of selective appropriate behaviors.

The goal of decreasing maladaptive behaviors may be accomplished through the implementation of *punishment* methods. Procedurally, punishment consists of establishing negative consequences for the display of target responses. Several types of punishment procedures exist. With *response cost*, a specified quantity of accumulated reinforcers is forfeited each time the undesired response occurs. *Time-out* consists of interrupting the availability of ongoing reinforcement and may be applied in a variety of ways: 1) removal of stimulus materials, 2) withdrawal of social attention, 3) removal of a discriminative stimulus for reinforcement, 4) exclusion from activities, or 5) isolation in a barren environment. *Overcorrection* represents another type of punishment procedure, the rationale of which is to have individuals assume responsibility for their maladaptive behaviors. Thus, contingent on a target response, one may be required to correct the environmental effects of his or her actions (termed *restitution*) and/or rehearse alternative ways of behaving (termed *positive practice*). Finally, response-contingent *aversive stimulation* includes the delivery of noxious stimuli as a consequence for undesirable behaviors. Types of aversive stimuli have consisted of foul odors (aromatic ammonia, valoric acid), distasteful solutions (lemon juice, mouthwash, pepper sauce), and stimulation applied to the skin (water spray, electric shock).

The second category of intervention techniques is *Behavioral Self-Control*. The strategy is oriented towards teaching individuals to self-manage therapeutic regimens. Within this general framework, three sets of treatment approaches may be defined. First, individuals can be taught to self-administer many of the contingency management procedures described previously. This would entail training one to identify the occurrence of a targeted behavior (self-monitoring) and then, to implement a predefined contingency plan. The second set of self-control strategies consists of *relaxation training*. The goal of relaxation training is to reduce tension and anxiety by lowering sympathetic arousal of the auto-nomic nervous system. Most typically, this is accomplished through variants of Jacobson's (1938) progressive muscle relaxation procedures. Once an indivi-dual has learned to induce relaxation, the state of disarousal may be conditioned to a distinct verbal cue such as, "Calm," or "Relax." In this way, such cues enable the individual to apply relaxation on a self-control basis outside of the training sessions. *Habit reversal* techniques represent another form of self-management. As developed by Azrin and Nunn (1973), these procedures are utilized to treat a variety of ritualistic responses such as tics, eye blinking, and mild forms of self-abuse (e.g., lip biting, tongue chewing, trichotillomania). When utilizing habit reversal, individuals learn to engage in isometric-like competing behaviors contingent on urges to perform or the actual expression of the problematic response.

In the third area, *Biofeedback*, therapeutic intervention is aimed at teaching individuals to discriminate normally undetectable physiological responses and to use this feedback as a method of controlling such responding in a clinically desir-able direction. There are several biofeedback training modalities available whose choice depends on the particular physiological response system that is afflicted and respective mode of action. For example, electromyographic (EMG) biofeed-back consists of attaching electrodes to specific body sites and recording the elec-trical discharges emanating from these locations. In cases of increased electrical output associated with high tension levels or spastic motor involvement, training would focus on lowering EMG levels; in cases where decreased electrical activity is recorded as with flaccid muscle tone, training would be directed at increasing EMG levels. Another biofeedback modality consists of training individuals to regulate their peripheral skin temperature, primarily as a method of treating vas-cular disorders such as migraine headache and Raynaud's disease. Small therm-istors are attached to skin sites and recorded temperatures are provided in the form of visual, digital displays. Finally, biofeedback procedures may be applied directly to responses of specific organ systems, for example, increasing rec-tosphincteric pressure of children with fecal incontinence (Whitehead, Parker, Masek, Cataldo, & Freeman, 1981).

There are several additional issues to consider in this discussion of treatment techniques. First, the majority of behavioral programs developed for clinical dis-orders are multicomponent in design. For example, intervention for a client with chronic ruminative vomiting might consist of altering the quantity and consis-tency of consumed foods, reinforcing the absence of emesis, and applying over-correction contingent on occurrences of the behavior. The implementation of so-called "treatment packages" is directed at producing the most robust interven-tion effect. Also, combined treatments enable the clinician to tailor therapeutic strategies to the individuality of the client and the complexity of the presenting problem(s). On a research level, a primary goal is to "dismantle" packaged interventions in an effort to tease out the individual influences of each component and identify the optimal combination of procedures.

A second issue closely aligned with treatment is generalization and maintenance. Generalization refers to the transfer of treatment across nontreated behaviors, settings, and change agents. Maintenance refers to the durability of behavior change once intervention has terminated (maintenance is sometimes described as generalization over time). Behavioral research has demonstrated consistently that generalization and maintenance are outcomes that must be *promoted* instead of expected (Marholin, Siegel, & Phillips, 1976). Imagine, for instance, an encopretic child who is treated within an inpatient hospital setting using a program of contingent token reinforcement. The successful management of the disorder in that environment is no indication that positive results will automatically transfer to the home upon discharge. At the same time, if the program is discontinued abruptly, it is probable that the problem behavior will reappear. To overcome these limitations, specific manipulations should be introduced during treatment. As suggested by Marholin and Siegel (1978), these include: 1) establishing contingencies of reinforcement in extra-treatment settings that are consistent with contingencies present in the treatment setting, 2) training significant others to implement effective contingencies in the natural environment, 3) establishing social stimuli as function reinforcers, 4) providing discriminative stimuli in the treatment setting that are likely to be encountered in extra-therapy locales, 5) fading from continuous to intermittent reinforcement schedules, 6) delaying the presentation of reinforcers, and 7) teaching self-management skills. Many examples of generalization and maintenance programming are cited in subsequent chapters.

Previously, the concept of social validity was defined as it relates to consumer satisfaction. A priority for behavioral psychologists is to design programs and procedures that are both acceptable to and easily managed by practitioners and clients. Any form of intervention that is difficult to implement or excessively time consuming is unlikely to be applied consistently. Overcorrection, as an example, is a multicomponent treatment strategy that has been criticized occasionally as being too procedurally complex and requiring extensive time for application. By conducting component and parametric analyses over the years, research studies have yielded information on how to employ overcorrection in a more cost-efficient manner (Marholin, Luiselli, & Townsend, 1980). Effective manipulation will be compromised further if the proposed techniques are distasteful to the recipient (as is the case frequently with aversive methods). Behavior therapists, then, have become increasingly aware of assessing the acceptability of treatment techniques and not just the magnitude of therapeutic change (Bornstein & Rychtarik, 1983). The issue of consumer acceptability is of significant concern in behavioral medicine since most physicians and allied health professionals have limited experiences with behavior therapy approaches.

Role of Behavioral Medicine in Developmental Disabilities

The classification of developmental disabilities featured in this volume includes children, adolescents, and adults afflicted with conditions that significantly affect adaptive functioning, intellectual abilities, and cognitive skills. In many cases, multiple impairments exist concurrently. The largest population covered in this regard are persons with various congenital disorders associated with mental retardation. Other categories consist of sensory impairments such as blindness and deafness, and neuromuscular deficits such as cerebral palsy and Tourette syndrome. Also included are individuals whose disabilities are traumatically induced as in the case of mental and motor dysfunction secondary to stroke.

The significance of behavioral medicine treatment and research with developmentally disabled individuals is apparent for several reasons. First, many handicapping conditions have associated physiological dysfunctions. Among mentally retarded and autistic individuals there exists a high prevalence of bladder and bowel problems, seizure disorders, and neuromuscular disturbances. Particular syndromes have well-established pathophysiological correlates such as self-mutilation in Cornelia de Lange and Lesch-Nyhan disease (Cataldo & Harris, 1982), obesity in Prader-Willi syndrome (Holm, Sulzbacher, & Pipes, 1981), and motor deterioration in mucopolysaccharide disorders such as Hurler and Hunter syndrome (Ampola, 1982). Chronic sensory and cognitive disabilities result from several congenital infectious diseases, for example, rubella, toxoplasmosis, and cytomegalovirus (Blackman, 1983).

Health-threatening behaviors (Chapter 6) represent another clinical concern for behavioral medicine intervention in developmental disabilities. The frequent occurrence of self-injury by handicapped children and adults is physically harmful in a variety of ways (e.g., body contusions, lacerations, infections, internal bleeding). Ruminative vomiting can lead to dehydration, malnutrition, weight loss, and even death. Pica, the ingestion of nonnutritive substances, may result in anemia, intestinal obstruction, and lead poisoning (Milar & Schroeder, 1983). These and other maladaptive behaviors demand carefully planned and systematically implemented management programs.

Finally, the life-styles of many disabled persons are not conducive to health maintenance. Teaching individuals to eat nutritious foods, engage in exercise, reduce coffee consumption, and eliminate cigarette smoking are meaningful goals. Promoting behaviors to improve personal hygiene such as dental (Horner & Keilitz, 1975) and menstrual care (Richman, Ponticas, Page, & Epps, 1986) represent additional examples. The design of effective technologies in primary prevention is a formidable challenge facing behavioral medicine treatment in developmental disabilities.

Summary

Behavioral medicine is the interdisciplinary field concerned with the integration of behavioral science and biomedical knowledge for the treatment of disease and the promotion of health. This chapter reviews some of the trends influencing the evolution of behavioral medicine as a specialty area, most notably, the attention of behavior therapists towards the treatment of somatic disorders, an emphasis in epidemiology from acute, infectious disease towards chronic illness, and the emerging technology of biofeedback. Various definitions of behavioral medicine are compared and contrasted and several commonalities are identified. Most descriptions stress an interdisciplinary team approach that encompasses therapeutic management and prevention efforts, including both basic and applied research. Behavior therapy is presented as a specialty discipline within behavioral medicine. The noteworthy features of a behavior therapeutic approach are its emphasis on assessment, utilization of clinically oriented, idiographic research design, and a commitment to empirically validated treatment strategies. Behavior therapy techniques within the categories of contingency management, self-control, and biofeedback are presented. As applied to developmentally disabled populations, behavioral medicine provides significant contributions towards the treatment of chronic disorders, risk reduction, primary prevention, and health maintenance.

References

Agras, W.S. (1975). Foreword. In R.C. Katz & S. Zlutnick (Eds.), *Behavior therapy and health care: Principles and applications*. New York: Pergamon Press.

Ampola, M.G. (1982). *Metabolic diseases in pediatric practice*. Boston: Little, Brown.

Azrin, N.H., & Nunn, R.G. (1973). Habit reversal: A method of eliminating nervous habits and tics. *Behaviour Research and Therapy, 11*, 619–628.

Barlow, D.H., Hayes, S.C., & Nelson, R.O. (1984). *The scientist practitioner: Research and accountability in clinical and educational settings*. New York: Pergamon Press.

Bernhardt, A.M., Hersen, M., & Barlow, D.H. (1972). Measurement and modification of spasmodic torticollis: An experimental analysis. *Behavior Therapy, 13*, 294–297.

Birk, L. (1973). *Biofeedback: Behavioral medicine*. New York: Grune & Stratton.

Blackman, J.A. (Ed.) (1983). *Medical aspects of developmental disabilities in children birth to three*. University of Iowa: Division of Developmental Disabilities, Iowa City.

Blanchard, E.B. (1982). Behavioral medicine: Past, present and future. *Journal of Consulting and Clinical Psychology, 50*, 795–796.

Blanchard, E.B., & Epstein, L.H. (1978). *A biofeedback primer*. Reading, MA: Addison-Wesley.

Borkovec, T.D. (1982). Insomnia. *Journal of Consulting and Clinical Psychology, 50*, 880–895.

Bornstein, P.H., & Rychtarik, R.G. (1983). Consumer satisfaction in adult behavior therapy: Procedures, problems, and future perspectives. *Behavior Therapy, 14*, 191–208.

Cataldo, M.F., & Harris, J. (1982). The biological basis of self-injury in the mentally retarded. *Analysis and Intervention in Developmental Disabilities, 2*, 21–39.

Cataldo, M.F., Jacobs, H.E., & Rogers, M.C. (1982). Behavioral/environmental considerations in pediatric in-patient care. In D.C. Russo & J.W. Varni (Eds.), *Behavioral pediatrics: Research and practice*. New York: Plenum Press.

Cataldo, M.F., Russo, D.C., & Freeman, J.M. (1979). A behavior analysis approach to high rate myoclonic seizures. *Journal of Autism and Developmental Disorders, 9*, 413–427.

Christophersen, E.R., & Abernathy, J.E. (1982). Research in ambulatory pediatrics. In D.C. Russo & J.W. Varni (Eds.), *Behavioral pediatrics: Research and practice* (pp. 299–332). New York: Plenum Press.

Elkin, T.E., Hersen, M., Eisler, R.M., & Williams, J.G. (1972). Modification of caloric intake in anorexia nervosa: An experimental analysis. *Psychological Reports, 32*, 75–78.

Epstein, L.H., & Cluss, P.A. (1982). A behavioral medicine perspective on adherence to long-term medical regimens. *Journal of Consulting and Clinical Psychology, 50*, 950–971.

Epstein, L.H., Katz, R.C., & Zlutnick, S. (1979). Behavioral medicine. In M. Hersen, R.M. Eisler, & P.M. Miller (Eds.), *Progress in behavior modification* (Vol. 7, pp. 117–170). New York: Academic Press.

Epstein, L.H., & LaPorte, R. (1978). Behavioral epidemiology. *AABT Newsletter, 1*, 3–5.

Epstein, L.H., Malone, D.R., & Cunningham, J. (1978). Feedback influenced EMG changes in stroke patients. *Behavior Modification, 2*, 387–402.

Ferguson, J.M., & Taylor, C.B. (Eds.). (1980). *Comprehensive handbook of behavioral medicine*. New York: Spectrum Books.

Hersen, M., & Barlow, D.H. (1976). *Single case experimental designs: Strategies for studying behavior change*. New York: Pergamon Press.

Hersen, M., & Bellack, A.S. (Eds.). (1981). *Behavioral assessment*. New York: Pergamon Press.

Holm, V.A., Sulzbacher, S.I., & Pipes, P.L. (Eds.). (1981). *Prader-Willi syndrome*. Baltimore: University Park Press.

Horner, R.D., & Keilitz, I. (1975). Training mentally retarded adolescents to brush their teeth. *Journal of Applied Behavior Analysis, 8*, 301–310.

Ince, L.P. (1976). *Behavior modification in rehabilitative medicine*. Springfield, IL: Thomas.

Jacobson, E. (1938). *Progressive relaxation*. Chicago: University of Chicago Press.

Kallman, M.W., Hersen, M., & O'Toole, D.H. (1975). The use of social reinforcement in a case of conversion reaction. *Behavior Therapy, 6*, 411–413.

Kazdin, A.E. (1977). Assessing the clinical or applied importance of behavior change through social validation. *Behavior Modification, 1*, 427–452.

Kazdin, A.E. (1982a). History of behavior modification. In A.S. Bellack, M. Hersen, & A.E. Kazdin (Eds.), *International handbook of behavior modification and therapy* (pp. 3–32). New York: Plenum Press.

Kazdin, A.E. (1982b). *Single case research designs: Methods for clinical and applied settings*. New York: Oxford.

Kazdin, A.E. (1984). *Behavior modification in applied settings*. Homewood, IL: Dorsey Press.

Keefe, F.J. (1982). Behavioral assessment and treatment of chronic pain: Current status and future directions. *Journal of Consulting and Clinical Psychology, 50*, 896–911.

Lichtenstein, E. (1982). The smoking problem: A behavioral perspective. *Journal of Consulting and Clinical Psychology, 50*, 804–819.

Luiselli, J.K. (1987). Behavioral medicine research and treatment in developmental disabilities. In R.P. Barrett & J.L. Matson (Eds.), *Advances in developmental disorders* (pp. 1–39). Greenwich, CT: JAI Press.

Marholin, D., II, Luiselli, J.K., & Townsend, N.M. (1980). Overcorrection: An examination of its rationale and treatment effectiveness. In M. Hersen, R.M. Eisler, & P.M. Miller (Eds.), *Progress in behavior modification* (Vol. 9, pp. 49–80). New York: Academic Press.

Marholin, D., II, & Siegel, L.J. (1978). Beyond the law of effect: Programming for the maintenance of behavioral change. In D. Marholin, II (Ed.), *Child behavior therapy* (pp. 397–415). New York: Gardner Press.

Marholin, D., II, Siegel, L.J., & Phillips, D. (1976). Treatment and transfer: A search for empirical procedures. In M. Hersen, R.M. Eisler, & P.M. Miller (Eds.), *Progress in behavior modification* (Vol. 3, pp. 293–342). New York: Academic Press.

Martin, J.E., & Dubbert, P.M. (1982). Exercise applications and promotion in behavioral medicine: Current status and future directions. *Journal of Consulting and Clinical Psychology, 50*, 1004–1017.

Masek, B.J., Epstein, L.H., & Russo, D.C. (1981). Behavioral perspectives in preventive medicine. In S.M. Turner, K.S. Calhoun, & H.E. Adams (Eds.), *Handbook of clinical behavior therapy* (pp. 475–499). New York: Wiley.

Matarazzo, J.P. (1980). Behavioral health and behavioral medicine: Frontiers for a new health psychology. *American Psychologist, 35*, 807–817.

Melamed, B.G., Robbins, R.L., & Graves, S. (1982). Preparation for surgery and medical procedures. In D.C. Russo & J.W. Varni (Eds.), *Behavioral pediatrics: Research and practice* (pp. 225–267). New York: Plenum Press.

Milar, C.R., & Schroeder, S.R. (1983). The effects of lead on retardation of cognitive and adaptive behavior. In J.L. Matson & F. Andrasik (Eds.), *Treatment issues and innovations in mental retardation* (pp. 129–158). New York: Plenum Press.

Mostofsky, D.I. (1981). Recurrent paroxysmal disorders of central nervous system. In S.M. Turner, K.S. Calhoun, & H.E. Adams (Eds.), *Handbook of clinical behavior therapy* (pp. 447–474). New York: Wiley.

Nelson, R.O., & Hayes, S.C. (1981). Nature of behavioral assessment. In M. Hersen & A.S. Bellack (Eds.), *Behavioral assessment* (pp. 3–37). New York: Pergamon Press.

Nidiffer, F.D., Iwata, B.A., Kelly, T.E., & Ward-Zimmerman, B. (1983). *Biochemical and behavioral assessment during the reduction of self-mutilation in a Lesch-Nyhan syndrome child.* Paper presented at Seventeenth Annual Convention, Association for Advancement of Behavior Therapy, Washington, DC.

Parker, L.H., Cataldo, M.F., Bourland, G., Emurian, C.C., Corbin, R.J., & Page, J.M. (1984). Operant treatment of orofacial dysfunction in neuromuscular disorders. *Journal of Applied Behavior Analysis, 17*, 413–428.

Parrish, J.M., Charlop, M.H., & Fenton, L.R. (1986). Use of a stated waiting list contingency and reward opportunity to increase appointment keeping in an outpatient pediatric psychology clinic. *Journal of Pediatric Psychology, 11*, 81–89.

Peterson, L. (1984). The "safe-at-home" game: Training comprehensive prevention skills in latch-key children. *Behavior Modification, 8*, 474–494.

Pomerleau, O.F. (1979). Behavioral medicine: The contribution of the experimental analysis of behavior to medical care. *American Psychologist, 34*, 654–663.

Pomerleau, O.F. (1982). A discourse on behavioral medicine: Current status and future trends. *Journal of Consulting and Clinical Psychology, 50*, 1030–1039.

Pomerleau, O.F., & Brady, J.P. (Eds.). (1979). *Behavioral medicine: Theory and practice.* Baltimore: Williams & Wilkins.

Redd, W.H., & Andresen, G.V. (1981). Conditioned aversion in cancer patients. *The Behavior Therapist, 4*, 3–4.

Richman, G.S., Ponticas, Y., Page, T.J., & Epps, S. (1986). Simulation procedures for teaching independent menstrual care to mentally retarded persons. *Applied Research in Mental Retardation, 7*, 21–35.

Rimm, R.C., & Masters, J.C. (1979). *Behavior therapy: Techniques and empirical findings.* New York: Academic Press.

Roberts, M.C. (1986). The future of children's health care: What do we do? *Journal of Pediatric Psychology, 11*, 3–14.

Roberts, M.C., & Turner, D.S. (1986). Rewarding parents for their children's use of safety seats. *Journal of Pediatric Psychology, 11*, 25–36.

Russo, D.C., Bird, B.L., & Masek, B.J. (1980). Assessment issues in behavioral medicine. *Behavioral Assessment, 2*, 1–18.

Russo, D.C., & Varni, J.W. (Eds.). (1982). *Behavioral pediatrics: Research and practice.* New York: Plenum Press.

Sandman, C.A., Datta, P.C., Barron, J., Hoehler, F.K., Williams, C., & Swanson, J.M. (1983). Naloxone attenuates self-abusive behavior in developmentally disabled clients. *Applied Research in Mental Retardation, 4*, 5–11.

Sarber, R.E., Halasz, M.M., Messmer, M.C., Bickett, A.D., & Lutzker, J.R. (1983). Teaching menu planning and grocery shopping skills to a mentally retarded mother. *Mental Retardation, 21*, 101–106.

Schwartz, G.E., & Weiss, S.M. (1978). Yale conference on behavioral medicine: A proposed definition and statement of goals. *Journal of Behavioral Medicine, 1*, 3–12.

Surwit, R.S., Feinglos, M.N., & Scovern, A.W. (1983). Diabetes and behavior: A paradigm for health psychology. *American Psychologist, 38*, 255–262.

Surwit, R.S., Williams, R.B., & Shapiro, D. (1982). *Behavioral approaches to cardiovascular disorders.* New York: Academic Press.

Varni, J.W. (1983). *Clinical behavioral pediatrics.* New York: Pergamon Press.

Wells, K.C., Turner, S.M., Bellack, A.S., & Hersen, M. (1978). Effects of cue-controlled relaxation on psychomotor seizures: An experimental analysis. *Behaviour Research and Therapy, 16*, 51–53.

Whitehead, W.E., Parker, L.H., Masek, B.J., Cataldo, M.F., & Freeman, J.M. (1981). Biofeedback treatment of fecal incontinence in patients with myelomeningocele. *Developmental Medicine and Child Neurology, 23*, 313–322.

Williams, R.B., & Gentry, W.D. (Eds.). (1977). *Behavioral approaches of medical treatment.* Cambridge, MA: Ballinger.

Wilson, G.T., & O'Leary, K.D. (1980). *Principles of behavior therapy.* Englewood Cliffs, NJ: Prentice-Hall.

Wolf, M.M. (1978). Social validity: The case for subjective measurement or how applied behavior analysis is finding its heart. *Journal of Applied Behavior Analysis, 2*, 203–214.

2
Behavioral Assessment

THOMAS R. LINSCHEID, L. KAYE RASNAKE, KENNETH J.
TARNOWSKI, AND JAMES A. MULICK

Introduction

The emergence of the interdisciplinary field of behavioral medicine has produced
the need to integrate assessment methodologies from such diverse areas as medicine, epidemiology, behavior analysis, and the physical sciences. Behavioral analysis methodologies are perhaps the most dissimilar of these various approaches.
Russo, Bird, and Masek (1980) suggest that the major characteristics that
differentiate behavioral assessment from traditional medical assessment are
its emphasis on direct observation of behavior, the reliability of measurement
over conceptual validity of the behavior measured, single-subject research
methodologies, and the importance of immediate functional relationships
between behavior and environment.

To ensure the contribution of behavior analysis to behavioral medicine it is
imperative that practitioners and researchers understand and integrate the
diverse procedural and philosophical differences in traditional behavioral and
medical assessment approaches. This integration must occur if the relationship
between behavior, environment, and health is to be understood to its fullest.

In this chapter the content is divided into two major areas. The first, *Behavioral
Assessment Techniques and Considerations*, discusses the need to combine
behavioral, self-report, and physiological data, describes direct observation
methods, examines the concepts of reliability and validity, and details single-
subject research methodologies. The second section, *Applications*, presents
examples of behavioral assessment methods as applied to specific medical
conditions. This section is not meant as a comprehensive review of behavioral
assessment applications, but rather will serve to highlight both common and
innovative applications of behavioral assessment strategies to medical problems. In some cases, the applications may not involve developmentally disabled individuals, but would be equally possible and appropriate with this
population.

Behavioral Assessment Techniques and Considerations

Purposes of Behavioral Assessment

The basic goals of behavioral assessment include identification and specification of: 1) client behaviors in need of modification, and 2) organismic and environmental variables (antecedent and consequent events) that control the occurrence of the behavior(s) of interest. Assessment procedures may be undertaken for purposes including diagnosis, design, and evaluation (Cone & Hawkins, 1977; Mash & Terdal, 1976; Mash & Terdal, 1982). *Diagnosis* refers to a description of the client's problem in terms of a behavioral taxonomy (Suinn, 1970) (e.g., behavioral deficits, behavioral excesses) or other nosological systems such as the *Diagnostic and Statistical Manual of Mental Disorders (DSM-III)* (American Psychiatric Association, 1980). *Design* refers to the collection of data relevant for client treatment. *Evaluation* refers to the ongoing monitoring of the effectiveness of intervention methods. Although a distinction is often made between diagnosis, design, and evaluation, these processes are not usually separate in the sense that initial assessment data are tied to choice of intervention strategy, the efficacy of which needs to be monitored on an ongoing basis.

Haynes (1977) has described other functions of behavioral assessment including: 1) obtainment of quantitative data on behavior (e.g., frequency, duration, etc.) and particular environmental events (e.g., staff attention to a client following aggressive episodes); 2) analysis of relevant historical data related to the target behavior(s); 3) behavior sampling [assessment of responses that may covary with changes in the main target behavior(s)] to assess generalization (across time, situations, and persons) and side effects of treatments; 4) analysis of mediation potential of environment (e.g., Can intervention be realistically carried out given staff, financial, other constraints?); and 5) assessment of cognitive and physiological components of the behaviors of interest.

Tripartite Assessment

Historically, behavioral assessors focused on the measurement of easily defined motor behaviors that were clearly observable (e.g., number of steps taken, bites of food consumed, etc.). Current behavioral assessment strategies are not limited to the observation of motor responding, and include a wide variety of methods for the assessment of responses from three response systems: motoric, cognitive-verbal, and physiological.

This focus has been referred to as triple response mode assessment or tripartite assessment. Although responses from these three systems may covary systematically, this need not be the case (Lang, 1968). In fact, several investigations have reported low to moderate correspondence between response systems (Bandura, Blanchard, & Ritter, 1969; Risley & Hart, 1968). For example, an individual might report feeling little to no pain following a distressful medical procedure, yet direct observation of the individual might yield conflicting data (e.g., observations of facial grimacing, moaning). On the other hand, Cataldo, Russo, and

Freeman (1979) demonstrated a high degree of correspondence between behaviorally and electrophysiologically recorded seizures in an epileptic patient. It can be seen that it is important to obtain assessment data for each response type as different controlling variables, both environmental and/or organismic, may be identified for each response system. Of course, the relative importance of data gleaned from each response system will vary as a function of client characteristics and nature of the presenting problem(s). A brief overview of these response systems is provided below.

MOTOR BEHAVIOR

The assessment of motor responding typically involves reliance upon observers who use established operational definitions to record the responses of one or more clients. Observers may be staff, parents, trained observers, or subjects themselves. Operational definitions recast general descriptions of behavior into clearly defined and observable aspects of behavior. The response of interest is quantified according to one or more of the following dimensions: frequency, duration, time, distance, occurrence per opportunity, or percentage of response components completed (Nelson & Hayes, 1979). Observations may be conducted in the natural environment (e.g., school), analogue setting (e.g., a room set up like a classroom), or lab setting (e.g., room with observational capabilities such as one-way mirror, etc.). The replicability of observations is established via interobserver reliability determinations whereby two or more observers code the same behavioral sequence and then calculate and quantify the extent of their agreement.

COGNITIVE-VERBAL

The most common methods of assessing client cognitive responding include interviews, questionnaires, and self-monitoring. Other means to assess cognitive responding include standardized IQ tests and the like. The problem here is that cognitive functioning is not directly observable and must be indexed by other means such as client verbal report. Unfortunately, the accuracy of client self-reports can be difficult to ascertain. As Nelson and Hayes (1979) have noted, given the lack of correspondence that may exist between cognitive and verbal behavior, assessors tend to rely on measurement of observable behavior whenever possible.

PHYSIOLOGICAL RESPONDING

Instrumentation is typically employed in the assessment of physiological responding. Biochemical (e.g., hemoglobin A_1Cs for diabetics), electrodiagnostic (e.g., electromyography, electrodermal), thermography (e.g., plethysmograph), and musculoskeletal (e.g., dynamometer) measures are commonly used (Varni, 1983). In addition to these more complicated measures, simple measures of physiological functioning are often available (e.g., heart rate, weight gain, temperature). Finally, recent technological advances have made telemetric physiological monitoring devices more readily available.

Thus, behavioral assessment methods encompass both indirect and direct means to measure client functioning. The indirect methods include interviews, self-report questionnaires, behavioral rating scales, peer ratings, and standard psychological tests. Behavioral observation procedures, self-monitoring, and frequency recording measures constitute direct assessment strategies. Self-report questionnaires and self-monitoring are likely to be of limited utility with very young children and with patients who are cognitively compromised (e.g., mentally retarded individuals). Permanent product measures (e.g., urinary output, kilograms of weight lost) are usually readily obtainable during the course of treatment or can be obtained from archival sources such as chart reviews. Thus, there are several means of directly and indirectly assessing client responding in each of the three response domains (motoric, cognitive-verbal, and physiological) described above. Readers are referred to Cone (1978) for a description of a detailed scheme for classifying behavioral measures according to contents, method, and types of generalizability.

Given the importance of direct observation procedures to behavioral assessment, we now turn to a description of direct observation methodologies and factors requiring consideration when selecting and using such measures.

Direct Observational Assessment

The most distinguishing feature of behavioral assessment is its emphasis on the measurement of overt behaviors (Kazdin, 1981). In the development of behavioral medicine in general and behavioral medicine assessment in particular, this is perhaps the single most important contribution from behavioral psychology. Direct observational assessment has several important features. First, by definition, it deals with observable and overt behaviors. Second, direct observational assessment usually deals with individualized behaviors that are operationally defined. Third, when using direct observational assessment, it is generally assumed that there is not an effort to generalize the behavior in question or changes in the behavioral pattern to large groups of individuals. Fourth, direct observational assessment is used not only to assess behavioral change, but can be used to assess and identify antecedent and consequent events through a functional analysis process. In other words, not only may targeted behaviors of the subject be measured but preceding environmental events (antecedents), and environmental consequent events may be defined and measured as well. This is most evident in behavioral interaction assessment (cf. Mash, Terdal, & Anderson, 1973).

Defining and Targeting Behaviors

The first and most crucial step in designing useful direct observational strategies is to ensure that the behavioral definition identifies specific, directly observable responses or actions. Every effort must be taken to avoid defining behavior in terms of internal states such as anger or frustration. It is not that these states or feelings do not exist but, rather, their expression behaviorally can vary from individual to individual and observers may have vastly different definitions of behaviors that they associate with conditions such as anger and frustration.

There are two guiding factors in selecting overt behavior to measure. The first pertains to obtaining reliable measurements. A measurement system is only as good as its ability to consistently measure the behavior in question. Thus, behavioral definitions must produce agreement between observers measuring the behavior. The second major factor relates to the validity of the measure. In other words, is it agreed that the actual observed behavior reflects what one seeks to measure? An inconsistency would occur, for example, if one chose to measure diabetic regimen compliance in a teenager by counting the number of times the teenager said "Yes sir." This is an extreme and rather silly example but does point out the need to evaluate operationally defined behaviors in terms of their treatment and social validity (Kazdin, 1977).

Hawkins and Dobes (1975) proposed that a response definition should meet three criteria: objectivity, clarity, and completeness. To be objective means that the definition should reference observable characteristics, behaviors, or environmental events. Terms such as aggressiveness, loyalty, and honesty are not directly observable. However, kicking, remaining beside a friend during a fight, and returning a found wallet might constitute behavioral expressions of those traits.

Definitions should also be clear. This means that individuals who hear or read the definition should be able to interpret it similarly. Ambiguity in meaning leads to lack of agreement between observers and should be avoided. The definition should make it clear as to what behaviors are to be included or excluded. Completeness suggests that the definition be broad enough to cover possible variations of the behavior so that observers can determine whether certain behavioral variations should be included or excluded.

FREQUENCY RECORDING

Frequency recording, which is essentially a running count of the occurrence of the target behavior(s), is the most easily understood and perhaps most widely used method for directly assessing behavior. Kazdin (1981) describes three desirable features of the frequency recording strategy. First, it is very simple to accomplish and to score, especially in natural settings. Essentially all that is required is a tally of behaviors. Second, frequency counts can readily reflect changes in the behavior over time. Third, frequency reflects the amount of behavior if the behavior is discrete and occurs with a consistent duration.

If the behavior under observation is variable in duration, it is possible that frequency recording may not accurately reflect the amount of behavior. As an example, during one observation period a behavior may occur with a very high frequency but for very short durations. In this instance, a high count would be obtained and would suggest a large quantity of behavior. During another observation period, the frequency may be low but duration of the behavior may have increased. With the high-frequency, short-duration pattern, there may actually have been less of the behavior during the observation interval than occurred when the behavior was characterized by low frequency, long duration.

The researcher or clinician should keep the frequency-duration consideration in mind when deciding to use frequency recording. It is possible that the responses could change in one dimension (frequency or duration) without changing in the other dimension. This could result in significant changes in the behavior that would not be reflected in the actual measure of the behavior or changes in the frequency of behavior without actual changes in the amount of behavior.

Frequency recording is commonly applied in behavioral medicine. Balaschak and Mostofsky (1981) suggest the use of simple frequency counts as a component in the behavioral assessment of seizure activity and as a means of assessing behavioral treatment efficacy. Azrin and Foxx (1971) used a frequency count of soilings per day to assess effectiveness of a toilet training program in the adults with mental retardation. Similarly, Cunningham and Linscheid (1976) used frequency counts of vomiting episodes in their treatment of an infant ruminator.

Frequency counts are often transformed into rate measures to control for varying lengths of observation periods. The total number of behaviors observed is divided by the length of the observation period to yield measures such as behaviors per minute, hour, and so forth.

DURATION RECORDING

For behaviors that vary in duration such as crying, on- or off-task, or the length of time to complete homework, simply measuring the length (duration) of the behavior may be an effective technique. As in frequency recording, duration recording is a conceptually simple form of measurement that requires only an adequate definition of the behavior and access to a timing device. Today many inexpensive electronic wristwatches have timing functions. With such devices the actual task of duration recording is quite simple. Frequency and duration recording can be combined so that the number of episodes and the duration of the episode are noted. For example, in the course of a 1-hour observation period, the number of times the behavior occurred and the proportion or the hour in which the behavior was occurring can be noted.

A variation of duration recording is the measurement of the length of time between when the behavior is supposed to occur and when it actually begins. For example, one measure of medical compliance could be the time differential between when a medication was scheduled to be taken and when it was actually taken.

INTERVAL RECORDING

Interval recording techniques have proven quite useful in behavioral assessment because they provide a nice blend of the advantages of both frequency and duration recording. With this technique, the observation interval is split into smaller time intervals and in each of these short intervals the occurrence or nonoccurrence of a previously targeted and defined behavior is scored. Two variations of the method, whole interval and partial interval, are often used. With the whole-interval method, the behavior must occur throughout the interval in order for that interval to be scored. When using the partial-interval method, the interval is scored for the behavior if it occurs at any time during the interval regardless of its duration.

The data yielded by interval recording techniques are denoted as either the number or percent of observation intervals in which the behavior occurs, as opposed to the number of behaviors in frequency recording or the total duration of the behavior in duration recording. For behaviors such as crying, that may begin and last for a long period of time or may begin and terminate after a short period of time, the interval technique is particularly useful.

Because interval recording does not require the observer to operate a stopwatch or to count absolute frequencies, it is easier to measure several behaviors simultaneously, especially when using the partial-interval method. When the observer simply places a plus or minus mark indicating whether or not the behavior occurred, multiple behavior recordings can be easily accomplished. If multiple behaviors are recorded, it is not uncommon to have, for example, a 10-second observation interval followed by a 5-second scoring interval, repeating this sequence throughout the entire observation period. During the scoring interval, the observer diverts attention from observation of the behavior to the score sheet in order to indicate presence or absence of the behavior during the previous observation interval. Elliot and Olson (1983) used this technique to measure 10 different pain behaviors in children undergoing a painful medical procedure (debridement).

The trick in interval recording is in the selection of the appropriate length of the intervals. Intervals that are too long can result in an insensitivity to behavior change, that is, behavior may reduce dramatically before it shows up in the actual number of intervals scored for the behavior. On the other hand, if the intervals are too short, while sensitivity is increased, ease in measurement as an advantage may be lost. The interval recording system can be used to obtain data from nurses, direct care staff, and other individuals involved in health care quite easily. For example, Touchette, MacDonald, and Langer (1985) describe the use of a scatter plot technique for assessing stimulus control variables. The technique is an interval recording procedure and uses a data grid composed of rows and columns. The columns represent successive days or treatment sessions and the rows represent sequential time intervals (e.g., 5 minutes, 1 hour, etc.). Observers fill in a grid cell with pen or colored pencil to indicate the occurrence of the behavior during that time interval. If the behavior does not occur, the cell is left blank. Depending on the behavior measured and its pattern, it is sometimes useful to indicate low rates (e.g., only one occurrence) by partially filling the cell or by use of a different color. By visual inspection of the data grid, temporal patterns of the behavior are easily seen and can potentially be related to environmental events such as meals, medication delivery, and so forth. The strengths of this technique include its ability to reveal relationships between behavior and environment and its ease of use by nurses, ward staff, and other nonbehaviorally trained observers. Indeed, the authors have found that nurses on a general pediatric unit, despite their numerous responsibilities, are quite willing and capable of using the system.

TIME SAMPLING

Another technique that may be thought of as a variation of interval recording is time sampling. With this method, at either preset or random times, an observer notes whether or not the target behavior is occurring. Time sampling does not require continuous observation on the part of the observer and for this reason can be of great advantage when there is insufficient manpower to use the previously mentioned techniques. In a recent study of the behavior of children on a pediatric burn unit, the authors used a time sampling procedure to observe patients for 1-minute observation periods at five randomly determined times throughout the day. The occurrence or nonoccurrence of 30 different behaviors was noted. The technique was also used by Cataldo, Bessman, Parker, Pearson, and Rogers (1979) to study children's responses to hospitalization on a pediatric intensive care unit.

As in interval recording, accuracy of measurement depends on the time sampling intervals chosen. When the behavior samples are separated by lengthy intervals, a true reflection of the behavior may not be obtained. If the intervals are too short, little advantage is gained over the interval, frequency, or duration recording techniques.

MEASUREMENT BY PRODUCTS

With this technique the behavior in question is not directly observed, but rather the product of the behavior. For example, rather than observing directly the intake of food by a patient on a weight loss program, a patient's weight can serve as a measure of eating behavior. Reductions in weight are assumed to be associated with reductions in calorie intake or increases in energy expenditure. In a more direct example, Tarnowski, Rosen, McGrath, and Drabman (1987) assessed reductions in trichotillomania (hair-pulling behavior) by actually measuring the size of hairless patches on the subject's head. The size of the patch served as an indirect measure of the hair-pulling behavior.

Concepts of Reliability and Validity

Once quantifiable behavioral measures are selected and methods for collecting the data of interest have been proposed, further thought must be devoted to assuring the believability and accuracy of the information to be obtained. These related concerns about the quality of measurement data are often referred to as validity and reliability. Threats to data quality differ as a result of the dimensions of behavior to be measured and the manner in which data are to be collected.

Validity refers to the extent to which a measurement value actually measures what it is intended to measure. Thus, any data recording system must be shown to be unambiguously and consistently related to its intended assessment function and to the true properties of the variable of interest along an appropriate dimension. Validity is potentially questionable when measures are combined to obtain derived scores, or in cases when observational categories are collapsed into broad summary categories. Such measures may be stable and consistent, but still fail to serve the original purposes of measurement. For example, a combined frequency of out-of-seat behavior, talking out, and touching classmates *may* reflect the construct of hyperactivity, the resulting score *may* even show a reliable response to a given dose of medication, but *may not* be useful in predicting the teacher's recommendation for special placement, which was based on these behaviors plus the student's low frequency of completion of assigned work and high frequency of fidgeting, pencil tapping, and noncompliance in the school playground during recess.

Consensus has been the traditional basis for establishing the accuracy or reliability of observational data. The basic rule has been, if two observers can consistently agree upon the occurrence of an event, then their reports are probably an accurate reflection of reality—that is, the event was most likely happening as recorded. Unfortunately, this basic concept is more difficult to demonstrate during some conditions of observation and with some data recording systems than others. Most applied researchers rely on an index of interobserver agreement.

Observational data are particularly prone to systematic and progressive measurement error due to problems associated with using humans to measure the behavior of other humans. There would be little need for a separate science of behavior if people behaved like mechanical toys, running off a fixed action sequence as long as they were wound up and turned on. If this were so, elementary physics alone would provide an adequate basis for understanding. The actuality is that humans are responsive to physical, biological, historical, and social influences, and not only provide interesting objects of study but also present interesting problems when used as measuring instruments.

Subjects may demonstrate *reactivity* by behaving in unusual ways as a result of their awareness of being observed, and may react in different ways as a function of the characteristics of the people observing or the observational technique used. The least obtrusive approach is obviously the best in order to minimize reactivity. Human observers, too, may demonstrate serious systematic recording error if they react to subjects or environmental contexts differentially as a result of prejudice or expectancy. Although often demonstrated and difficult to completely rule out, *observer bias* can be partially controlled by stringent observer training, employing observers with no knowledge of expected results or critical historical and procedural information, and using unambiguous behavioral definitions in the observational recording system.

Two other problems are noteworthy in observational measures. Observers may gradually respond differently to the events they intend to record, with consequent changes in consistency or accuracy of data as time passes. These effects can occur within and between recording sessions, and can change in direction of effect. This *observer drift* (Johnson & Bolstad, 1973) can develop through the influence of an evolving expectancy, progressive alteration of category definitions to encompass small or novel variations in behavioral topography, fatigue, or boredom. Observer drift can be partially controlled through periodic retraining of observers, by recalibrating decision rules against videotapes previously scored during initial training, and by using additional observers to periodically check the ratings of the primary observers.

Finally, observers may knowingly fabricate data or falsify selected portions of a data set due to real or imagined influences including employer expectations, funding requirements, and personal prejudice. Here too, periodic independent verification or data samples is a way to control for this infrequent but serious problem.

When mechanical or electronic instruments are used to collect data, human sources of poor data quality are minimized. Instruments may require periodic recalibration, however, and this should be made a routine procedure when necessary. A more serious threat to validity when instrumentation or permanent products are used as data involves the extent to which these measures actually reflect the behavioral variable of interest. For example, how accurately does the weight of the food left on a plate at the end of a meal reflect the amount of food consumed by the client? This question can be addressed through recording multiple, logically related variables, such as correlated body weight over time or using observational probe sessions to get a concurrent performance criterion measure.

It is prudent to assess interobserver agreement frequently during an intervention; some 20% to 40% of the total sessions is a common range. It is necessary to sample agreement across all experimental or treatment conditions, because observers may be differentially reactive to the conditions or the behavior may change in topography or frequency in ways that affect recording accuracy. Finally, covert reliability assessment (e.g., a second observer records data through a one-way mirror without knowledge of the primary observer) provides a better check on data accuracy than does overt assessment, because primary observers may react differentially to the presence of the second observer.

Various statistics have been proposed to portray the degree of consensus between observers. The statistics include weighted versions of percent agreement divided for categorical data (most often, the number of exact agreements divided by the number of agreements plus disagreements) and correlational statistics for examination of session totals as the unit of analysis (Hartman, 1977). The range of statistics useful in conveying interobserver agreement and accuracy is great, and has been covered in many extensive methodological reviews (e.g., Kent & Foster, 1977; Rojahn & Schroeder, 1983).

Single-Subject Designs

To establish functional relationships between behavior and environment, behavioral psychologists have developed single-subject designs. These designs were developed for use with individual subjects and provide a format for determining the effect of an environmental manipulation (treatment) upon behavior. Practitioners and researchers are painfully aware of multiple sources of variability that may cause broad fluctuations in a patient's clinical course. Use of single-subject designs promotes the acceptance of broad variability and allows for direct measurement of clinically relevant target behaviors and experimental evaluation of treatment interventions. Single-subject designs recognize the necessity of repeated, frequent measurement as an avenue for discovering the sources of variability. Measurements are repeated over extended periods of time using standard conditions (i.e., measurement devices, personnel, times, instructions) (Barlow & Hersen, 1984).

The initial measurement period for most single-subject designs is a baseline period, which involves repeated measurement of the natural frequency of occurrence of the target behavior(s). This is generally designated as the "A phase" of the paradigm. Baseline observations provide an assessment of the behavior prior to intervention, which can then be used for comparison following initiation of treatment. Determination of the length of baseline measurement is an essential component of single-subject design construction. Typically, baseline measurement continues until a stable behavior pattern is observed (Baer, Wolf, & Risley, 1968). However, in clinical practice, ethical and logistical issues may preclude continuing the baseline until a stable pattern is established. Generally, a minimum of three separate baseline points is mandated (Barlow & Hersen, 1973).

The simplest of all single-subject designs is the A-B design. Once a target behavior is clearly specified, the baseline (A) phase is conducted, followed by the treatment phase (B). A major disadvantage of this design is that it is difficult to ascertain whether changes during the B phase are the result of treatment or have simply occurred coincidentally. Thus, the A-B design results in weak conclusions and at best should be used as a last resort when circumstances do not allow for the use of better controlled designs.

Designs that allow the researcher or clinician to make stronger conclusions about treatment effectiveness have been developed. The reversal design is the most commonly used single-subject design. In its simplest form, the A-B-A design, it utilizes baseline (A), treatment (B), and return to baseline (A) conditions. If improvement is noted after treatment is initiated but the behavior returns to baseline levels with the withdrawal of the intervention, one can conclude with acceptable confidence that the treatment produced the observed behavioral changes. However, this design is flawed in that it ends on a baseline phase rather than a treatment phase, a problem that is unacceptable in clinical practice.

The A-B-A-B design, a slightly more complex design, follows the procedures of the A-B-A design but prescribes termination in a treatment phase. It also creates increased confidence in the conclusion by demonstrating the effect of the treatment on two occasions.

The B-A-B design is an additional single-subject design that can be used to evaluate treatment effectiveness. This design is more acceptable in clinical practice since it ends on a treatment phase. However, the A phase in this design may not represent the pretreatment baseline rate of the target behavior.

Multiple treatment interventions can be assessed using variations of reversal designs. One might desire to assess three treatment interventions and do so with an A-B-A-C-A-D design, with the letters B, C, and D representing three different treatments. A confound may be introduced, however, since the treatments must be introduced sequentially. Thus, the effects of each individual treatment are clouded by the effects of the sequential application of the treatments. Of the designs presented, the A-B-A-B design is recognized as the preferred design (Barlow & Hersen, 1973).

Reversal designs can present problems in clinical settings, both ethically and practically. When treatment has been effective in reducing a seriously problematic behavior (i.e., self-injurious behavior), the withdrawal of the treatment may be unacceptable even for very brief periods of time. Designs have been developed for use in situations that do not permit the use of reversal designs. The multiple-baseline design and the alternating treatment design are the two most commonly used single-subject designs that do not involve treatment removal.

The multiple-baseline design requires identification of several behaviors that can be measured over time. Treatment is applied to each behavior sequentially, while the remaining behaviors are simply measured (ongoing baseline measurement). If improvement is noted in each behavior following initiation of the treatment while nontreated behaviors remain at baseline rates, one can conclude that the treatment has been effective in creating behavioral change. A basic assumption of this design is that the multiple behaviors are independent from one another (Barlow & Hersen, 1984). If this independence is not the case, the controlling effects of the treatment cannot be determined conclusively and the alternating treatments design may be more appropriate. The multiple-baseline design is considered weaker than the reversal design since the effect of treatment is identified via comparative observation of untreated behaviors. Thus, it is generally recommended that three or four independent behaviors, settings, or individuals be monitored. The evaluation of several behaviors at the same time makes the information potentially more naturalistic and generalizable.

There are three basic types of multiple-baseline designs: multiple-baseline design across behaviors (one subject, multiple behaviors), multiple-baseline design across settings (one behavior, multiple settings), and multiple-baseline design across individuals. The selection of each design depends on the specific case for study.

The final design to be discussed, the alternating treatments design, can be useful in situations that do not permit use of reversal designs. This design involves the alternation of two or more treatments or conditions within a single subject. Of concern when using this design are order effects and carry-over effects. Order effects occur when the effect of one treatment is related to the order of its presentation relative to the other treatments. Carry-over effects suggest that a treatment has differential effects related to which other treatment precedes it. It is important to randomize the presentation of the various treatments to control for sequential confounding. Counterbalancing (randomizing) the order of treatments and separating the treatments with a reasonable time interval can help to reduce the problem of carry-over effects.

Applications

In this section, the application of behavioral assessment is examined in several behavioral medicine areas, namely, medical regime compliance, pain management, and pharmacotherapy. This review is not exhaustive, but is meant to highlight certain applications of behavioral assessment technology to medically related problems. In addition, a discussion of technological advances in assessment capabilities is included in order to emphasize what the authors feel will be a significant contribution to the field in the future.

Compliance

Failure to comply with a medically prescribed regime is a widespread problem in both adult and pediatric populations. In a review of the literature, Dunbar (1983) concluded that noncomplicance rates range from 25% to 80% with overall noncomplicance estimated at 50%. Noncompliance makes treatment evaluation difficult if not impossible and results in less than optimal treatment effectiveness in those patients for whom the appropriate and proven treatment is prescribed.

In the developmentally disabled (DD) population, the issue of compliance is especially complicated. The degree to which a DD person can be expected to be responsible for compliance can vary with physical or intellectual limitations. Frequently, in the DD population someone other than the patient (e.g., nurse, direct care worker, dietician) is responsible for compliance with the prescribed treatment regime. The following assessment strategies were designed for individuals who were responsible for their own compliance, but can be modified to assess the compliance of treatment staff as well.

In a 1977 study, Magrab and Papadopoulou used a measurement by products technique to assess dietary compliance in children on hemodialysis. Instead of directly observing what foods the children ate between dialysis sessions, their weight and two blood test indices were used as measures of calorie, sodium, and potassium intake.

Another behavioral measure of compliance is the use of pill counts to assess the degree to which patients are taking medication as prescribed. While this method can easily be invalidated if the patient wants to fool the physician, variations of the technique have proven helpful in assessing compliance. For example, Epstein et al. (1981) used a modification of the technique with diabetic children who were instructed to test their own urine glucose levels. This involved the addition of a reagent pill to a solution of 2 drops of urine and 10 drops of water. The reagent causes the urine-water solution to change color and the amount of glucose in the urine is determined by comparing the solution to a color chart. Epstein et al. added a set number of visually identical but inert pills to each bottle of reagent pills. When the inert pills were added to the urine-water solution, no color change occurred. Children were instructed to record the number of inert pills found during their self-testing. At the end of each week, parents tested the remaining reagent pills, added the number of inert pills they found to the number reported by the child, and compared this number to the number originally placed in the bottle. If the children did not report finding the correct number of inert pills, it was assumed that they were not conducting the number of tests requested.

Another interesting example in the area of diabetic compliance and a technological advance is described by Wilson and Endres (1986). Children with insulin-dependent diabetes mellitus were supplied with blood glucose reflectance meters that had electronic memory capabilities. The meters could not only store in memory whether a test was conducted, but could record time, date, and results. The children's diabetic regime required that they conduct blood glucose tests three to four times daily and record the results in a diary. Compliance was determined by the correspondence between the reported testing and results and the actual number, time, and results of each test as stored in memory. Interestingly, compliance did improve when subjects were told of the devices' memory capabilities, but noncompliance remained at about 16% despite the subjects' knowledge that the accuracy of their self-recording was being monitored.

Pharmacology

Behavioral strategies can be invaluable in the assessment of the effects of pharmacological agents. Numerous reports published in the last 10 to 15 years have attempted to document the prevalence rate of drug use in the mentally retarded population. Most investigations have focused on the use of psychoactive drugs with mentally retarded populations in institutional and community settings. Calculated rates of use range from a high of 76% (Sprague, 1977) to a low of 20% to 24% (Erickson, Bock, Young, & Silverstein, 1981). More recent interest in drug utilization in persons with mental retardation has focused on the appropriateness of the administration of drugs and the benefits obtained from the drugs prescribed (Bates, Smeltzer, & Arnoczky, 1986). Considering the multiple side effects that can occur from use of psychoactive medications (e.g., tardive dyskinesia, interference with learning, increase of problem behaviors, paradoxical excitement) and recent ethical and legal challenges to drug use with the mentally retarded population, objective assessment of the effects of pharmacological agents is a necessity (Barron & Sandman, 1985; Briggs, Hamad, Garrard, & Wills, 1984).

Behavior analytic techniques used to assess the effects of drugs were first mandated by court proceedings in 1974 (Briggs et al., (1984). In this case, the court required that the target behavior be clearly described, baseline frequencies of the behavior be obtained, and ongoing recordings be made to note frequency changes. With the appearance of litigations addressing the use and assessment of psychoactive drugs with mentally retarded individuals, a series of reports noted efforts to evaluate drug effects with the mentally retarded population (Ferguson, Cullari, Davidson, & Breuning, 1982; Fielding, Murphy, Reagan, & Peterson, 1980; Inoue, 1982). Most of these reports discuss use of comprehensive assessment techniques to reduce the use of drugs in large residential centers. Each study used an idiosyncratic means of assessing drug effects and benefits, including use of objective frequency counts of maladaptive behaviors, interdisciplinary team reviews, and direct care staff interviews.

Fielding et al. (1980) used a daily frequency count of prespecified maladaptive behaviors to assess the benefits of psychoactive drugs with institutionalized mentally retarded individuals. Clients participated in a 50-day assessment period consisting of 20 days during which they received medications and 30 days when no medications were administered. At the end of 30 medication-free days, those individuals whose specific behavior rates did not increase to twice that exhibited while receiving medications were no longer given psychoactive drugs. Ferguson et al. (1982) used a combination of a monthly interdisciplinary team review and graphic presentations of maladaptive behavior frequencies to assess the benefits of psychoactive medications. Mean daily frequencies, mean deviations scores, and trendlines were computed. When the trendline was stable, the medication dosage was decreased. If the trendline was decreasing, no changes were made. When the trendline was increasing, an increase in medication dosage was made. Numerous studies have documented a behavioral approach to the assessment and use of psychoactive drugs in the mentally retarded population. For a detailed review of this literature, the reader is referred to Briggs et al. (1984).

Although the literature predominately contains reports of the use of behavioral techniques to assess the effects of psychoactive agents, behavioral assessment techniques are appropriate for use with other pharmacological agents such as medication for epileptic disorders. Briggs et al. (1984) propose a behavioral model that, in general, is useful for evaluating pharmacological agents. If the medication is a psychoactive agent and is being prescribed to decrease unacceptable behavior, it is essential that the behavior be clearly defined and the baseline frequency be established. Since medications are generally not selectively effective, it is recommended that several behaviors be observed in order to clearly assess the effects and side effects of the drugs. Treatment teams should be identified to regularly review the medication administered, behavior changes noted via objective data collection (e.g., frequency counts, interval recording, etc.), and evidence of side effects. Staff expectancy problems and interobserver reliability measures must also be considered.

Pain

Unfortunately, there are few research data available on the use of behavioral assessment methods in the treatment of pain and stress in DD populations. Of course, DD individuals present with medical disorders and are subjected to the same medical protocols as are non-DD individuals. The reasons for the lack of information on pain-stress assessment in DD individuals is unclear. However, one might speculate that there continues to be gross misunderstanding of the biological and psychological functioning of these individuals (e.g., the belief that retarded individuals have decreased pain responsivity), resulting in the lack of clinical and research data for this population. For this reason, examples of tripartite pain assessment studies are presented that have employed non-DD subjects. Without doubt, the use of these methods can be generalized to DD populations with perhaps minor modification.

Objective direct observational coding schemes for the assessment of pain have been developed only recently. Although there exist several indices of behavioral distress/pain used in adult populations (e.g., Fordyce, 1976), pediatric examples are presented here with the belief that they may hold more potential for adaptation to DD populations. Adult measures often emphasize patient verbal responses and thus may have restricted application.

First, it should be noted that the constructs of pain and anxiety are probably inextricably intertwined (e.g., Katz, Kellerman, & Siegel, 1981; Shacham & Daut, 1981). That is, from an observational viewpoint it is not possible to easily distinguish between anxiety and pain responses evidenced either as a function of a specific medical disorder (e.g., rheumatoid arthritis) or administration of aversive medical procedures (e.g., injections, bone marrow aspiration, burn debridement, etc.). At this time, one often encounters the compromise term *behavioral distress* in reference to medically related pain and anxiety responses.

Many of the observational methods of recording pain responses or behavioral distress are based on some modification of the observational scale originally developed by Katz, Kellerman, and Siegel (1980). The scale consists of operationally defined responses, such as flinching, screaming, crying, and so on that reflect aspects of the patient's motor and verbal responses to an aversive medical procedure (bone marrow aspiration in this case). Similar coding schemes or modification of the Katz et al. code have since been used successfully with hematology-oncology patients (Jay, Ozolins, Elliott, & Caldwell, 1983) and pediatric burns (Kelley, Jarvie, Middlebrook, McNeer, & Drabman, 1984; Tarnowski, McGrath, Calhoun, & Drabman, 1987). The use of these observational scales typically involves observing patients either during specific medical procedures or in specific care settings (e.g., physical therapy) and noting patient responses via the use of a time sampling or interval recording procedure. Molecular patient responses (e.g., crying, screaming, verbal requests to stop a procedure, etc.) are then collapsed to produce some type of molar response summary index such as verbal or motoric pain.

Most often, the use of direct observational codes are accompanied by the use of self-report measures. Such measures typically involve obtaining ratings from the patient concerning subjective reports of distress. Rating forms consisting of Likert scales are often used for this purpose. These forms ask patients to indicate the degree of distress subjectively experienced on a 5- or 7-point scale. Typically, such scales are anchored on each end by descriptors that range from "no discomfort at all" to "the most severe pain I have ever experienced." For individuals with limited language abilities, visual analogue scales (Stewart, 1977) (e.g., pain thermometers) may be helpful. It should be noted, that oftentimes staff who are working with patients are asked to complete these same self-report scales. For example, Kelley et al. (1984) observed the behavioral distress of two young children who were undergoing debridement (removal of devitalized tissue) via a variant of the Katz et al. (1980) observational coding scheme. In addition, children were asked to rate their subjective distress on a pictorial rating scale. Finally, parents and staff were asked to provide ratings of the children's cooperation, fear, and so forth. Hilgard and LeBaron (1982) employed similar behavioral observational and self-report procedures in their analysis of childhood cancer patients' behavioral distress in response to bone marrow aspirations. These measures hold the promise of generalized application to a wide variety of medical procedures and disorders that induce patient distress.

Finally, physiological measures are often collected in the attempt to better assess patient progress. Such measures may include electromyographic recordings, galvanic responses, palmar sweat index, heart rate, blood pressure, and the like. Oftentimes, physiological correlates of patient behavioral distress are readily available in medical charts but often overlooked. For example, time out of bed, food intake, steps taken in physical therapy, time to complete procedures, decreased analgesic intake, and so forth are often very helpful in assessing patient status. Again, these variables may or may not systematically covary with behavioral and self-report data.

For more detailed review of the tripartite pain assessment literature, interested readers may refer to the reviews by Jay et al. (1983), Katz, Varni, and Jay (1984), and Varni, Jay, Masek, and Thompson (1986).

Technology

Improvements in data quality can result from the use of modern technology in behavioral assessment. Examples will vary over time with advances in technology, but the role of technology in behavioral assessment can be summarized as follows: technology is useful to the extent that it brings the decision-making process of the clinician or experimenter under better stimulus control of real changes in the behavior of interest. There are three ways in which technology can accomplish this: 1) by improving our ability to detect certain responses, 2) by increasing the reliability of the data to be analyzed, and 3) by speeding data analysis through partial processing of the data as it is collected and, as a result, decreasing the time required to draw conclusions from it.

Behavior of clinical or educational interest may be difficult to detect. First, detection via direct observation may be inconvenient because of response rate characteristics, the absence of observer availability at relevant times, or the need for behaviorally intrusive detection procedures. Inappropriate urination is an example of a response with these characteristics, and treatment has been facilitated through the use of simple electronic moisture detection devices (Azrin, Sneed, & Foxx, 1974; Hansen, 1979) and by the simpler technology of blue litmus paper that turns pink when urine touches it (Foxx & Azrin, 1973). Rugh and Schwitzgebel (1977) provide a comprehensive discussion of various response detection systems. Another reason for the need to use technology for response detection is the response hypothesized to be of greatest relevance may be of low intensity or represent a private event. Electrophysiological responses fall in this second category.

Self-injurious behavior is typically assessed by direct observation, but this technique increases the risk of allowing an uncontrolled episode to begin, with the resulting risk of serious injury to the client. Schroeder, Peterson, Solomon, and Artley (1977) used an electromyogram (EMG) signal, voltage increases in the right trapazius muscle that seemed to occur prior to head banging in two mentally retarded subjects, as an early warning to therapists that a head-banging episode was about to begin. Similarly, Lang and Melamed (1969) recorded EMG from under the chin and from throat muscles of a 4-year-old ruminative vomiter. The EMG tracings recorded on a polygraph were discriminably different from other response patterns such as crying, and were used to confirm the occurrence of the target vomiting response.

Many researchers have hypothesized that aberrant behavior, such as aggression or self-injury and even fear or abnormal tension, would be incompatible with a state of relaxation. Relaxation has been defined in terms of certain presumably correlated electrophysiological response patterns. Relaxation was defined with EMG signals in a study of the use of biofeedback-assisted relaxation training in the treatment of aggression by Hughes and Davis (1980). Other examples of relaxation training with and without biofeedback are reviewed by Luiselli (1980). A note of caution, however, was sounded by Parker et al. (1984), who demonstrated that the behavioral topography of abnormal orofacial responses could be therapeutically shaped by environmental contingencies for visually detected responses without any consistent changes in the EMG signal for those muscle groups that would have been affected had biofeedback training been used.

Examples of increasing the reliability of behavioral data include the use of permanent audio and video recordings of behavioral samples, permanent product data such as a record of answers stored with a computerized testing system, and any technique for transducing the behavior of an individual in an experimental setting. Tiller, Stygar, Hess, and Reimer (1982) used a mercury switch to operate an audible alarm signal device to reliably detect certain abnormal postures in a subject with Down syndrome. Another example is the use of EEG recordings to verify that observed behavior thought to reflect seizures actually did so (Cataldo, Russo, et al., 1979). Neill and Alvares (1986) used a radiotelemetered EEG video recording system to determine the relationship between behavior thought to signify seizures and abnormal electrical brain activity. Their system allowed precise temporal relationships to be established between the two measures, and both seizures and pseudoseizures could be demonstrated clearly. Finally, noise intensity was measured by Tiller, Masek, and Walker (1974) in an EMR classroom. Noise level is a good example of a behavioral event that is most reliably recorded electronically because human observers would be subject to effects of either masking or habituation within and between sessions.

The last set of examples to be considered represents partial processing of the data during its collection. Any computer-based testing paradigm has the potential to accomplish partial analysis of subject data during the recording session. Ditallo (1986) used a microcomputer to record and present sensory stimuli in a study designed to demonstrate a reliable method to derive a reinforcer preference hierarchy in youngsters with severe and profound retardation. Schroeder (1972a, 1972b) described a system in which the use of tools by workers in a sheltered workshop could be recorded by electromechanical equipment. The tools completed electrical connections when they were touched against the work on an assembly line, and cumulative recorders provided experimenters with an accuate representation of their rate of work as it was being done. Linscheid, Feiner, and Sostek (1984) used time-lapse video recording to measure the activity level of a hyperactive retarded child in an open-field test. Their system greatly reduced the time needed to derive an activity score when compared with scoring real-time tapes, and the grid used to measure activity was superimposed on the video image, not marked on the floor as is usually done, thereby eliminating a potential source of subject reactivity.

These examples simply provide an overview of the many ways to use technology to enhance assessment. A more extensive review of devices and instrumentation in assessment and intervention for this population is provided by Mulick, Scott, Gaines, and Campbell (1983).

Summary

This chapter describes the basis of behavioral assessment and highlights selected applications. The usefulness of behavioral assessment as a tool in behavioral medicine research lies in its ability to reveal functional relationships between behavior, medical condition, and medical and behavioral treatments for individuals. This contrasts with traditional, medically oriented group research that attempts to establish more generalized relationships between variables. For example, a hypothetical finding might be that psychoactive drugs are of benefit in treating behavior problems in 80% of developmentally disabled clients. What is lost in the above example, of course, is information on which type of behaviors are changed, the degree of change, and the specification of other environmental factors that may be functionally related to the noted behavior change.

The discussion of tripartite assessment, emphasizes the need to examine assessment data from direct observation, self-report, and physiological sources in order to fully understand their interrelatedness. To be sure, data obtained from these dimensions often do not correlate even though they are assumed to be measurements of the same thing.

Direct observational techniques are central to behavioral assessment. Knowledge of frequency, duration, interval, and time sampling techniques is essential for the behavioral medicine clinician and researcher. This is especially true with a developmentally disabled population where verbal self-report may be impossible or of questionable validity because of motor or cognitive impairments.

Single-subject designs provide the mechanism whereby functional relationships can be determined. In addition, they allow for increased confidence that observed functional relationships indeed do exist and are not due to chance or other extraneous variables.

Concepts of reliability and validity are of importance in any measurement schema. With behavioral assessment, where human observers are often used, reliability of measurement is of foremost concern. Interobserver agreement forms the basis for establishing behavioral observation reliability. Reliability estimates are an essential component of behavioral assessment and behavioral medicine intervention.

As the field continues to develop, a wider variety of behavioral assessment techniques will emerge. It is the feeling of these authors that technological advances will lead to improved reliability and more sophisticated assessment, reducing the role of the human observer while yielding reliable and meaningful information.

References

American Psychiatric Association. (1980). *Diagnostic and statistical manual of mental disorders: DSM-III.* Washington, DC: Author.

Azrin, N.H., & Foxx, R.M. (1971). A rapid method for toilet training the institutionalized retarded. *Journal of Applied Behavior Analysis, 4,* 89–99.

Azrin, N.H., Sneed, T.J., & Foxx, R.M. (1974). Dry-bed training: Rapid elimination of childhood enuresis. *Behavior Research and Therapy, 12,* 147–156.

Baer, D.M., Wolf, M.M., & Risley, T.R. (1968). Some current dimensions of applied behavior analysis. *Journal of Applied Behavior Analysis, 1,* 91–97.

Balaschak, B.A., & Mostofsky, D.I. (1981). Seizure disorders. In E.J. Mash & L.G. Terdal (Eds.), *Behavioral assessment of childhood disorders* (pp. 602–638). New York: Guilford Press.

Bandura, A., Blanchard, E.B., & Ritter, B. (1969). Relative efficacy of desensitization and modeling approaches for inducing behavioral, affective, and attitudinal changes. *Journal of Personality and Social Psychology, 13,* 173–199.

Barlow, D.H., & Hersen, M. (1973). Single case experimental designs: Uses in clinical research. *Archives of General Psychiatry, 29,* 319–325.

Barlow, D.H., & Hersen, M. (1984). *Single case experimental designs: Strategies for studying behavior change.* New York: Pergamon Press.

Barron, J.B., & Sandman, C. (1985). Paradoxical excitement to sedative-hypnotics in mentally retarded clients. *American Journal of Mental Deficiency, 90,* 124–129.

Bates, W.J., Smeltzer, D., & Arnoczky, S. (1986). Appropriate and inappropriate use of psychotherapeutic medications for institutionalized mentally retarded persons. *American Journal of Mental Deficiency, 90,* 363–370.

Briggs, R., Hamad, C., Garrad, S., & Wills, F. (1984). A model for evaluating psychoactive medication use with mentally retarded person. In J.A. Mulick & B. Mallory (Eds.), *Transitions in mental retardation* (Vol. 1, pp. 229–248). Norwood, NJ: Ablex Publishing Corp.

Cataldo, M.F., Bessman, C.A., Parker, L.H., Pearson, J.E., & Rogers, M.C. (1979). Behavioral assessment for pediatric intensive care units. *Journal of Applied Behavior Analysis*, *12*, 279–281.

Cataldo, M.F., Russo, D.C., & Freeman, J.M. (1979). A behavioral analysis approach to high-rate myoclonic seizures. *Journal of Autism and Developmental Disabilities*, *9*, 413–427.

Cone, J.D. (1978). The behavioral assessment grid (BAG): A conceptual framework and taxonomy. *Behavior Therapy*, *9*, 882–888.

Cone, J.D., & Hawkins, R.P. (1977). *Behavioral assessment: New directions in clinical psychology.* New York: Brunner/Mazel.

Cunningham, C.E., & Linscheid, T.R. (1976). Elimination of chronic infant rumination by electric shock. *Behavior Therapy*, *7*, 231–234.

Ditallo, J. (1986). Computerized assessment of preference for severely handicapped individuals. *Journal of Applied Behavior Analysis*, *19*, 445–448.

Dunbar, J. (1983). Compliance in pediatric populations. In P.J. McGrath & P. Firestone (Eds.), *Pediatric and adolescent behavioral medicine: Issues in treatment* (pp. 210–230). New York: Springer.

Elliot, C., & Olson, R. (1983). The management of children's distress in response to painful medical treatment of burns. *Behavior Research and Therapy*, *21*, 675–683.

Epstein, L.H., Beck, S., Figueroa, J., Farkas, G., Kazdin, A.E., Daneman, D., & Becker, D. (1981). The effects of targeting improvements in urine glucose on metabolic control in children with insulin dependent diabetes. *Journal of Applied Behavior Analysis*, *14*, 365–375.

Erickson, E., Bock, W., Young, R., & Silverstein, B. (1981). Psychotropic drug use in Title XIX (ICF-MR) facilities for the mentally retarded in Minnesota. In R. Young & J. Kroll (Eds.), *The use of medications in controlling the behavior of mentally retarded: Proceedings* (pp. 82–88). Minneapolis: University of Minnesota.

Ferguson, D., Cullari, S., Davidson, N., & Breuning, S. (1982). Effects of data-based interdisciplinary medication reviews on the prevalence and pattern of neuroleptic drug use with institutionalized mentally retarded persons. *Education and Training of the Mentally Retarded*, *17*, 103–108.

Fielding, L., Murphy, R., Reagan, M., & Peterson, T. (1980). An assessment program to reduce drug use with the mentally retarded. *Hospital and Community Psychiatry*, *31*, 771–773.

Fordyce, W.E. (1976). *Behavioral methods for chronic pain and illness.* St. Louis: C.V. Mosby.

Foxx, R.M., & Azrin, N.H. (1973). *Toilet training the retarded: A rapid program for day and nighttime independent toileting.* Champaign, IL: Research Press.

Hansen, G.D. (1979). Enuresis control through fading, escape, and avoidance training. *Journal of Applied Behavior Analysis*, *12*, 303–307.

Hartman, D.P. (1977). Consideration in the choice of interobserver reliability estimates. *Journal of Applied Behavior Analysis*, *10*, 103–116.

Hawkins, R.P., & Dobes, R.W. (1975). Behavioral definitions in applied behavior analysis: Explicit or implicit. In B.C. Etzel, J.M. LeBlanc, & D.M. Baer (Eds.), *New developments in behavioral research: Theory, methods and applications. In honor of Sidney W. Bijou* (pp. 167–188). Hillsdale, NJ: Lawrence Erlbaum.

Haynes, S.N. (1977). *Principles of behavioral assessment.* New York: Gardner Press.

Hilgard, J.R., & LeBaron, S. (1982). Relief of anxiety and pain in children and adolescents with cancer: Quantitative measures and clinical observations. *International Journal of Clinical and Experimental Hypnosis*, *30*, 417–442.

Hughes, H., & Davis, R. (1980). Treatment of aggressive behavior: The effect of EMG response discrimination biofeedback training. *Journal of Autism and Developmental Disorders, 10,* 193–202.

Inoue, F. (1982). A clinical pharmacy service to reduce psychotropic drug use in an institution for mentally handicapped persons. *Mental Retardation, 20,* 70–74.

Jay, S.M., Ozolins, M., Elliott, C.M., & Caldwell, S. (1983). Assessment of children's distress during painful medical procedures. *Health Psychology, 2,* 133–147.

Johnson, S.M., & Bolstad, O.D. (1973). Methodological issues in naturalistic observation: Some problems and solutions for field research. In L.A. Hamerlynck, L.C. Handy, & E.J. Mash (Eds.), *Behavior change: Methodology, concepts, and practice* (pp. 7–67). Champaign, IL: Research Press.

Katz, E.R., Kellerman, J., & Siegel, S.E. (1980). Behavioral distress in children with cancer undergoing medical procedures: Developmental considerations. *Journal of Consulting and Clinical Psychology, 48,* 356–365.

Katz, E.R., Kellerman, J., & Siegel, S.E. (1981). Anxiety as an affective focus in the clinical study of acute behavioral distress: A reply to Shacham and Daut. *Journal of Consulting and Clinical Psychology, 49,* 470–471.

Katz, E.R., Varni, J.W., & Jay, S.M. (1984). Behavioral assessment and management of pediatric pain. In M. Hersen, R.M. Eisler, & P.M. Miller (Eds.), *Progress in behavior modification* (Vol. 18, pp. 163–193). Orlando, FL: Academic Press.

Kazdin, A.E. (1977). Assessing the clinical and applied importance of behavior change through social validation. *Behavior Modification, 1,* 427–452.

Kazdin, A.E. (1981). Behavioral observation. In M. Hersen & A.S. Bellack (Eds.), *Behavioral assessment: A practical handbook* (pp. 101–124). New York: Pergamon Press.

Kelley, M.L., Jarvie, G.L., Middlebrook, J.L., McNeer, M.F., & Drabman, R.S. (1984). Decreasing burned children's pain behavior: Impacting the trauma of hydrotherapy. *Journal of Applied Behavior Analysis, 17,* 147–158.

Kent, R.N., & Foster, S.L. (1977). Direct observational procedures: Methodological issues in naturalistic settings. In A.R. Ciminero, K.S. Calhoun, & H.E. Adams (Eds.), *Handbook of behavioral assessment* (pp. 279–328). New York: Wiley.

Lang, P.J. (1968). Fear reduction and fear behavior: Problems in treating a construct. In J.M. Schlien (Ed.), *Research in psychotherapy* (Vol. 3). Washington, DC: American Psychological Association.

Lang, P.J., & Melamed, B.G. (1969). Avoidance conditioning therapy of an infant with chronic ruminative vomiting. *Journal of Abnormal Psychology, 74,* 1–8.

Linscheid, T.R., Feiner, J.M., & Sostek, A.M. (1984). Use of time-lapse video recording for the direct measurement of behavior in the mentally retarded. *Applied Research in Mental Retardation, 5,* 317–327.

Luiselli, J.K. (1980). Relaxation training with the developmentally disabled: A reappraisal. *Behavior Research of Severe Developmental Disabilities, 1,* 191–213.

Magrab, P.R., & Papadopoulou, Z.L. (1977). The effects of a token economy on dietary compliance for children on hemodialysis. *Journal of Applied Behavior Analysis, 10,* 573–578.

Mash, E.J., & Terdal, L.G. (1976). *Behavior therapy assessment: Diagnosis, design, and evaluation.* New York: Springer.

Mash, E.J., & Terdal, L.G. (1982). *Behavioral assessment of childhood disorders.* New York: Guilford Press.

Mash, E.J., Terdal, L.G., & Anderson, K. (1973). The response-class matrix: A procedure for scoring parent-child interactions. *Journal of Consulting and Clinical Psychology, 40*, 163–164.

Mulick, J.A., Scott, F.D., Gaines, R.F., & Campbell, B.M. (1983). Devices and instrumentation for skill development and behavior change. In J.L. Matson & F. Andrasik (Eds.), *Treatment issues and innovations in mental retardation* (pp. 515–580). New York: Plenum Press.

Neill, J.C., & Alvarez, N. (1986). Differential diagnosis of epileptic versus pseudoepileptic seizures in developmentally disabled persons. *Applied Research in Mental Retardation, 7*, 285–298.

Nelson, R.O., & Hayes, S.C. (1979). Some current dimensions of behavioral assessment. *Behavioral assessment, 1*, 1–16.

Parker, L.H., Cataldo, M.F., Bourland, G., Emurian, C.S., Corbin, R.J., & Page, J.M. (1984). Operant treatment of orofacial dysfunction in neuromuscular disorders. *Journal of Applied Behavior Analysis, 17*, 413–428.

Risley, T.R., & Hart, B. (1968). Developing correspondence between the non-verbal and verbal behavior of preschool children. *Journal of Applied Behavior Analysis, 1*, 267–281.

Rojahn, J., & Schroeder, S.R. (1983). Behavioral assessment. In J.L. Matson & J.A. Mulick (Eds.), *Handbook of mental retardation* (pp. 227–244). New York: Pergamon Press.

Rugh, J.D., & Schwitzgebel, R.L. (1977). Instrumentation for behavioral assessment. In A.R. Ciminero, K.S. Calhoun, & H.E. Adams (Eds.), *Handbook of behavioral assessment* (pp. 79–113). New York: Wiley.

Russo, D.C., Bird, B.L., & Masek, B.J. (1980). Assessment issues in behavioral medicine. *Behavioral Assessment, 2*, 1–18.

Schroeder, S.R. (1972a). Automated transduction of sheltered workshop behaviors. *Journal of Applied Behavior Analysis, 5*, 523–525.

Schroeder, S.R. (1972b). Parametric effects of reinforcement frequency, amount of reinforcement, and required response force on sheltered workshop behavior. *Journal of Applied Behavior Analysis, 5*, 431–441.

Schroeder, S.R., Peterson, C.R., Solomon, L.J., & Artley, L.J. (1977). EMG feedback and the contingent restraint of self-injurious behavior among the severely retarded: Two case examples. *Behavior Therapy, 8*, 738–741.

Shacham, S., & Daut, R. (1981). Anxiety of pain: What does the scale measure? *Journal of Consulting and Clinical Psychology, 49*, 468–469.

Sprague, R. (1977). Overview of psychopharmacology for the retarded in the United States. In P. Mittler (Ed.), *Research to practice in mental retardation: Biomedical aspects* (Vol. 3, pp. 199–202). Baltimore: University Park Press.

Stewart, M.L. (1977). Measurement of clinical pain. In A. Jacox (Ed.), *Pain: A sourcebook for nurses and other health professionals* (pp. 107–137). Boston: Little, Brown.

Suinn, R.M. (1970). *Fundamentals of behavior pathology.* New York: Wiley.

Tarnowski, K.J., McGrath, M., Calhoun, B., & Drabman, R.S. (1987). Self- versus therapist-mediated debridement in pediatric thermal injury. *Journal of Pediatric Psychology, 12*, 567–579.

Tarnowski, K.J., Rosen, L.A., McGrath, M., & Drabman, R.S. (1987). Application of a modified habit reversal procedure to a recalcitrant case of trichotillomania. *Journal of Behavior Therapy and Experimental Psychiatry, 18*, 157–163.

Tiller, J., Stygar, M.K., Hess, C., & Reimer, L. (1982). Treatment of functional chronic stooped posture using a training device and behavior therapy. *Physical Therapy, 62,* 1597–1600.

Tiller, J.E., Masek, B.J., & Walker, L.C. (1974). A system for monitoring and modifying noise levels in the classroom. *Behavioral Engineering, 1,* 20–23.

Touchette, P.E., MacDonald, R.F., & Langer, S.N. (1985). A scatter plot for identifying stimulus control of behavior problems. *Journal of Applied Behavior Analysis, 18,* 343–351.

Varni, J.W. (1983). *Clinical behavioral pediatrics: An interdisciplinary approach.* New York: Pergamon Press.

Varni, J.W., Jay, S.M., Masek, B.J., & Thompson, K.L. (1986). Cognitive-behavioral assessment and management of pediatric pain. In A.D. Holzman & D.C. Turk (Eds.), *Pain management: A handbook of psychological treatment approaches* (pp. 168–192). New York: Pergamon Press.

Wilson, D.P., & Endres, R.K. (1986). Compliance with blood glucose monitoring in children with Type I diabetes mellitus. *Journal of Pediatrics, 108,* 1022–1024.

3
Feeding Disorders

LORI A. SISSON AND VINCENT B. VAN HASSELT

Introduction

Problems relating to feeding occur in approximately one out of four children. The prevalence of eating disorders is even higher among developmentally disabled individuals. For example, it has been estimated that 80% or more of these persons exhibit maladaptive feeding behaviors that can lead to undesirable consequences for physical, social, and educational/vocational development (Perske, Clifton, McClean, & Stein, 1977). More conservative figures are reported by Jones (1982), who summarized findings from a number of researchers indicating that 19% to 61% of mentally retarded clients at inpatient or outpatient centers experience eating problems.

At least four feeding-related problems have been identified. First, a major area of concern is acquisition and maintenance of independent self-feeding behavior. There are mentally retarded persons who cannot scoop food onto a spoon and bring it to their mouths (O'Brien, Bugle, & Azrin, 1972) or who do not exhibit socially acceptable table manners (O'Brien & Azrin, 1972). Second, disruptive mealtime responses, such as stereotypic behavior, throwing a tantrum, and stealing food, also have received much investigative attention (Barton, Guess, Garcia, & Baer, 1970). These may occur throughout the day (Sisson & Dixon, 1986b) or may be specific to mealtimes (Horton, 1987). A third target in feeding research is the rate at which food is ingested. Some clients eat too fast (Favell, McGimsey, & Jones, 1980), while others eat too slowly (Luiselli, 1988). A fourth set of feeding disorders involves dietary inadequacies in which the total amount of food consumed is insufficient, or the variety of foods accepted is severely limited from a nutritional standpoint. Many individuals with developmental disabilities display highly selective food preferences, and in some cases, almost total food refusal (Luiselli & Gleason, 1987).

Rumination and vomiting, as well as obesity, also are frequent among mentally retarded children and adults. Although feeding-related problems, these disorders will not be addressed in the present review since they are covered in other chapters in this book (Fox, Meyer, & Rotatori, Chapter 5, this text; Luiselli, Chapter 6, this text). The interested reader also is referred to two other excellent reviews for information pertaining to rumination and vomiting (Starin & Fuqua, 1987) and obesity (Burkhart, Fox, Rotatori, 1985) in the developmentally disabled population.

The causes for mealtime problems are diverse. Neuromotor dysfunction may contribute to inability to manage utensils and interfere with chewing and swallowing (Utley, Holvoet, & Barnes, 1977). Such dysfunction may be characterized by: 1) spasticity or increased muscle tone resulting in stiffness, 2) athetosis or fluctuating muscle tone evidenced in uncontrolled movements, 3) hypotonia or decreased muscle tone appearing as flaccidity, or 4) oral hypersensitivity or hyposensitivity. Sensory or physical impairments, such as blindness, muscular dystrophy, paralysis, cleft lip or palate, deformities of the digestive tract, and multiple food allergies, also may account for an individual's failure to self-feed or accept certain foods (Jones, 1978). Finally, inadequate exposure to a variety of foods, insufficient feeding skills training, and inappropriate contingencies for mealtime behaviors can explain the abnormal eating behaviors of some developmentally delayed clients (Jones, 1982). Despite the deleterious effects of neuromotor dysfunction and physical limitations on feeding, it has been suggested that caregiver mismanagement plays a pivotal role in most eating problems and that nearly 20% of all cases may be explained by environmental influences alone (Palmer & Horn, 1978).

There are numerous deleterious consequences of feeding disorders. Persons who are not independent feeders, who eat slowly, or who refuse to eat may consume insufficient amounts of food. This places them at high risk for a number of difficulties, including excessive weight loss, lethargy, malnutrition, diminished function, and growth retardation (Martin, 1973; Riordan, Iwata, Finney, Wohl, & Stanley, 1984; Wurtman & Wurtman, 1977). In addition, the increased caregiver time required to assist in feeding may prohibit these individuals from placement in community residential, educational, and vocational settings (Ohwaki & Zingarelli, 1988; Reid, Wilson, & Faw, 1983). Eating too quickly or stealing food may result in increased calorie intake and obesity and are socially unacceptable (Reid, 1983). Rapid eating also may result in health problems such as vomiting or aspiration (Favell et al., 1980). Disruptive behaviors are especially troublesome at mealtimes when caregivers often are responsible for managing large groups of clients with special needs. These responses not only interfere with adequate food intake, but also pose a danger to individuals and property, such as when the person becomes aggressive or destructive (Barton et al., 1970). Finally, mealtimes provide many opportunities to facilitate social and communication skills in developmentally delayed individuals. Unfortunately, the client with a feeding problem usually fails to benefit from positive interpersonal interactions and training efforts in these crucial areas (Reid et al., 1983).

Treatments for feeding disorders have included psychotherapy for the individual and his or her family, positioning and therapeutic exercises, liquifying meals, and tube feeding (Jones, 1982). Further, the past two decades have yielded a significant body of research demonstrating the efficacy of procedures derived from operant conditioning principles in the treatment of mealtime problems. The purpose of this chapter is to review the behavioral treatment approaches employed with developmentally disabled individuals who have feeding disorders. Included is an examination of both clinical and experimental efforts to remediate the aforementioned feeding problems. Unfortunately, many reports are case studies and program descriptions that lack experimental rigor. Such papers are included because they represent pioneering work in the area and suggest future directions for controlled research. At this point, they comprise a large portion of the literature addressing treatment of developmentally disabled clients; to exclude them would result in an incomplete representation of the field.

Promoting Self-Feeding Behavior

Since the mid-1960s, there has been a proliferation of endeavors documenting the effectiveness of behavior modification techniques in teaching self-help and social competency skills to severely and profoundly mentally retarded persons. One emphasis of this work was the establishment of appropriate self-feeding responses to encourage independence (Reid, 1983) and increase social acceptability (Barton et al., 1970). Although it is difficult to ascertain the number of developmentally disabled individuals who do not feed themselves, it has been estimated to be quite large (Jones, 1982; Reid et al., 1983). Concern for the development of this self-help skill is reflected in the large number of commercially available training programs and curricula that have been developed for use with mentally retarded individuals (Reid, 1983).

Several reports describe general behavioral approaches to training a variety of adaptive behaviors in institutionalized mentally retarded persons. In these, techniques to promote feeding skills are but one component of a broad spectrum of self-help skills training strategies. Alternatively, behavioral programs specifically designed to develop independent feeding behavior have been discussed. These two groups of studies are presented below.

Self-Help Skills Training Programs

Early self-help skills training efforts generally involved four elements: 1) environmental improvements, 2) increases in staff-to-client ratios, 3) staff training in reinforcement and response shaping, and 4) implementation of these techniques with participants at all levels of mental retardation and across a wide range of behaviors and settings (Bensberg, Colwell, & Cassel, 1965; Colwell, Richards, McCarver, & Ellis, 1973; Gorton & Hollis, 1965; Pursley & Hamilton, 1965; Roos, 1965). In these investigations, the utility of behavioral treatment was inferred from improved ratings of subjects' independent living skills on assessment instruments that covered several disparate responses including feeding (Reid et al., 1983). In addition, anecdotal information suggested that staff were more satisfied with their jobs (Bensberg et al., 1965) and that residents demonstrated gains in areas not directly addressed, such as greater behavioral control and higher overall IQ scores (Colwell et al., 1973).

Subsequent work evaluated the confounding effects of environmental changes and increased attention from ward staff by including control groups that experienced these improvements alone in addition to experimental subjects who received these conditions combined with behavior therapy. Results of these studies revealed that operant conditioning increased independent self-care skills to a greater degree than environment and staffing upgrades alone (Gray & Kasteler, 1969; Kimbrell, Luckey, Barbuto, & Love, 1967; Roos & Oliver, 1969). Further, improved physical and social environments were shown to be about equal to existing ward conditions in fostering independent feeding, dressing, and grooming (Murphy & Zahm, 1975, 1978). Other investigations demonstrated that gains in self-help skills were maintained for 4 (Lawrence & Kartye, 1971) or 7 (Leath & Flournoy, 1970) months, despite termination of formal training programs. The success of these early efforts was in large part responsible for promoting the use of behavioral interventions with severely and profoundly mentally retarded individuals.

Feeding Skills Training Programs

As mentioned earlier, other studies focused specifically on training feeding skills as opposed to teaching several self-help skills simultaneously. Approaches to teaching self-feeding can be roughly categorized in terms of the techniques employed. These include: 1) behavior shaping, 2) graduated guidance, and 3) treatment packages including instructions, modeling, physical guidance, behavior rehearsal, and performance feedback. A summary of investigations that targeted acquisition of independent self-feeding skills in developmentally disabled individuals is provided in Table 3.1.

BEHAVIOR SHAPING

In behavior shaping, the process of self-feeding is viewed as a sequence of responses and is task analyzed into discrete behavioral components. Then, training procedures are employed in which successively larger combinations of separate behaviors are systematically reinforced in order to form more complex skills. Chaining of feeding responses can be in a forward format by sequentially training each behavior in the order in which it normally occurs or in a backward format by teaching the steps in a reverse order. Prompting usually is necessary to elicit required behaviors. Prompts are provided according to a hierarchy of increasing intrusiveness. First, verbal instructions are given. If ineffective, gestures or modeling are used to communicate the desired behavior. Finally, physical guidance may be instituted. Forward and backward chaining in self-help skills training programs are discussed in detail by Watson and Uzzell (1981).

One early case study provides an example of forward chaining with a profoundly mentally retarded adolescent who did not feed herself (Whitney & Barnard, 1966). In this approach, the subject was fed a small piece of food from her meal when she displayed more and more advanced behavior. That is, bites of the

TABLE 3.1. Summary of behavioral research on acquisition of self-feeding skills

Primary treatment[a]	Reference	Subject[b]	Target[c]	Design
Behavior shaping: Forward chaining	Whitney & Barnard, 1966	1 PMR adolescent	Spoon-feeding	None
	Wilson, Reid, Phillips, & Burgio, 1984	4 PMR adolescents	Family-style eating: Setting place, passing and serving food, clearing place	Multiple baseline with 4-month follow-up
Behavior shaping: Backward chaining	Berkowitz, Sherry, & Davis, 1971	14 PMR children	Spoon-feeding	None
	Lemke & Mitchell, 1972	1 PMR child	Spoon-feeding	None
	McDonald, McCabe, & Mackle, 1977	5 PMR children	Spoon-feeding & other mealtime compliance	None
	Miller, Patton, & Henton, 1971	1 PMR child	Spoon-feeding & finger foods	None
	O'Brien, Bugle, & Azrin, 1972	1 PMR child	Spoon-feeding	None
	Song & Gandhi, 1974	4 PMR children	Spoon-feeding	None with 8-month follow-up
	Zeiler & Jervey, 1968	1 PMR adolescent	Spoon-feeding	None
Graduated guidance	Albin, 1977	3 PMR children	Spoon-feeding	None with 18-month follow-up
	Azrin & Armstrong, 1973	22 PMR adults	Use of all utensils, drinking from a cup	Compared to "best effort" training
	Richmon, Sonderby, & Kahn, 1980	6 SMR children	Use of fork	Multiple baseline with 6-month follow-up
Treatment packages: Instructions, modeling, physical guidance, feedback	Matson, Ollendick, & Adkins, 1980	40 Mo, S, & PMR adults	26 mealtime behaviors: Loading tray, table manners, clearing place, etc.	Compared to no treatment
	Nelson, Cone, & Hanson, 1975	24 Mo, S, & PMR adolescents	Use of all utensils	None
	O'Brien & Azrin, 1972 (Study 1)	6 Mi, Mo, S, & PMR adults	Use of all utensils, table manners	Compared to no treatment
	O'Brien & Azrin, 1972 (Study 2)	6 Mo, S & PMR adults	Use of all utensils, table manners	Compared to no treatment
	Sisson & Dixon, 1986a	6 Mo, S, & PMR children	Use of all utensils, table manners	Multiple baseline with 1-month follow-up
	Sisson & Dixon, 1986c	4 Mi and Mo MR children	Use of all utensils, table manners	Multiple baseline

[a] Studies are categorized according to primary treatment as determined by the description of procedures. This is not necessarily the only treatment employed.
[b] Level of mental retardation was determined as closely as possible from subject descriptions and is represented by Mi = Mild, Mo = Moderate, S = Severe.
[c] Primary or representative target behaviors are listed, as determined by the description of procedures. These are not necessarily the only behaviors treated.

meal served as reinforcers for increasingly complex feeding responses. Initially, she merely had to *look* at her spoon. Next, she was required to *look* at and *reach* for the spoon. Then, *looking* at, *reaching* for, and *grasping* the spoon were required before food was forthcoming. Additional behaviors in the chain were not described but no doubt included: scooping, bringing food to her mouth, placing food in her mouth, and chewing and swallowing the food. Results showed that independent spoon-feeding was acquired in only five feeding sessions.

A recent investigation used forward chaining to develop more advanced family-style dining skills (e.g., setting place, passing and serving food, clearing place) in profoundly mentally retarded adolescents (Wilson, Reid, Phillips, & Burgio, 1984). This study used a multiple-baseline experimental design to demonstrate the controlling effects of the intervention. Training effects were immediate, and they were maintained over a 16-week follow-up period.

Results of several reports attest to the success of backward chaining in teaching feeding skills to developmentally disabled clients (see Table 3.1). In one of these (Berkowitz, Sherry, & Davis, 1971), 14 profoundly handicapped boys were trained to feed themselves with a spoon. The self-feeding process was divided into seven discrete steps, with reinforcement occurring naturally when food entered the mouth:

1. Aide, holding child's hand with spoon in child's hand, makes entire feeding cycle, from plate (scooping food) to mouth and back to plate.
2. Aide makes entire feeding cycle, but partially releases child's hand (still holding spoon with food on it) 2–3 inches below child's mouth. Child lifts spoon these last few inches himself.
3. Aide releases child's hand approximately six inches from child's mouth. Child lifts spoon about six inches.
4. Aide scoops food, releases child's hand at plate level. Child lifts spoon from plate to mouth.
5. Aide brings child's hand to plate, releasing hand. Child scoops food, and lifts spoon to mouth.
6. Aide releases hand after child has emptied spoon. Child brings spoon down to plate, scoops food, and lifts to mouth.
7. Child executes entire self-feeding cycle by himself (p. 64).

With this approach, all participants demonstrated independent feeding following 2 to 60 days of training, depending on the severity of their handicaps and associated behavior disorders. Similar effects have been replicated in other investigations, thus suggesting the efficacy of backward chaining in promoting appropriate eating skills (e.g., O'Brien et al., 1972; Zeiler & Jervey, 1968).

GRADUATED GUIDANCE

Graduated guidance is a highly sophisticated strategy with several defining characteristics. First, clients are taught using a forward sequencing format. Second, gentle manual guidance is employed to ensure that each response is completed correctly. The trainer begins by molding his or her hand around the subject's hand and guiding the entire self-feeding response. As the client learns to grasp the utensil, guidance is progressively reduced at the hand to a gentle touch. The locus of guidance then is faded up the arm to the forearm, elbow, upper arm, shoulder, and upper back. Finally, guidance is withdrawn completely.

High-density reinforcement is a third important characteristic of the graduated guidance approch. Clients receive verbal and physical reinforcement (e.g., praise, pats, hugs) almost continuously during training. In addition, primary and secondary reinforcers are administered upon completion of each training trial. Fourth, meals often are divided into several smaller portions to permit several training sessions per day and to control for satiation. Fifth, restitutional and positive practice overcorrection procedures are utilized to correct errors. For example, when spilling occurs, the client must clean up the area (restitution) and demonstrate the correct form of the response across several practice trials (positive practice).

Graduated guidance was developed by Azrin and Armstrong (1973), who taught 11 low-functioning institutionalized adults to eat properly in an average of 5 days. Replications with children (e.g., Richmon, Sonderby, & Kahn, 1980; Stimbert, Minor, & McCoy, 1977) have confirmed the effectiveness of the procedure.

TREATMENT PACKAGES

With few exceptions (Wilson et al., 1984), behavior shaping and graduated evidence have been used to foster very elementary eating behaviors, such as spoonfeeding. Once early skills are mastered, other strategies often are employed to produce more advanced responses. For example, Sisson and Dixon (1986c) trained multiple utensil use and table manners (chewing with mouth closed, wiping with a napkin, and sitting appropriately) in four hospitalized mentally retarded, psychiatrically disordered children. At the beginning of each training session, the therapist offered individualized verbal instructions and modeled each participant's target behavior(s). Then, praise, token reinforcement, and access to food were provided when subjects engaged in desired responses. On occurrences of inappropriate behaviors, an instructional sequence of verbal prompts, modeling, and physical guidance was carried out to ensure demonstration of positive feeding-related behaviors. This procedure was effective in improving objective assessments of level of target behaviors as well as subjective impressions by independent judges of subjects' overall feeding skills.

Instructions, modeling, physical guidance, rehearsal, and feedback are the basic elements of the treatment packages employed in the other investigations listed in Table 3.1. In a particularly ambitious project, 26 types of eating behaviors were treated in 40 institutionalized mentally retarded adults (Matson, Ollendick, & Adkins, 1980). Adaptations of the above-mentioned treatment package for use with such a large number of experimental subjects included adding self-evaluation and monitoring, as well as peer social reinforcement. Results indicated that treatment enhanced mealtime skills of participants when compared to ratings of individuals who had not received the intervention. Several additional reports have shown the efficacy of various behavioral treatment packages in teaching more complex feeding-related behaviors, such as grocery shopping (Wheeler, Ford, Nietupski, Loomis, & Brown, 1980), cooking (Martin, Rusch, James, Decker, & Trtol, 1982), and ordering meals at fast-food restaurants (van den Pol et al., 1981).

Decreasing Disruptive Mealtime Behavior

Although the previously discussed research focused primarily on teaching appropriate self-feeding skills, many of the treatment programs also incorporated a mild punishment component to reduce inappropriate responses during meals. For example, O'Brien et al. (1972) interrupted inappropriate feeding behaviors; Sisson and Dixon (1986a, 1986c) removed subjects' trays for a short period when disruptive or maladaptive responses occurred; and Miller, Patton, and Henton (1971) used brief time-out or dismissal from the meal to manage tantrumming.

A second group of investigations were carried out specifically to evaluate the ineffectiveness of deceleration strategies in eliminating unacceptable mealtime behaviors. Information pertaining to the number of mentally retarded individuals who exhibit behavior problems at meals is unavailable. Although estimates vary, the incidence of behavior disorders is higher in disabled than in nondisabled populations, and may exceed 50% (Jacobson, 1982a, 1982b). In general, interventions that have proven useful in managing maladaptive behaviors of developmentally delayed clients in other settings have been adapted for mealtimes. These studies are discussed in terms of the various behavioral treatments employed: 1) contingent-interrupted auditory stimulation, 2) interruption, 3) time-out, and 4) facial screening. Investigations targeting reduction of inappropriate mealtime responses are summarized in Table 3.2.

Contingent-Interrupted Auditory Stimulation

Despite a growing emphasis on positive approaches to behavior management with developmentally delayed individuals (Reese, 1982), only one study used a reinforcement-based procedure to eliminate undesirable mealtime responses. In this investigation, severe self-injurious behaviors (self-hitting and eye gouging) of a 10-year-old multihandicapped girl were treated (Sisson & Dixon, 1986b). Self-injury occurred in situations other than mealtime. However, mealtime provided a setting to test the value of an intervention that eventually could be applied across the day. Treatment involved continuous presentation of audiotaped stories when self-injurious behaviors were not observed. The stories were read by the child's mother, and anecdotal observations revealed that the young girl calmed and oriented toward the sound when the tape recording was played. The story tape was turned off when self-injury was noted. Evaluation of treatment using a withdrawal design demonstrated the effectiveness of this procedure. Once

TABLE 3.2. Summary of behavioral research on decreasing disruptive mealtime behavior

Primary treatment[a]	Reference	Subject[b]	Target[c]	Design
Contingent-interrupted auditory stimulation	Sisson & Dixon, 1986b	1 SMR, blind child	Self-injury	Withdrawal
Interruption	Henrickson & Doughty, 1967	4 PMR children	Disruptive behaviors: throwing, hitting, stealing	None
	Luiselli, in press (Study 1)	1 SMR, deaf-blind child	Self-stimulation	Withdrawal
Time-out: Brief tray removal	Christian, Hollomon, & Lanier, 1973	28 S & PMR adults	Stealing, messiness, eating with fingers	None
	Cipani, 1981	1 SMR adolescent	Spilling	Withdrawal with 3-month follow-up
	Martin, McDonald, & Omichinski, 1971	4 PMR children & adolescents	Messiness	Withdrawal
Time-out: Removal from meal	Barton, Guess, Garcia, & Baer, 1970	16 S & PMR children & adults	Stealing, messiness, eating with fingers	Multiple baseline
	Edwards & Lilly, 1966	26 PMR adolescents & adults	Stealing	None
	Groves & Carrocio, 1971	60 S & PMR adolescents & adults	Eating with fingers	None
	Hamilton & Allen, 1967	59 S & PMR adolescents & adults	Disruptive behaviors: Throwing, out of seat, stealing	None
	Thompson, 1977	1 Mo MR child	Disruptive behavior: Crying, throwing, self-injury	None
Facial screening	Horton, 1987	1 SMR child	Banging	Withdrawal with 19-month follow-up

[a] Studies are categorized according to primary treatment as determined by description of procedures. This is not necessarily the only treatment employed.
[b] Level of mental retardation was determined as closely as possible from subject descriptions and is represented by Mo = Moderate, S = Severe, and P = Profound.
[c] Primary or representative target behaviors are listed, as determined by the description of procedures. These are not necessarily the only behaviors treated.

self-injury was under control, appropriate use of napkin and utensils was trained using praise and access to food for appropriate behavior and brief time-out plus instructions for inappropriate responding. Desired mealtime responses were more frequent following initiation of behavioral programming.

Interruption

A slightly more restrictive treatment was used by Henrickson and Doughty (1967) to suppress several disruptive mealtime responses, including stealing and throwing food and hitting others. Subjects were four severely and profoundly mentally retarded boys. Whenever a child began to display one of the misbehaviors, he was told, "That's bad boy!" If inappropriate responding continued, it was interrupted by holding the boy's arms at his sides for 3 seconds. Daily monitoring for 13 weeks revealed that instances of maladaptive behavior requiring physical interruption decreased to near-zero levels, despite a change from specialized to natural settings at 11 weeks.

Time-Out

The most popular treatment for inappropriate mealtime behavior has been time-out or some variant. If food consumption is assumed to be reinforcing for the individual, then its removal (i.e., time-out from reinforcement) contingent on unwanted behaviors should decrease those responses. In one version of time-out, trainers simply deny access to food for a brief period of time, usually by moving subjects' trays away from them, whenever maladaptive behavior occurs. Alternatively, the individual is dismissed from the dining area and placed in a separate time-out room.

An example of the use of the former technique is provided by Cipani (1981), who modified food spilling by a 16-year-old severely mentally retarded female through the use of brief time-out. Whenever spilling occurred, the subject was required to place her spoon down on her tray, which was removed from her reach for 30 seconds. In addition, appropriate feeding behavior was reinforced through presentation of a preferred drink following gradually increasing numbers of correct feeding responses. A withdrawal design demonstrated the efficacy of treatment, and improved eating behavior was recorded during follow-up probes at 1, 2, and 3 months.

Time-out also was evaluated with 16 severely and profoundly handicapped individuals who displayed a variety of unacceptable eating habits (Barton et al., 1970). In this study, messiness was followed by a 15-second tray time-out, similar to that utilized by Cipani (1981). However, for stealing food and eating with fingers, subjects were removed from the table and placed in a unit time-out room for the remainder of the meal. These treatments were applied to target behaviors in a sequential and cumulative fashion according to the multiple-baseline design. Reduction of each inappropriate response was observed when the time-out procedure was initiated for that behavior. As Table 3.2 indicates, several replications of each time-out procedure have documented the utility of this approach with developmentally delayed clients (e.g., Hamilton & Allen, 1967; Martin, McDonald, & Omichinski, 1971).

Facial Screening

Horton (1987) examined the efficacy of facial screening as a treatment to reduce repetitive spoon banging by an 8-year-old, severely mentally retarded girl. In baseline, each episode of spoon banging was terminated by the trainer saying "No bang" while gently grasping the subject's wrist and returning her hand to a scoop dish. Treatment consisted of saying "No bang" and pulling a terry-cloth bib over the child's entire face for 5 seconds. Results of a withdrawal design indicated high frequencies of spoon banging during nontreatment conditions. In contrast, levels of disruptive banging rapidly decelerated when facial screening was in effect. Follow-up data at 6-, 10-, 15-, and 19-month intervals showed that gains were maintained.

Altering Rate of Eating

Rapid eating by developmentally delayed individuals is one of the most prevalent mealtime problems. One group of investigators (reported in Favell et al., 1980) surveyed two residential units for 60 severely and profoundly mentally retarded clients. Twenty-eight percent were reliably rated as "fast eaters." While individuals considered to eat at normal rates took approximately 8 bites of food per minute and consumed a meal within 15 to 20 minutes, clients judged as fast eaters consumed food at rates sometimes exceeding 20 bites per minute and finished their meal within 1 to 3 minutes. Despite the high frequency of pacing problems among mentally retarded individuals, there is a paucity of remediation efforts. A summary of the five investigations that have addressed this problem appears in Table 3.3.

One report (Kaufman, LaFleur, Hallahan, & Chanes, 1975) describes the use of imitation of rapid and sloppy eating as a punishment for eating too fast. However, the primary treatment has been a combination of physical prompting to slow down and positive reinforcement for adequate pauses between bites of food. For example, in a recent investigation, Lennox, Miltenberger, and Donnelly (1987) treated three profoundly mentally retarded adults who exhibited high-rate eating behaviors. First, any feeding response that occurred within 15 seconds of the previous one was prevented by guiding the subject's hand to the table. Second, the absence of an attempted bite for an entire 15-second interval was required before an eating response was permitted. Third, a competing behavior was prompted via a graduated guidance procedure following each eating response (whether permitted or interrupted). That is, subjects were physically guided to place utensils on their tray and hands in their laps. A multiple-baseline analysis showed that this multicomponent procedure increased the interval

TABLE 3.3. Summary of behavioral research on altering rate of eating

Primary treatment[a]	Reference	Subject[b]	Target[c]	Design
Imitation	Kauffman, LaFleur, Hallahan, & Chanes, 1975	1 Mo MR child	Rapid eating	Withdrawal
Prompts and reinforcement	Favell, McGimsey, & Jones, 1980	4 PMR adolescents	Rapid eating	Multiple baseline
	Knapczyk, 1983	1 SMR child	Rapid eating	Withdrawal with 1-month follow-up
	Lennox, Miltenberger, & Donnelley, 1987	3 PMR adults	Rapid eating	Multiple baseline with 5-month follow-up
	Luiselli, 1988	3 SMR sensory impaired children & adolescents	Rapid eating (1 subject), slow eating (2 subjects)	Withdrawal

[a] Studies are categorized according to primary treatment as determined by description of procedures. This is not necessarily the only treatment employed.
[b] Level of mental retardation was determined as closely as possible from subject descriptions and is represented by Mo = Moderate, S = Severe, and P = Profound.
[c] Primary or representative target behaviors are listed, as determined by the description of procedures. These are not necessarily the only behaviors treated.

between bites, or decelerated the rate of eating responses. Treatment effects were durable for 5 months.

Luiselli (1988) extended paced prompting treatment by employing it with three multihandicapped youths, one of whom ate too fast and two of whom ate too slowly. In the adapatation of paced prompting for slow eaters, subjects were guided through a feeding response whenever the pause between bites became too great. Again, results were positive, and the controlling effects of intervention were demonstrated with the withdrawal design.

Increasing Amount and Variety of Foods Consumed

Food selectivity and refusal have received much attention from the medical and psychiatric communities. This is largely due to the realization that, in extreme forms, these disorders are clearly life threatening. One review places the incidence of multiple food dislikes at higher than one third of the disabled population (Jones, 1982). Food intake may be limited by texture, where no solid foods are accepted, or by taste, where a severely limited range of foods is consumed. In addition, food acceptance, when it does occur, often is under very restricted stimulus control. That is, a child who routinely consumes baby food from a bottle may reject the same product when it is presented on a spoon.

Typical medical methods for treating food refusal include hyperalimentation (e.g., dietary supplementation, forced feeding), intravenous feeding, and the use of oral-gastric, nasogastric, or gastrostomy tubes. In cases of immediate risk from dehydration or severe malnutrition, these procedures often serve an essential stabilizing function. On the other hand, artificial feeding methods are undesirable as long-term strategies, for they do not actively promote effective feeding behavior and are themselves associated with additional health risks (Raventos, Kralemann, & Gray, 1982). Behavioral techniques offer an alternative to such interventions, and the available research suggests that operant procedures are promising with developmentally delayed individuals. Typically, this approach requires that preferred foods are delivered contingent upon eating nonpreferred ones. Several additional components have been added to this general strategy, including: 1) pacing, 2) texture fading, and 3) temporal limits for meals. Other researchers have evaluated overcorrection procedures and forced feeding to increase food intake. These studies are presented in Table 3.4 and described below.

Positive Reinforcement

Riordan and her colleagues (Riordan et al., 1984; Riordan, Iwata, Wohl, & Finney, 1980) used positive reinforcement procedures to increase the amount and variety of foods consumed by disabled children hospitalized for feeding problems. In these studies, foods were selected for training on the basis of extremely low percentages of acceptance or high rates of expulsion during baseline meals.

TABLE 3.4. Summary of behavioral research on increasing the amount and variety of foods consumed

Primary treatment[a]	Reference	Subject[b]	Target[c]	Design
Edible and social reinforcement	Palmer, Thompson, & Linscheid, 1975	1 BMR child	Food selectivity	None with 4-month follow-up
	Riordan, Iwata, Finney, Wohl, & Stanley, 1984	4 Handicapped children	Food selectivity	Multiple baseline with 30-month follow-up
	Riordan, Iwata, Wohl, & Finney, 1980	2 Mo MR children	Food selectivity	Multiple baseline with 2-month follow-up
	Sisson & Dixon, in press	1 Mo MR adolescent	Food selectivity	Withdrawal and multiple baseline
Edible reinforcement & pacing	Luiselli, in press a (Study 2)	1 SMR, deaf-blind child	Food selectivity	Withdrawal
Sensory reinforcement & texture fading	Luiselli & Gleason, 1987	1 SMR, deaf-blind child	Food refusal	None with 12-month follow-up
Edible reinforcement & texture fading	Leibowitz & Holcer, 1974	1 Mo MR child	Food selectivity and self-feeding	None with 5-month follow-up
Edible reinforcement & temporal limits	Luiselli, Evans, & Boyce, 1985	1 Mo, deaf-blind MR child	Food selectivity and oppositional behavior	Withdrawal with 1-month follow-up
Overcorrection: functional movement training	Duker, 1981	1 SMR child	Food refusal	Withdrawal with 6-month follow-up
Forced feeding, negative reinforcement, edible and social reinforcement	Ives, Harris, & Wolchik, 1978	1 SMR child	Food refusal	Multiple baseline

[a] Studies are categorized according to primary treatment as determined by description of procedures. This is not necessarily the only treatment employed.
[b] Level of mental retardation was determined as closely as possible from subject descriptions and is represented by B = Borderline, Mo = Moderate, and S = Severe.
[c] Primary or representative target behaviors are listed, as determined by the description of procedures. These are not necessarily the only behaviors treated.

In addition, a nutritionist indicated a need to increase consumption of target foods. At the onset of treatment, a small amount of a preferred food and social praise was delivered contingent upon the child feeding himself or herself a bite of the selected food. Over subsequent meals, the number of bites required prior to delivery of the preferred food item was systematically increased, whereas social praise continued to be delivered after each bite. This treatment was extended across several food groups (including meat, vegetable, and fruit) in multiple-baseline fashion, and proved to be effective in increasing the number of bites taken as well as the number of grams of the target foods consumed. Follow-up assessments indicated that these gains were durable with continued treatment carried out by parents following discharge of the children from the hospital.

As mentioned above, the efficacy of reinforcement for eating presumably has been enhanced with the addition of a variety of other procedures. In a recent study by Luiselli (1988), a pacing strategy was incorporated in training with a severely handicapped deaf-blind boy who was an independent feeder, but for breakfast foods only (cereal, pancakes, and toast). In this procedure, one bite of nonpreferred food at a time was placed on the youngster's plate. This discouraged playing with food and provided a distinct cue for reinforcement. When this bite was consumed, candy was delivered and another bite was offered. A withdrawal design demonstrated the controlling effects of treatment.

Luiselli and Gleason (1987) combined reinforcement and texture fading procedures to treat a 4-year-old deaf, visually impaired, and severely handicapped child whose consumption of food was limited to milk and, occasionally, pureed baby food. Since preferred edibles could not be identified, sensory reinforcement was employed. This consisted of the contingent presentation of bright light and rocking motion following consummatory responses. Texture fading entailed gradually increasing food composition from strained baby food to thickened baby food to soft foods to finely diced foods. These procedures appeared to be effective in increasing the number and kinds of foods accepted by the child. Eventually, the cumbersome sensory reinforcement procedures were faded and discontinued. Texture fading also was used by Leibowitz and Holcer (1974), who offered an increasing variety of foods along with a small amount of ice cream to their multi-handicapped subject.

In another variation, edible reinforcement was supplemented with a procedure whereby the feeding session was terminated after 25 minutes, signaled by a timer, regardless of the amount of food consumed (Luiselli, Evans, & Boyce, 1985). The 11-year-old deaf-blind participant responded positively to these contingencies, as indicated by withdrawal experimental design procedures. Further, follow-up assessment at 1 month showed maintenance of improved eating behaviors.

Overcorrection

In a unique approach to food refusal, Duker (1981) used overcorrection training with a young multihandicapped boy who only accepted some cereals and baby food at the start of the study. When presented with a spoonful of other types of food, the child clenched his teeth, turned away, and attempted to push the spoon away from his face. During intervention phases, these behaviors were followed by overcorrection exercises that consisted of guiding the subject's arms through four positions. His arms were held for 5 seconds in each position. The positions included maintaining his arms outstretched above his head, out at right angles to his body, down at his sides, and down in front of him. Because of his physical disability, manual guidance was necessary to obtain these positions. The overcorrective functional movement training proved to be an effective method for decreasing the frequency of the child's food refusal behaviors. Use of the withdrawal design showed that food intake was controlled by the application of the treatment, and follow-up assessments demonstrated the durability of treatment effects.

Forced Feeding

Ives, Harris, and Wolchik (1978) evaluated a multiple-component treatment for food refusal by a severely mentally retarded, sensory impaired child. Treatment initially involved offering the child a piece of food. Upon refusal, he was placed on his back on a mat, held still, and food was put into his mouth. If necessary, chewing movements were physically prompted, and spitting was prevented by placing one or two fingers over his mouth. As soon as the youngster began to chew, the therapist released the restraint and praised eating behavior. When the food was swallowed, the boy was cuddled enthusiastically and given a sip of breakfast drink. Thus, the full procedure involved forced feeding (putting food in the subject's mouth and preventing expulsion), negative reinforcement (restraint), and edible and social positive reinforcement (breakfast drink and praise). Later, the continuous reinforcement schedule gradually was weaned and an increasing variety of foods presented. Results of a multiple-baseline design across school and home settings attested to the effectiveness of treatment. Anecdotal follow-up reports indicated continued progress at 6 months.

Forced feeding is quite intrusive and difficult to implement. Further, it can produce gagging and choking. Although effective with the child in the Ives et al. (1978) study, this extreme intervention is not recommended except in cases of complete food refusal (Riordan et al., 1980), and then only after positive reinforcement and texture fading approaches have been attempted.

Issues in Research and Practice

The previous sections provide a summary of the behaviorally oriented treatments that have been applied to remediate feeding disorders in mentally retarded and multihandicapped persons. A number of procedures have been developed and evaluated for teaching independent feeding skills, decreasing undesirable mealtime behaviors, adjusting eating rate, and dealing with food selectivity and refusal. The successful treatment of skills deficits and problem behaviors related to feeding fosters a degree of optimism with regard to training developmentally delayed individuals to be more independent. However, this is not to suggest that few research questions remain regarding amelioration of feeding disorders in this population. Indeed, the success of previous research has set the stage for: 1) more rigorous evaluations of current procedures, 2) development of innovative treatment strategies that are relevant to the clinical applied needs of clients and caregivers, and 3) assessment of the extent to which interventions significantly correct referral problems. The remainder of this chapter addresses the current status of the research with regard to these issues and presents suggestions for future investigations.

Methodological Considerations

ASSESSMENT

Repeated and direct observations of one or more target behaviors (e.g., bites of food consumed, instances of disruptive behavior) documented the utility of behavioral treatments in the majority of studies. Most researchers recorded each occurrence of the target response during a feeding session (e.g., Cipani, 1981; Favell et al., 1980), which produces a frequency count of the behavior under investigation. Some experiments coded whether a specified response was displayed during a number of predefined time intervals (Sisson & Dixon, 1986a, 1986b, 1986c), yielding an estimate of the percentage of time the behavior was exhibited. Lennox et al. (1987) measured the duration of the response of interest (i.e., the pause between each bite of food). Finally, estimates of the amount of food consumed served as the dependent measure in one study (Luiselli et al., 1985). Occasionally, indirect assessment of progress in treatment supplemented frequency, interval, or duration recording. The number of grams of food consumed (Riordan et al., 1980) and weight of the subject (Duker 1981; Riordan et al., 1984) are examples of such measures.

When behavioral observations are used to measure target responses, the reliability of the data must be ascertained for meaningful interpretation of results. As used here, reliability refers to the extent to which two independent raters agree on the occurrence and/or nonoccurrence of a behavior. The majority of investigations conducted in the 1960s and 1970s provided insufficient information concerning data collection procedures or interrater agreement to determine whether data were reliable. Notable exceptions are studies by Azrin and his colleagues (Azrin & Armstrong, 1973; O'Brien et al., 1972; O'Brien & Azrin, 1972), Barton et al. (1970), Ives et al. (1978), Nelson, Cone, and Hanson (1975), and Stimbert et al. (1977). Growing sophistication with regard to behavioral assessment is reflected in investigations carried out since 1979. In these, interrater agreement was assessed at least once per experimental phase, and levels of agreement were acceptable.

TREATMENT INTEGRITY

A related methodological issue is the accuracy with which treatment procedures are implemented. As Salend (1984) cogently contends: "If the experimental conditions are not administered as intended, the findings are susceptible to multiple interpretations" (p. 309). Maintaining treatment integrity may be facilitated by carefully defining treatments (Berkowitz et al., 1971), using uncomplicated, easily applied procedures (Luiselli, 1988), and training and supervising behavior change agents (Barton et al., 1970; Cipani, 1981). However, because of their special relationship with the client as teacher, parent, or experimenter, trainers may have expectations about treatment outcome and other, simultaneous responsibilities. These may lead to inaccurate treatment administrations. This concern led Kazdin (1978) to recommend that behavioral researchers report data showing the extent to which the intervention was carried out as prescribed.

Four recent reports address this issue by rating trainer as well as subject behaviors and measuring accuracy of implementation of various treatment components (Horton, 1987; Sisson & Dixon, 1986b, 1986c; Wilson et al., 1984). In each of these cases, trainer compliance with treatment procedures was exemplary. For example, Sisson and Dixon (1986c) cued the trainer to observe each subject and deliver reinforcement and/or instructions at preprogrammed variable intervals. Observers (a) recorded whether the trainer actually attended to the child within 10 seconds of the cue, and (b) described trainer attention as "appropriate" (praise and tokens were delivered for desired behaviors or an instructional sequence followed feeding errors) or "inappropriate" (praise and tokens were given when the child exhibited problematic responses or instructions occurred subsequent to positive target behaviors). Analysis of these data indicated that the trainer attended to children within 10 seconds of the cue on 93% of occasions, with 97% of these attends of the appropriate nature.

EVALUATION

A final methodological point concerns determination of treatment efficacy. Experimental control was demonstrated in 24 of the 43 (56%) studies reviewed (see Tables 3.1 to 3.4). In three cases, the performance of subjects who received training was compared to that of subjects who did not receive training using a traditional group comparison format (Azrin & Armstrong, 1973; Matson et al., 1980; O'Brien & Azrin, 1972). However, unavailability of sufficient subject pools, extreme heterogeneity with regard to the nature and degree of disabilities, and reluctance to withhold treatment for control subjects make group comparison studies difficult or impossible to carry out with developmentally delayed populations. Single-case experimental design strategies (Barlow & Hersen, 1984; Van Hasselt & Hersen, 1981) provide an alternative to group designs for evaluating treatment outcome with these individuals. In this approach, experimental control is established through timely initiations and terminations of treatments delivered to a single subject. Thus, the above-mentioned drawbacks of group research are circumvented. Further, single-case methodology is especially suited to applied clinical research since effects are carefully monitored on an ongoing basis to ensure that interventions are achieving the desired effects.

Twenty-one investigations employed withdrawal or multiple-baseline single-case experimental designs to assess the effects of treatment. In the former strategy, baseline and treatment conditions are alternated, while in the latter design, interventions are applied sequentially and cumulatively to behaviors, subjects, or settings. The essence of the single-case approach is that behavior change can be attributed to the treatment if it occurs in the desired direction when and only when treatment is applied. As with the assessment of interrater agreement, demonstration of experimental control was more frequent in studies conducted since 1979.

Clinical Application

LEAST RESTRICTIVE INTERVENTION

Litigation, legislation, and standards established by professional organizations and advocacy groups require that behavior-change agents employ the least restrictive, but effective, approach in the treatment of disabled individuals. Often this is interpreted to mean that if procedures can be conceptualized on a continuum of aversiveness, the least aversive strategy should be attempted first (Reese, 1982). Consistent with this directive, the majority of studies comprising the feeding literature have assessed the efficacy of reinforcement-based programs. In one area, however, there has been an overreliance on punitive methods. Inappropriate mealtime activities frequently are reduced with aversive techniques, despite the growing literature supporting the effectiveness of positive approaches to behavior management with developmentally delayed clients.

Interventions need not be aversive to be restrictive. Clinical researchers must employ simple techniques likely to be executed accurately but unobtrusively in the natural environment over more elaborate, or arbitrary, strategies. Often, due to the severity of disability in the developmentally delayed client, interventions initially are intense. Treatments may require extra personnel, occur at high rates, appear unusual, or otherwise elicit attention and interfere with everyday activities. With behavior shaping and graduated guidance programs, interventions are faded naturally as the client becomes more independent and requires fewer prompts. With other interventions however, techniques must be systematically modified for implementation during daily classroom, residential, and other rehabilitative programming. For example, in one study, an elaborate reinforcement procedure consisting of bright light and rocking was discontinued after eating responses were well established (Luiselli & Gleason, 1987). In several others, continuous reinforcement schedules were changed to intermittent ones as the investigation progressed (e.g., Cipani, 1981; Riordan et al., 1984). Finally, a number of early investigations carefully faded trainer presence during feeding sessions and/or changed the training setting from a special one to the natural dining area (e.g., Albin, 1977; Christian, Hollomon, & Lanier, 1973; Henrickson & Doughty, 1967). However, in several reports, high-density reinforcement and prompting procedures, often requiring one-to-one attention from staff, were maintained throughout the course of the investigation (e.g., Lennox et al., 1987; Luiselli, in press; Sisson & Dixon, 1986b).

Cost Effectiveness

Treatments with the greatest utility are those that: 1) produce multiple positive effects across a number of behaviors (Voeltz & Evans, 1982), 2) result in changes that transfer to nontreatment settings (Stokes & Baer, 1977), and 3) foster gains that are maintained over time (Stokes & Baer, 1977). However, only two investigations included systematic assessment of nontargeted behaviors (Barton et al., 1970; Wilson et al., 1984). Barton et al. documented that as inappropriate use of fingers declined, messy utensil behavior increased. Later, as messy utensil behavior declined, neat utensil behavior increased. Wilson et al. found that training family-style dining skills did not impact on communication, messiness, or rate of eating. Similarly, two investigations incorporated measurement of target behaviors in a nontreatment setting (Lennox et al., 1987; Sisson & Dixon, 1986c). These data showed that skills trained in a quasi-analogue session transferred to natural dining situations with (Lennox et al., 1987) and without (Sisson & Dixon, 1986c) application of behavioral contingencies in the natural environment.

Seventeen (40%) of the studies listed in Tables 3.1 to 3.4 included follow-up assessments to document the durability of behavioral gains once formal interventions were discontineud. Eight studies demonstrated maintenance of improved feeding for 6 months or longer. It should be noted that several methods were employed to program generalization and maintenance of new feeding behaviors. These included conducting assessments and interventions in the natural environment (e.g., Luiselli, 1988; Matson et al., 1980) and training teachers, aides, and parents to carry out programs (e.g., Duker, 1981; Groves & Carroccio, 1971).

Target Behaviors

Early feeding-related research primarily focused on training very elementary skills, such as eating with a spoon. Also, severely disruptive responses were reduced. Later, the range of target behaviors was expanded to include multiple utensil use, table manners, and other dining skills. Now, with the national movement toward normalizing living environments and deinstitutionalization, independent self-feeding may be a necessary but insufficient goal. More complex responses must be shaped. Awareness of this need is reflected in the burgeoning body of research examining the community adjustment of developmentally disabled individuals. These persons have been taught to shop for groceries (Matson

& Long, 1986; Wheeler et al., 1980), prepare food (Bellamy & Clark, 1977; Martin et al., 1982; Robinson-Wilson, 1977), order food at restaurants (Marholin, O'Toole, Touchette, Berger, & Doyle, 1979; van den Pol et al., 1981), and converse appropriately at the table (Halle, Marshall, & Spradlin, 1979; Schepis et al., 1982).

Social Validity

The preceding sections evaluate feeding research with regard to methodological considerations and clinical utility. The third area to be examined is the extent to which interventions promote more adequate functioning in the natural environment. Proponents of behavior therapy have been particularly active in emphasizing this as a criterion for evaluating overall treatment efficacy (Kazdin, 1977; Van Houten, 1979; Wolf, 1978). However, few investigators specify the clinical criterion or use such a standard to evaluate behavior change.

A technology for determining the clinical significance of behavior change has been available since the early 1970s, at which time Wolf and his colleagues recommended that applied interventions be socially validated (Maloney et al., 1976; Minkin et al., 1976; Phillips, Phillips, Wolf, & Fixen, 1973). This is accomplished by assessing the functioning of the subject in a relevant social context before and after treatments have been implemented. Social comparison or subjective evaluation methods are then used to ascertain the clinical significance of behavior change (Kazdin, 1977; Kazdin & Matson, 1981). These methods are elaborated in the following sections.

SOCIAL COMPARISON

In social comparison, performance of the client before and after treatment is compared with that of peers who did not require intervention. Through this approach, there is an attempt to determine whether the behavior of the subject at these two points is distinguishable from that of his or her peers. If the subject's pretreatment behavior does not fall within the normative range, there is justification for implementation of an intervention. The goal of treatment is to bring the individual's performance closer to that of the peer group. Then, if the client's posttreatment level of behavior does not deviate dramatically from that of the normative group, the intervention is considered a success. The social comparison method was used in four feeding studies to evaluate treatment outcome.

In the first investigation, O'Brien and Azrin (1972) trained eating skills in residents at an institution for mentally retarded persons. Prior to treatment, subjects rarely used utensils, frequently spilled food on themselves, stole food from others, and ate food previously spilled on the floor. Employing an intense program of prompts, verbal praise, and food reinforcement, inappropriate eating behaviors were markedly decreased. To determine whether improvement was clinically significant, the investigators compared responses of the group that received training with eating habits of customers at a local restaurant. These normative data on eating skills were unobtrusively obtained by staff from the institution. Pretreatment assessment revealed that the mentally retarded residents were much higher in their number of inappropriate behaviors than the mean level of the restaurant patrons. After training, the residents ate more appropriately than nonretarded customers at the restaurant. Thus, the magnitude of changes achieved with training brought the behavior to acceptable community standards. Similar social validation procedures were employed by Azrin and Armstrong (1973) and Cipani (1981), except that in these studies, subjects' eating responses were compared with those exhibited by hospital employees. Lennox et al. (1987) established a criterion rate of consumption for their subjects by observing the mealtime behavior of "socially appropriate" residents at the same institution.

SUBJECTIVE EVALUATION

Another means of assessing the clinical significance of treatment effects is the subjective evaluation method. In this strategy, the behaviors altered in training are evaluated by individuals who are likely to have contact with the subject, or who are in a special position to judge the targeted behavior by virtue of their expertise or relationship to the client. The question examined by this method of validation is whether behavior changes have led to qualitative differences in how the person is viewed by others.

In two studies, Sisson and Dixon (1986a, 1986c) altered various eating behaviors displayed by hospitalized mentally retarded, behaviorally disordered children. A multiple-component training package consisting of instructions, modeling, physical guidance, behavior rehearsal, and positive reinforcement was effective in increasing appropriate utensil use, chewing, napkin use, and posture. Also, videotaped segments were randomly chosen from baseline and treatment sessions and shown to research assistants and special education teachers familiar with multihandicapped children. Baseline and treatment sessions were ordered randomly across viewers and subjects. Judges were blind as to the phase from which the segments were obtained. Immediately after watching each session, viewers rated the child's overall eating skills on a 7-point Likert scale (1 = very poor, 4 = acceptable, 7 = excellent). Treatment consistently improved behavior ratings to at least the "acceptable" level in all cases but one. Further, comparisons of mean pre- and post-treatment ratings of each child's feeding behaviors indicated a large improvement in overall skills for all children except one.

Luiselli (1988) used a different method of obtaining subjective evaluations of treatment efficacy. In his study, various paced-prompting procedures were used to alter feeding rates in multihandicapped subjects. Following intervention, five staff members who had applied the techniques were presented with a questionnaire to obtain information concerning treatment acceptability and effectiveness.

Their ratings revealed that treatment was considered "very effective" and they were "very satisfied" with results.

Future Directions

There is a trend toward increased methodological rigor in studies of feeding disorders in the mentally retarded population. Unfortunately, most of the early investigations evaluated forward and backward chaining strategies for teaching self-feeding. Although a substantial number of clinical replications are available, no methodologically sound report has appeared to substantiate the effectiveness of these approaches. Better controlled evaluations of other skills training methods (graduated guidance, multi-element treatment packages) and procedures to ameliorate problematic mealtime responses have been conducted. Yet, replications and extensions across all areas are necessary to advance the education and care of developmentally delayed individuals. In these efforts, heightened attention to experimental methodology will enhance confidence in results. In addition, investigators are encouraged to utilize available research designs to compare treatments so that the most efficacious approaches can be determined. The single-case strategy most appropriate for comparing the differential effectiveness of two or more interventions is the alternating treatments design. In this procedure, disparate treatments are applied across various stimulus conditions, and levels of responding associated with each treatment indicate differences or similarities between them.

Future research on feeding disorders also must incorporate positive approaches to behavior change, particularly for decreasing maladaptive responding at the table. In many instances, the availability of food at mealtimes promotes the unobtrusive use of primary reinforcement in a natural setting. However, for some individuals, edibles do not serve as reinforcers, and events such as access to preferred free-time activities (Riordan et al., 1984) or sensory stimulation (Luiselli & Gleason, 1987) must be programmed contingently. It is likely that positive treatments will be increasingly accepted and implemented by caregivers. In addition, systematically altering behavior change strategies so that they fit into the ongoing routine will encourage their adoption in applied situations. Regardless, once an effective intervention is found, its impact across behaviors, settings, and time must be assessed. Further, continued investigation of the administration of behavioral treatment strategies to advanced feeding-related skills is necessary. In this research, efforts must be made to include individuals functioning in the severe-to-profound ranges of mental retardation as well as those with serious physical handicaps.

Finally, attention to the extent to which skills deficits or problem mealtime behaviors actually are remediated, as evaluated by clinical as well as experimental criteria, should be assessed. It is significant that a number of investigations presently reviewed utilized social validity procedures to ascertain the significance of results obtained. Developmentally disabled individuals are best served when interventions produce changes in behavior that are observable by others and that foster responding at levels acceptable in community environments.

Acknowledgments. Preparation of this chapter was facilitated by Grant G008530258 from Special Education Programs of the U.S. Department of Education and Grant MH18269 from the National Institute of Mental Health.

References

Albin, J.B. (1977). Some variables influencing the maintenance of acquired self-feeding behavior in profoundly retarded children. *Mental Retardation, 15,* 49–52.

Azrin, N.H., & Armstrong, P.M. (1973). The "mini-meal"—A method for teaching eating skills to the profoundly retarded. *Mental Retardation, 11,* 9–13.

Barlow, D.H., & Hersen, M. (1984). *Single-case experimental designs: Strategies for studying behavior.* New York: Pergamon Press.

Barton, E.S., Guess, D., Garcia, E., & Baer, D.M. (1970). Improvement of retardates' mealtime behaviors by timeout procedures using multiple baseline techniques. *Journal of Applied Behavior Analysis, 3,* 77–84.

Bellamy, G.T., & Clark, G. (1977). Picture recipe cards as an approach to teaching severely and profoundly retarded adults to cook. *Education and Training of the Mentally Retarded, 12,* 69–73.

Bensberg, G.J., Colwell, C.N., & Cassel, R.H. (1965). Teaching the profoundly retarded self-help activities by behavior shaping techniques. *Americal Journal of Mental Deficiency, 69,* 674–679.

Berkowitz, S., Sherry, P.J., & Davis, B.A. (1971). Teaching self-feeding skills to profound retardates using reinforcement and fading procedures. *Behavior Therapy, 2,* 62–67.

Burkhart, J.E., Fox, R.A., & Rotatori, A.F. (1985). Obesity of mentally retarded individuals: Prevalence, characteristics, and intervention. *American Journal of Mental Deficiency, 90,* 303–312.

Christian, W.P., Hollomon, S.W., & Lanier, C.L. (1973). An attendant operated feeding program for severely and profoundly retarded females. *Mental Retardation, 11,* 35–37.

Cipani, E. (1981). Modifying food spillage behavior in an institutionalized retarded client. *Journal of Behavior Therapy and Experimental Psychiatry, 12,* 261–265.

Colwell, C.N., Richards, E., McCarver, R.B., & Ellis, N.R. (1973). Evaluation of self-help habit training of the profoundly retarded. *Mental Retardation, 11,* 14–18.

Duker, P.C. (1981). Treatment of food refusal by the overcorrective functional movement training method. *Journal of Behavior Therapy and Experimental Psychiatry, 12,* 337–340.

Edwards, M., & Lilly, R.T. (1966). Operant conditioning: An application to behavioral problems in groups. *Mental Retardation, 4,* 18–20.

Favell, J.E., McGimsey, J.F., & Jones, M.L. (1980). Rapid eating in the retarded: Reduction by nonaversive procedures. *Behavior Modification, 4,* 481–492.

Gorton, C.E., & Hollis, J.H. (1965). Redesigning a cottage unit for better programming and research for the severely retarded. *Mental Retardation, 3,* 16–21.

Gray, R.M., & Kasteler, J.M. (1969). The effects of social reinforcement and training on institutionalized mentally retarded children. *American Journal of Mental Deficiency*, *74*, 50–56.

Groves, I.D., & Carroccio, D.F. (1971). A self-feeding program for the severely and profoundly retarded. *Mental Retardation*, *9*, 10–12.

Halle, J.W., Marshall, A.M., & Spradlin, J.E. (1979). A technique to increase language use and facilitate generalization in retarded children. *Journal of Applied Behavior Analysis*, *12*, 431–439.

Hamilton, J., & Allen, P. (1967). Ward programming for severely retarded institutionalized residents. *Mental Retardation*, *5*, 22–24.

Henrickson, K., & Doughty, R. (1967). Decelerating undesired mealtime behavior in a group of profoundly retarded boys. *American Journal of Mental Deficiency*, *72*, 40–44.

Horton, S.V. (1987). Reduction of disruptive mealtime behavior by facial screening: A case study of a mentally retarded girl with long-term follow-up. *Behavior Modification*, *11*, 53–64.

Ives, C.C., Harris, S.L., & Wolchik, S.A. (1978). Food refusal in an autistic type child treated by a multi-component forced feeding procedure. *Journal of Behavior Therapy and Experimental Psychiatry*, *9*, 61–64.

Jacobson, J.W. (1982a). Problem behavior and psychiatric impairment within a developmentally disabled population. I: Behavior frequency. *Applied Research in Mental Retardation*, *3*, 121–139.

Jacobson, J.W. (1982b). Problem behavior and psychiatric impairment within a developmentally disabled population. II: Behavior severity. *Applied Research in Mental Retardation*, *3*, 369–381.

Jones, A.M. (1978). Overcoming the feeding problems of the mentally and physically handicapped. *Journal of Human Nutrition*, *32*, 359–367.

Jones, T.W. (1982). Treatment of behavior-related eating problems in retarded students: A review of the literature. In J.H. Hollis & C.E. Meyers (Eds.), *Life threatening behavior: Analysis and intervention* (pp. 3–26). Washington, DC: American Association on Mental Deficiency.

Kaufman, J.M., LaFleur, N.K., Hallahan, D.P., & Chanes, C.M. (1975). Imitation as a consequence for children's behavior: Two experimental case studies. *Behavior Therapy*, *6*, 535–542.

Kazdin, A.E. (1977). Assessing the clinical or applied importance of behavior change through social validation. *Behavior Modification*, *1*, 427–452.

Kazdin, A.E. (1978). Methodological and interpretive problems of single-case experimental designs. *Journal of Consulting and Clinical Psychology*, *46*, 629–642.

Kazdin, A.E., & Matson, J.L. (1981). Social validation in mental retardation. *Applied Research in Mental Retardation*, *2*, 39–53.

Kimbrell, D.L., Luckey, R.E., Barbuto, P.F.P., & Love, J.G. (1967). Operation dry pants: An intensive habit-training program for severely and profoundly retarded. *Mental Retardation*, *5*, 32–36.

Knapczyk, D.R. (1983). Use of teacher-paced instruction in developing and maintaining independent self-feeding. *The Journal of the Association for the Severely Handicapped*, *8*, 10–16.

Lawrence, W., & Kartye, J. (1971). Extinction of social competency skills in severely and profoundly retarded females. *American Journal of Mental Deficiency*, *75*, 630–634.

Leath, J.R., & Flournoy, R.L. (1970). Three year follow-up of intensive habit-training program. *Mental Retardation*, *3*, 32–34.

Leibowitz, J.M., & Holcer, P. (1974). Building and maintaining self-feeding skills in a retarded child. *American Journal of Occupational Therapy, 28*, 545–548.

Lemke, H., & Mitchell, R.D. (1972). Controlling the behavior of a profoundly retarded child. *The American Journal of Occupational Therapy, 26*, 261–264.

Lennox, D.B., Miltenberger, R.G., & Donnelly, D.R. (1987). Response interruption and DRL for the reduction of rapid eating. *Journal of Applied Behavior Analysis, 20*, 279–284.

Luiselli, J.K. (1988). Improvement of feeding skills in multihandicapped students through paced-prompting interventions. *Journal of the Multihandicapped Person, 1*, 17–30.

Luiselli, J.K. (in press). Behavioral feeding intervention with deaf-blind, multihandicapped children. *Child and Family Behavior Therapy.*

Luiselli, J.K., Evans, T.P., & Boyce, D.A. (1985). Contingency management of food selectivity and oppositional eating in a multiply handicapped child. *Journal of Clinical Child Psychology, 14*, 153–156.

Luiselli, J.K., & Gleason, D.J. (1987). Combining sensory reinforcement and texture fading procedures to overcome chronic food refusal. *Journal of Behavior Therapy and Experimental Psychiatry, 18*, 149–155.

Maloney, D.M., Harper, T.M., Braukmann, D.J., Fixen, D.L., Phillips, E.L., & Wolf, M.M. (1976). Effects of training predelinquent girls on conversation and posture behaviors by teaching-parents and juvenile peers. *Journal of Applied Behavior Analysis, 9*, 371–390.

Marholin, D., II, O'Toole, K.M., Touchette, P.E., Berger, P.L., & Doyle, D.A. (1979). "I'll have a Big Mac, large fries, large coke, and apple pie" . . . or teaching adaptive community skills. *Behavior Therapy, 10*, 236–248.

Martin, G.H., McDonald, S., & Omichinski, M. (1971). An operant analysis of response interactions during meals with severely retarded girls. *American Journal of Mental Deficiency, 76*, 68–75.

Martin, H.P. (1973). Nutrition: Its relationship to children's physical, mental, and emotional development. *American Journal of Clinical Nutrition, 16*, 766–775.

Martin, J.E., Rusch, F.R., James, V.L., Decker, P.J., & Trtol, K.A. (1982). The use of picture cues to establish self-control in the preparation of complex meals by mentally retarded adults. *Applied Research in Mental Retardation, 3*, 105–119.

Matson, J.L., & Long, S. (1986). Teaching computation/shopping skills to mentally retarded adults. *American Journal of Mental Deficiency, 91*, 98–101.

Matson, J.L., Ollendick, T.H., & Adkins, J (1980). A comprehensive dining program for mentally retarded adults. *Behavior Research and Therapy, 18*, 107–112.

McDonald, G., McCabe, P., & Mackle, B. (1977). Mealtime behaviour in the profoundly subnormal. *British Journal of Mental Subnormality, 23*, 29–35.

Miller, H.R., Patton, M.E., & Henton, K.R. (1971). Behavior modification in a profoundly retarded child: A case report. *Behavior Therapy, 2*, 375–384.

Minkin, N., Braukmann, D.J., Minkin, B.L., Timbers, G.D., Timbers, G.J., Fixen, D.L., Phillips, E.L., & Wolf, M.M. (1976). The social validation and training of conversation skills. *Journal of Applied Behavior Analysis, 6*, 343–353.

Murphy, M.J., & Zahm, D. (1975). Effects of improved ward conditions and behavioral treatment on self-help skills. *Mental Retardation, 13*, 24–26.

Murphy, M.J., & Zahm, D. (1978). Effect of improved physical and social environment on self-help and problem behaviors of institutionalized retarded males. *Behavior Modification, 2*, 193–210.

Nelson, G.L., Cone, J.D., & Hanson, C.R. (1975). Training correct utensil use in retarded children: Modeling vs. physical guidance. *American Journal of Mental Deficiency, 80,* 114–122.

O'Brien, F., & Azrin, N.H. (1972). Developing proper mealtime behaviors of the institutionalized retarded. *Journal of Applied Behavior Analysis, 5,* 389–399.

O'Brien, F., Bugle, C., & Azrin, N.H. (1972). Training and maintaining a retarded child's proper eating. *Journal of Applied Behavior Analysis, 5,* 67–72.

Ohwaki, S., & Zingarelli, G. (1988). Feeding clients with severe multiple handicaps in a skilled nursing care facility. *Mental Retardation, 26,* 21–24.

Palmer, S., & Horn, S. (1978). Feeding problems in children. In S. Palmer & S. Ekvall (Eds.), *Pediatric nutrition in developmental disorders* (pp. 325–347). Springfield, IL: Thomas.

Palmer, S., Thompson, R.J., & Linscheid, T.R. (1975). Applied behavior analysis in the treatment of childhood feeding problems. *Developmental Medicine and Child Neurology, 17,* 333–339.

Perske, R., Clifton, A., McClean, B.M., & Stein, J.I. (Eds.). (1977). *Mealtimes for severely and profoundly handicapped persons: New concepts and attitudes.* Baltimore: University Park Press.

Phillips, E.L., Phillips, E.A., Wolf, M.M., & Fixen, D.L. (1973). Achievement Place: Development of the elected manager system. *Journal of Applied Behavior Analysis, 6,* 541–561.

Pursley, N.B., & Hamilton, J.W. (1965). The development of a comprehensive cottage-life program. *Mental Retardation, 3,* 26–29.

Raventos, J.M., Kralemann, H., & Gray, D.B. (1982). Mortality risks of mentally retarded and mentally ill patients after a feeding gastrostomy. *American Journal of Mental Deficiency, 86,* 439–444.

Reese, M. (1982). Helping human rights committees and clients balance intrusiveness and effectiveness: A challenge for research and therapy. *The Behavior Therapist, 5,* 95–99.

Reid, D.H. (1983). Trends and issues in behavioral research on training, feeding and dressing skills. In J.L. Matson & F. Andrasik (Eds.), *Treatment issues and innovations in mental retardation* (pp. 213–240). New York: Plenum Press.

Reid, D.H., Wilson, P.G., & Faw, G.D. (1983). Teaching self-help skills. In J.L. Matson & J.A. Mulick (Eds.), *Handbook of mental retardation* (pp. 429–442). New York: Pergamon Press.

Richmon, J.S., Sonderby, T., & Kahn, J.V. (1980). Prerequisite vs. in vivo acquisition of self-feeding skill. *Behavior Research and Therapy, 18,* 327–332.

Riordan, M.M., Iwata, B.A., Finney, J.W., Wohl, M.K., & Stanley, A.E. (1984). Behavioral assessment and treatment of chronic food refusal in handicapped children. *Journal of Applied Behavior Analysis, 17,* 327–341.

Riordan, M.M., Iwata, B.A., Wohl, M.K., & Finney, J.W. (1980). Behavioral treatment of food refusal and selectivity in developmentally disabled children. *Applied Research in Mental Retardation, 1,* 95–112.

Robinson-Wilson, M.A. (1977). Picture recipe cards as an approach to teaching severely and profoundly retarded adults to cook. *Education and Training of the Mentally Retarded, 12,* 69–73.

Roos, P. (1965). Development of an intensive habit-training unit at Austin State School. *Mental Retardation, 3,* 12–15.

Roos, P., & Oliver, M. (1969). Evaluation of operant conditioning with institutionalized retarded children. *American Journal of Mental Deficiency, 74*, 325–330.

Salend, S.J. (1984). Integrity of treatment in special education research. *Mental Retardation, 22*, 309–315.

Schepis, M.M., Reid, D.H., Fitzgerald, J.R., Faw, G.D., van den Pol, R.A., & Welty, P.A. (1982). A program for increasing manual signing by autistic and profoundly retarded youth within the daily environment. *Journal of Applied Behavior Analysis, 15*, 363–380.

Sisson, L.A., & Dixon, M.J. (1986a). A behavioral approach to the training and assessment of feeding skills in multihandicapped children. *Applied Research in Mental Retardation, 7*, 149–163.

Sisson, L.A., & Dixon, M.J. (1986b). Improving mealtime behaviors of a multihandicapped child using behavior therapy techniques. *Journal of Visual Impairment and Blindness, 80*, 855–858.

Sisson, L.A., & Dixon, M.J. (1986c). Improving mealtime behaviors through token reinforcement: A study with mentally retarded behaviorally disordered children. *Behavior Modification, 10*, 333–354.

Sisson, L.A., & Dixon, M.J. (in press). Multiply disabled children. In M. Hersen & V.B. Van Hasselt (Eds.), *Psychological aspects of developmental and physical disabilities: A casebook*. Newbury Park, CA: Sage Publications.

Song, A.Y., & Gandhi, R. (1974). An analysis of behavior during the acquisition and maintenance phases of self-spoon-feeding skills of profound retardates. *Mental Retardation, 12*, 25–28.

Starin, S.P., & Fuqua, R.W. (1987). Rumination and vomiting in the developmentally disabled: A critical review of the behavioral, medical, and psychiatric treatment research. *Research in Developmental Disabilities, 8*, 575–605.

Stimbert, V.E., Minor, J.W., & McCoy, J.F. (1977). Intensive feeding training with retarded children. *Behavior Modification, 1*, 517–530.

Stokes, T.F., & Baer, D.M. (1977). Discriminating a generalization technology: Recommendations for research in mental retardation. In P. Mittler (Ed.), *Research to practice in mental retardation: Education and training* (pp. 331–336). Baltimore: University Park Press.

Thompson, R.J. (1977). Applied behavior analysis in the treatment of mealtime tantrums and delay in self-feeding in a multihandicapped child. *Journal of Clinical Child Psychology, 6*, 52–54.

Utley, B.L., Holvoet, J.F., & Barnes, J. (1977). Handling, positioning, and feeding the physically handicapped. In E. Sontag (Ed.), *Educational programming for the severely and profoundly handicapped* (pp. 119–132). Reston, VA: Division on Mental Retardation Council for Exceptional Children.

van den Pol, R.A., Iwata, B.A., Ivancic, M.T., Page, T.J., Neef, N.A., & Whitley, F.P. (1981). Teaching the handicapped to eat in public places: Acquisition, generalization, and maintenance of restaurant skills. *Journal of Applied Behavior Analysis, 14*, 61–69.

Van Hasselt, V.B., & Hersen, M. (1981). Application of single-case designs to research with visually impaired individuals. *Journal of Visual Impairment and Blindness, 77*, 199–203.

Van Houten, R. (1979). Social validation: The evolution of standards for competency for target behaviors. *Journal of Applied Behavior Analysis, 12*, 581–591.

Voeltz, L.M., & Evans, I.M. (1982). The assessment of behavioral interrelationships in child behavior therapy. *Behavioral Assessment, 4*, 131–165.

Watson, L.S., & Uzzell, R. (1981). Teaching self-help skills to the mentally retarded. *Handbook of behavior modification with the mentally retarded* (pp. 151–175). New York: Plenum Press.

Wheeler, J., Ford, A., Nietupski, J., Loomis, R., & Brown, L. (1980). Teaching moderately and severely handicapped adolescents to shop in supermarkets using pocket calculators. *Education and Training of the Mentally Retarded, 15,* 105–112.

Whitney, L.R., Barnard, K.E. (1966). Implications of operant learning theory for nursing care of the retarded child. *Mental Retardation, 4,* 26–29.

Wilson, P.G., Reid, D.H., Phillips, J.F., & Burgio, L.D. (1984). Normalization of institutional mealtimes for profoundly retarded persons: Effects and noneffects of teaching family-style dining. *Journal of Applied Behavior Analysis, 17,* 189–201.

Wolf, M.M. (1978). Social validity: The case for subjective measurement or how applied behavior analysis is finding its heart. *Journal of Applied Behavior Analysis, 11,* 203–215.

Wurtman, R.J., & Wurtman, J.J. (Eds.). (1977). *Nutrition and the brain.* New York: Raven Press.

Zeiler, M.D., & Jervey, S.S. (1968). Development of behavior: Self-feeding. *Journal of Consulting and Clinical Psychology, 32,* 164–168.

4
Bladder and Bowel Incontinence

LOUIS D. BURGIO AND KATHRYN LARSEN BURGIO

Bladder and bowel incontinence are potentially devastating conditions that can adversely affect psychological well-being and social functioning. These conditions have also been associated with an array of medical problems, including urinary tract infection and decubitus ulcers. Incontinence is seen in individuals of all ages, including normally developing children, adults of normal intelligence, and the elderly. Although prevalence figures exist for incontinence in some populations, it has not been surveyed adequately in the developmentally disabled population. Still, it is commonly acknowledged to be a significant problem, particularly in severely and profoundly retarded individuals (Whitman, Sciback, & Reid, 1983).

One problem that exists in characterizing incontinence in this population is inconsistent terminology. For example, *incontinence* and *enuresis* are often used interchangeably, while the term *enuresis* is also used to describe nighttime wetting exclusively. In an attempt to remediate this problem, the International Continence Society has established definitions for use by investigators and clinicians. The Society prefers the term *incontinence* over enuresis, and defines it as "a condition in which involuntary loss of urine is a social or hygienic problem and is objectively demonstrable" (International Continence Society, 1977). The definition in its present form is somewhat problematic due to the inclusion of the term *involuntary*. Assessing volition requires an inference regarding the individual's intentions—an exercise not welcomed by environmental determinists. Simply excluding the term involuntary tightens the definition considerably without detracting from its descriptive function. Finally, adding the word *feces* yields a more comprehensive definition; thus, "incontinence is a condition in which the loss of urine or feces is a social or hygienic problem and is objectively demonstrable." Individuals may experience daytime or nighttime incontinence, or both. Similarly, they may display urinary or fecal incontinence or double incontinence.

Many of the behavioral training procedures discussed in this chapter can be used for either bowel or bladder incontinence. This chapter focuses on urinary incontinence because it is much more prevalent than fecal incontinence. However, selected treatment studies for fecal incontinence are briefly reviewed in a latter section of the chapter. Following a synopsis of the causes of urinary incontinence, behavioral treatment procedures are described and suggestions for future research are outlined.

Causes of Urinary Incontinence

A reflex arc at the level of the sacral spinal cord permits the bladder to relax while filling to a threshold volume of approximately 200 ml, and then causes the bladder to contract and empty. Continence is achieved through modulation of this reflex arc from the cerebral cortex, or more specifically, one must perceive when the bladder is distended and inhibit reflex bladder contraction when the social setting is inappropriate for urination. One must also constrict the bladder outlet during transient pressure rises associated with coughing or movement. Finally, one must relax the pelvic floor muscles and the bladder must contract for normal voiding to occur.

Failure to emit these responses at the appropriate times can result in these three types of incontinence: 1) *urge incontinence*, in which bladder contractions are not inhibited; 2) *stress incontinence*, in which the urethra is not effectively closed off during transient pressure rises; and 3) *overflow incontinence*, in which urine is lost from a chronically full bladder. This occurs when the bladder does not contract (atonic bladder), when the periurethral muscles do not relax during bladder contractions (bladder-sphincter dyssynergia), or because the bladder outlet is obstructed mechanically (usually by fecal impaction or an enlarged prostate). The majority of incontinence in the normal adult population results from these types of bladder or sphincter dysfunction. The contributions of these factors to incontinence in the developmentally delayed population have not been evaluated, but it is quite possible that they play a role in this population as well.

A variety of organic conditions can interfere with the normal operation of the genitourinary system, causing bladder or sphincter dysfunction. Diseases such as diabetes mellitus, multiple sclerosis, tumors, urinary tract infection, atrophic vaginitis and urethritis in women, and prostatic enlargement in men can contribute to incontinence (Wendland & Ouslander, 1986). Incontinent episodes can also result from urinary retention, bladder stones, fecal impaction, and polyuria (increased urine flow).

Abnormalities of the central nervous system or in the innervation of the genitourinary tract may also affect continence, and it has been reported that soiling and bed-wetting among severely retarded persons is correlated highly with the degree of damage to the central nervous system (Hundziak, Maurer, & Watson, 1965). An extreme example of central nervous system (CNS) involvement in incontinence is myelomeningocele, a severe form of spina bifida (Whitehead & Schuster, 1985). In this disorder, the vertebrae fail to close, permitting the spinal cord and nerves to herniate out and become tangled. Closure of this herniation necessitates cutting some nerve fibers. Because the nerves innervating the external anal sphincters and puborectalis muscle exit the spinal cord in the lowest segment, myelomenigocele often involves bowel and bladder incontinence.

TABLE 4.1. Drugs that can affect continence[a]

Drug	Potential effects	Drug	Potential effects
Diuretics		Antidepressants	
Furosemide (Lasix)	⎱ Increased urine flow (polyuria, frequency, and urgency)	Amitriptyline (Elavil, others)	Sedation, as above
Thiazides (Hydrodiuril, Dyazide, Zaroxolyn, others)		Doxepin (Sinequan)	
		Imipramine (Tofranil)	Anticholinergic (urinary retention, overflow incontinence)
		Tjazodone (Desyrel)	Constipation, fecal impaction
Antipsychotics		Analgesics (Narcotic)	
Haloperidol (Haldol)	Sedation (diminished awareness of toilet needs)	Codeine (Tylenol #3, #4)	Sedation, as above
Thioridazine (Mellaril)	Rigidity (diminished ability to get to and use toilet)	Hydromorphone (Dilaudid)	Bladder relaxation, urinary retention
Thiothixene (Navane)	Anticholinergic (urinary retention and overflow incontinence)	Meperidine (Demerol)	Constipation, fecal impaction
		Morphine	
Sedatives/Hypnotics		Others	
Alprazolam (Xanax)	Sedation, as above	Amantadine (Symmetrel)	Anticholinergic (urinary retention)
Chloral hydrate (Noctee, others)		Diphenhydramine (Benadryl)	
Flurazepam (Dalmane)		Disopyramid (Norpace)	
Lorazepam (Ativan)			
Temazepam (Restoril)	Muscle relaxation (bladder outlet relaxes)	Methyldopa (Aldomet)	Bladder outlet (relaxation incontinence)
Triazolam (Halcion)		Hydroxyzine (Atarax)	
		Prazosin (Minipress)	

[a] From *A rehabilitative approach to urinary incontinence in long-term care: Monograph for nurses* by C.J. Wendland and J.G. Ouslander, 1986, South Pasadena: The Beverly Foundation. Copyright 1986 by C.J. Wendland and J.G. Ouslander. Adapted by permission.

An important factor often ignored by persons working with developmentally delayed individuals is the potential effect of drugs on urinary function. Table 4.1 lists a number of medications that can affect normal urinary function or interfere with toilet training. Trainers should be aware of the medication regimen of their clients before initiating a toilet training program. Every attempt should be made to administer the lowest effective dosage of a medication. Clinicians should also investigate recent changes in medications when previously continent patients display a bowel or bladder problem, and alternative medications should be investigated.

In addition to incontinence caused by bladder or sphincter dysfunction, there is a fourth type of incontinence, functional incontinence, in which loss of urine is associated with an inability or unwillingness to use the toilet appropriately. Many individuals with developmental disabilities also suffer physical or mental impairments that interfere with normal toileting. For example, some may have normal bladder function, but because they are unable to walk or transfer from a wheelchair to the toilet, urinary accidents occur. For these individuals, the physical environment is an important factor in their ability to stay dry. Convenient bathroom or toilet equipment, such as handrails, and adequate space in the bathroom and doorway can be significant contributions to continence and should be considered in any analysis of incontinence.

Environmental factors play an important role in the establishment and maintenance of continence in physically normal individuals as well. To establish continence, individuals must learn a chain of behaviors that constitute appropriate toileting. After toileting skills have been learned, the environment must provide contingencies that maintain these responses in natural settings. Natural contingencies, such as the embarrassment associated with accidents, are usually sufficient to maintain appropriate toileting. Among the developmentally disabled population however, many are unaffected by the usual social consequences of incontinence and more stringent or contrived contingencies are often required.

Although complete independence in toileting is the goal for most developmentally disabled individuals, limitations in mobility or dexterity due to physical disability can render this impossible. For these individuals, appropriate toileting may consist of the resident notifying staff of the need for assistance in toileting and delaying voiding until he or she receives assistance.

Behavioral Treatments

Toilet Training

Ellis (1963) was the first to describe a behavior analysis of toileting. Although his paradigm was described within a S-R drive-reduction model, an operant analysis can easily be derived from his description. To summarize, Ellis suggested that prior to toileting training, an appropriate toileting response, voiding, is under the control of the internal cues or discriminative stimuli (SD) of a distended bladder or visceral stimuli arising from the rectum. As a result of toilet training, the individual no longer voids solely in response to internal SDs. These cues now result in an approach response or a request for assistance in toileting. Voiding now occurs in association with cues associated with a toilet or an appropriate toileting device (e.g., a portable commode), in combination with internal distention cues.

Ellis' analysis has spawned numerous operant approaches to toilet training. Two distinct methods of toilet training have been articulated in recent years: timed toileting and regular toileting. Both are indebted to Ellis' original conceptualization, but differ on the point of emphasis within the model. Proponents of timed toileting (Van Wagenen, Meyerson, Kerr, & Mahoney, 1969) intervene at the stimulus of bladder distension. Individuals are trained at the times of actual or predicted incontinence in an effort to associate bladder distension with the toilet. An alternative approach, often referred to as regular toileting, ignores the hypothesized times of bladder fullness and trains the individual at arbitrarily set intervals of time (Azrin & Foxx, 1971).

TIMED TOILETING

Ellis' original description of toilet training placed considerable emphasis on the individual's natural schedule of elimination. The focus of the program was on defecation, not on urination, because defecation, according to the author, was more orderly and easier to predict. Individuals are taken to the toilet at the time they are considered most likely to defecate. This prediction is based on a 30-day baseline period during which frequency and time of defecation are recorded. If the client defecates while on the toilet, the staff administers reinforcement. If a client's clothes are found to be soiled, a 15-minute delay is imposed before the clothes are changed. Staff assistance in toileting is gradually weaned and greater independence in toileting is reinforced. Finally, a delay in the schedule of toileting is imposed to instigate self-initiated toileting. External reinforcement is faded as regular toileting habits are established. Ellis' goal was to establish a behavior analysis of toileting; data are not presented on the efficacy of the intervention.

Baumeister and Klosowski (1965) attempted to apply the procedures suggested by Ellis (1963), including the timed toileting component. Eleven severely retarded subjects with an average age of 18 were trained, as a group, over a 70-day period. Subjects were placed on a special unit and their frequency and times of urination and defecation were observed for a 30-day period. Initially, subjects were taken to the toilet at the time they were expected to defecate. As the program progressed, staff were reportedly able to identify behaviors that were reliable precursors to defecation, and patients were taken to the toilet when these behaviors were detected. Food and other material reinforcers were delivered contingent upon appropriate voiding and, as Ellis suggested, soiled clothing was not changed until at least 15 minutes after detection of an accident. By the 20th day of training, the frequency of appropriate elimination was 62% for defecation and 57% for urination. Baseline performance was not reported, although the authors report progress for all patients due to training.

Later in training a decision was made to allow the patients to go into the playground for a brief period each day. At this time all patients regressed to pretraining levels of performance.

Two controlled group studies of the timed toileting procedure have been conducted. Kimbrell, Luckey, Barbuto, and Love (1967) treated 20 severely or profoundly retarded children with timed toileting and compared them with 20 similar subjects who were exposed to "a conventional method of treatment." Experimental subjects were directed to the bathroom on a schedule according to their individual habits of elimination. The authors do not report whether they included both bowel and bladder elimination. Social and edible reinforcement was provided for appropriate toileting, and edibles were gradually withdrawn after 3 months following treatment. Results show that soiled laundry was reduced by half for the experimental group by the 5th week of treatment. No differences were reported for the conventional treatment control group.

Tierney (1973) compared 18 profoundly retarded trainees with 18 no-treatment controls. The author states that the experimental patients were toileted to accommodate their baseline pattern of elimination (especially fecal), but also describes the toileting sessions as increasing from about 3 to 10 occurrences as training progressed. The toileting sequence was broken down into a series of smaller steps and indigenous nursing staff were taught to use a shaping procedure with contingent social and edible reinforcement. Fourteen of the 18 experimental patients displayed a reduction in incontinence and acquisition of the toileting response at various levels. Also, the amount of laundry used was decreased for these patients. The control group showed minimal improvement.

The timed toileting procedure reached a higher level of sophistication in two studies conducted by Van Wagenen and colleagues. Van Wagenen et al. (1969) noted that most of the previous timed toileting studies employed a backward chaining procedure where the terminal response of voiding in the toilet was the first response to be trained. The authors reasoned that it would be preferable to teach the toileting components in the same temporal sequence as will be required when training is completed. This is referred to as forward training, or in more traditional terminology, forward chaining.

Similar to prior timed toileting studies, Van Wagenen et al. (1969) felt that individuals would learn more efficiently to initiate urination in a proper receptacle if they were trained at those times when reflex voiding occurred. Instead of relying on estimates of likely voiding times or discriminable behavioral precursors to voiding, the authors developed a sensor that was attached to the child's pants, and was triggered if the child urinated.

When voiding in the pants occurred, the signal was activated. The trainer then approached the patient, said "stop," took the trainee by the hand and guided him or her to the toilet. The trainee was placed in an appropriate voiding position, and the trainer rewarded the child if appropriate voiding occurred. As the child learned to reliably emit the first steps in the toileting sequence (i.e., approaching the toilet before voiding), the signal device was removed. Cotton briefs were introduced and removing and replacing the pants were prompted. Finally, the child was urged to drink additional liquids to increase voiding and the number of practice trials.

Van Wagenen et al. (1969) field-tested this procedure with nine profoundly retarded children who ranged in age from 4 to 9 years. Performance was assessed by a rating scale classifying six mutually exclusive response categories (e.g., urinates on floor, walks to toilet). Results indicate that the nine subjects were trained to toilet independently within 5 to 22 days. Anecdotal reports for seven of the children suggest that appropriate toileting was maintained at an acceptable level.

In a second study, Mahoney, Van Wagenen, and Meyerson (1971) noted that increasing fluid intake still did not provide a sufficient number of training trials. In this study, five severely/profoundly retarded subjects were trained to walk to the commode in response to an auditory signal triggered by the experimenter — not in response to a voiding response as in the earlier study. After the entire toileting sequence was learned, voiding was allowed to trigger the signal. All other aspects of the procedure were identical to Van Wagenen et al.'s (1969) study. Results show that four of the five subjects were taught to independently toilet after an average of 29 hours of training.

REGULAR TOILETING

Timed and regular toileting procedures share many features. The major distinction between the two procedures is that in regular toileting, patients are toileted on a rigid schedule (every 15 minutes to 2 hours), irrespective of their natural temporal patterns of voiding. Regular toileting procedures also rely more heavily on fluid loading in an effort to affect the patients' voiding patterns and increase the opportunities for training (cf. Van Wagenen et al., 1969). Both procedures have employed pants alarms. However, in timed toileting the alarm elicits a training sequence; the alarm in regular toileting programs results in a consequence for wet pants (usually time-out and/or overcorrection).

Dayan (1964) described an early informal attempt at regular toileting. As a result of attending conferences on toilet training, a direct care worker initiated his own program in a cottage for 25 severely/profoundly retarded children. The clients were placed on the toilet every 2 hours and rewarded for appropriate elimination. The author reported a decrease in laundry associated with the toileting program.

A toileting schedule was used by Giles and Wolf (1966) but the specific time interval was not reported. Subjects received their first six meals while sitting on the toilet. Material and social reinforcers were made contingent upon appropriate elimination, and toileting accidents produced a mildly aversive consequence. Independent toileting was gradually shaped by restraining the patients to the toileting area for the major part of the day. Giles and Wolf employed this procedure for five severely retarded children for 60 days. At the end of the study, three of the children displayed independent toileting and virtually no toileting accidents. The remaining two children required staff prompting but displayed almost no soiling.

Hundziak et al. (1965) compared a regular toileting procedure with conventional training and a no-treatment control group of severely retarded boys. Subjects in the regular toileting and conventional training groups were taken to the toilet every 2 hours or whenever overt signs of impending elimination were intercepted. The regular toileting group received immediate edible reinforcement for appropriate elimination, through the use of an electronically operated candy dispenser located beside the toilet. The conventional training group occasionally received reinforcement but also occasionally were scolded for toileting accidents. The authors report significant differences in favor of the regular toileting group; however, due to improvement displayed by the control group and the manner in which the data are reported, these results are difficult to interpret.

Regular toileting procedures have been further articulated in two more recent studies conducted by Azrin and colleagues. Azrin, Bugle, and O'Brien (1971) provided liquids and toileted four profoundly retarded children every ½ hour (the children were toileted every 2 hours during baseline). Appropriate elimination was reinforced with social and edible reinforcers. Urine alarm devices were used to detect urine in the toilet bowl and in the children's pants. If the pants alarm sounded as a result of a toileting accident, the trainer administered a single spank and a 10-minute time-out. If necessary, manual guidance was provided to teach the children to dress and undress. Results indicated that the number of wet pants per day reduced to zero soon after training was initiated.

This procedure was elaborated considerably by Azrin and Foxx (1971). It differed from the earlier study in several ways. Trainees were still toileted every ½ hour, but now they were regularly required to stay seated on the toilet for 20 minutes or until an appropriate void. Appropriate toileting was still reinforced, but now, residents were given edible and social reinforcers every 5 minutes while dry. Also, the consequences for a toileting accident were altered in this latter study. Trainees were now required to do cleanliness training contingent upon an accident (i.e., they changed their clothes, cleansed themselves, and washed their soiled clothing). In addition, a 1-hour time-out component was used. Finally, an elaborate maintenance procedure was developed that included abbreviated versions of many of the components used during training.

Azrin and Foxx (1971) initially treated four residents and, after a delay, trained five additional residents. Results showed that there were significantly fewer accidents during the experimental phase, and that all nine subjects showed a significant decrease in the number of accidents per day. The residents completed training (i.e., they were virtually accident free) in a median of 4 days and a mean of 6 days.

The Azrin-Foxx method of regular toileting has been replicated in a number of small studies (Barton 1975; Bettison, Davison, Taylor, & Foxx, 1976; Dixon & Smith, 1976; Sadler & Merkert, 1977; Singh, 1976; Smith, 1983; Trott, 1977). Many of these authors have commented upon the complexity of the procedure and the amount of staff time and effort required. Consequently, efforts have been made to modify the Azrin-Foxx procedure to render it more practical. Smith, Britton, Johnson, and Thomas (1975) removed the cleanliness training component of the Azrin-Foxx procedure and reduced the 1-hour time-out to ½ hour. Ando (1977) and Richmond (1983) further modified the procedure by eliminating fluid loading, the ½-hour pants checks, and reinforcement. Both authors also altered the consequence for a toileting accident. Richmond (1983) responded to an accident by delivering a verbal reprimand and requiring restitution; Ando (1977) administered a spank plus a 10-minute time-out. All three studies reported success in toilet training with these simplified procedures. None of the results is as clear or impressive as those obtained in Azrin and Foxx (1971).

COMPARISON OF TIMED AND REGULAR TOILET TRAINING METHODS

We have recognized the similarities in timed and regular toileting procedures; however, the differences are sufficiently noteworthy to warrant some discussion. Both procedures are relatively complex and staff intensive. The strategy of teaching the toileting sequence in the presence of internal cues of a distended bladder (timed toileting) is conceptually appealing. Unfortunately, there appear to be practical problems with determining the presence of these internal cues. Researchers have relied on baseline records of natural toileting events (Kimbrell et al., 1967) and behavioral precursors (Baumeister & Klosowski, 1965) to identify the presence of these cues. Both of these procedures rely upon a considerable amount of clinical intuition, which may affect the precision of the procedure. Individual variation in temporal voiding patterns can also introduce logistical complications in applying timed toileting on an institutional scale. The procedure developed by Van Wagenen and colleagues avoids some of these problems by using a pants alarm to signal training sessions. Such dependence on an electronic device can be worrisome, considering their expense and occasional unreliability. Finally, few researchers have used the Van Wagenen procedure (e.g., Litrownik, 1974) leaving its wide-scale efficacy untested.

One study has been conducted that directly compares the efficacy of timed and regular toileting procedures. Smith (1983) compared the procedures with groups of five severely/profoundly retarded children. Although the results show no differences in these groups, the author reports that timed toileting was more difficult to apply than regular toileting (e.g., Azrin & Foxx, 1971). The staff also expressed a clear preference for regular toileting, and it was suggested that strong superiority of timed toileting would need to be demonstrated before its use could be justified.

Special Considerations

Irrespective of method of toilet training, a very relevant practical issue is the use of group versus individual training. In individual training, one resident is trained at a time by one trainer (e.g., Azrin & Foxx, 1971; Van Wagenen et al., 1969). In a group training situation, one trainer attempts to train several children or adults at once (Baumeister & Klosowski, 1965; Dayan, 1964). Logic dictates that individual training would be more intensive and, thus, more effective. Smith

(1983) compared small groups of retarded children trained individually or in a group. As expected, the author found that individual training was not only clinically more effective, but also more cost effective.

Another issue of importance is the use of water loading in toilet training procedures (Thompson & Hanson, 1983). If water loading is exercised to an extreme, it can result in nausea, emesis, or grand mal seizures. Overhydration is a risk with developmentally delayed individuals who may be less able to self-regulate water intake during training. If an electrolyte imbalance ensues, the trainee can experience hyponatremia (low serum sodium), a condition that can be life threatening. The authors noted that most practitioners appear to use overhydration cautiously; however, guidelines for its use are needed. Thompson and Hanson suggested that liquid intake should be limited to 85 to 125 ml per hour for children weighing 60 to 100 pounds and 165 ml per hour for adolescents and adults weighing 100 to 150 pounds (for a maximum of 12 hours per 24 hours). Also, because water loading is contraindicated with many medical conditions common to developmentally delayed individuals (e.g., seizure disorders), they strongly urged that all candidates for toilet training be evaluated by a physician prior to training.

IRREGULAR INCONTINENCE

Occasionally, developmentally delayed individuals will display incontinence on a sporadic basis after self-initiated toileting has been established. Applying full timed or regular toileting procedures for this problem is unwarranted because the procedures are time consuming and because the trainees already have the skills necessary for self-initiation. Barmann, Katz, O'Brien, and Beauchamp (1981) developed a treatment procedure that excluded the bladder training phase and emphasized the overcorrection component. Subjects were three moderate to severely retarded children. Their pants were checked hourly and they received praise if the pants were found dry. If the subjects' pants were found wet, they were required to clean themselves and to put on dry clothes. Immediately following restitution, the children were required to engage in the toileting sequence 10 times in rapid succession. The authors report that this procedure took approximately 20 minutes. Results showed a rapid and substantial improvement in the rate of accidents. Training required a mean of 10 days for complete elimination of incontinence, although the number of accidents was reduced by 50% or more after the first 5 days of training.

HYGIENIC TOILETING

After trainees acquire the toileting sequence, some individuals may experience difficulty in using proper hygiene. Proper hygiene includes appropriate wiping, and washing the hands after toileting. Neither of these very important components has been given proper attention by researchers. In applied settings, these behaviors are often ignored or staff completes the activity for the resident. This is unfortunate because with proper training, developmentally delayed individuals can be taught to engage in proper toileting hygiene.

Another hygienic problem is misdirected urination from the standing position by retarded males. Siegel (1977) attempted to modify misdirected urination in nine moderately retarded male children and adolescents. The author developed a practical procedure that required very little staff time. A small floating target was placed in the toilet bowl so that subjects could "track" the target with their stream of urine. This procedure significantly and rapidly reduced the number of misdirected urinations. The use of verbal instructions to hit the target appeared to facilitate the procedure.

TOILETING PHOBIA

Researchers have stated that developmentally delayed individuals display phobias typical of intellectually average children of 7 or 8 years of age (Sternlicht, 1979). As described by Luiselli (1977), these fears can extend to toileting and can interfere with the performance of appropriate toileting in individuals who have previously displayed this skill. Luiselli (1977) reported on a 15-year-old severely retarded male who suddenly displayed avoidance responses in the presence of toileting stimuli. Using a case-study design, the attendant staff regularly prompted toileting and delivered tokens contingent upon appropriate use of the toilet. Tokens were exchanged for a preferred activity. Toileting accidents were followed by a 40-minute time-out in one area of the ward. Later in the training phase, self-recording was employed and tokens were delivered intermittently. Results show that toileting accidents immediately decreased by two-thirds (the baseline rate was 15 accidents per week), and they maintained at this low rate for about 4 months. By the 6-month follow-up, accidents had been eliminated and the resident was found to be completely dry at the 1-year follow-up.

Nighttime Incontinence

Surveys by Sugaya (1967) and Azrin, Sneed, and Foxx (1973) indicate the incidence of nighttime incontinence in institutionalized, severely retarded persons to be about 70%. Daytime toilet training does not usually affect nighttime continence, and the former should be established before the latter is attempted. The same social reinforcement and inhibitory influences operating in daytime incontinence contribute to nighttime incontinence. Nighttime incontinence is further influenced by the resident's reduced state of alertness at this time and the greater delay of social reactions to accidents at night.

The first study to address nighttime incontinence was a presentation of 30 case studies reported by Mowrer and Mowrer (1938). These authors connected a urine-alarm device to the child's bed. If the child wet the bed, he or she was taken to the bathroom. No additional consequences were applied. If the child awakened during the night, he or she was toileted regardless of the presence of an urge. All of the 30 children were successfully treated. One of the subjects was mildly retarded, and the authors reported that this child also responded satisfactorily to treatment.

with myelomeningocele frequently have both megacolon and weak external anal sphincters. Consequently, their treatment procedure combined biofeedback with habit training (regular toileting) and contingent rewards to teach children to self-initiate bowel movements. This combined treatment program resulted in at least a 50% reduction in the frequency of incontinence for 65% of the children. The majority of the studies involved in this brief review were conducted with normal children. Generalization to a developmentally delayed population should be made with caution.

Suggestions for Future Research

In a recent review of the self-help literature for the developmentally disabled population, Konarski and Diorio (1985) found that "toileting skills" was the behavioral subcategory most represented in the literature between 1962 and 1982. This publication trend is continuing unabated; moreover, the experimental quality of the research is steadily improving. Still, the authors concluded that only 25% of these toileting studies used acceptable reliability and design. Only 47% of the studies looked at the issue of maintenance to some degree, and none of the studies assessed the social validity of their training procedures.

Both timed and regular toileting procedures have been examined; however, the comparative efficacy of these procedures has not been sufficiently established. Nevertheless, the issue may be moot. Practitioners have largely ignored or are unaware of the Van Wagenen timed toileting procedure. The Azrin-Foxx regular toileting procedures have become standard fare, particularly in institutional settings. This may be due to the authors' publication of their comprehensive training manual (Foxx & Azrin, 1973). Furthermore, it may be more important to determine the relative contributions of the several treatment components, especially in view of the fact that the full procedure is so time intensive.

A large clinical trial of the Azrin-Foxx procedure could provide some very valuable information. It would be useful to know the overall success rate of this procedure. A large clinical trial can also isolate predictor variables that may help clinicians tailor their treatments to the needs of individual residents. Pfadt and Sternlicht (1980) discussed a large group study using the Azrin-Foxx procedures. The results of their report showed that 50% of trainees became fully continent; however, the study is still in progress and subsequent results have not appeared.

Konarski and Diorio (1985) found that only 13% of toileting studies reviewed involved parents, and only 6% involved teachers as behavior-change agents (e.g., Barmann et al., 1981; Drabman, Spitalnik, Hagamen, & Van Witsen, 1973). Considering the recent emphasis on less restrictive environments for developmentally disabled individuals, more emphasis needs to be placed on training parents and teachers to apply behavioral interventions for incontinence.

The effects of medications as a contributing factor in incontinence have not yet been examined with the developmentally delayed population. This is unfortunate considering the numerous medications received by many of these individuals.

Another area receiving very little attention is the use of medication as an adjunct to behavioral treatment. Combining medication and behavior therapy for the treatment of incontinence has been examined in elderly populations (Ouslander & Sier, 1986). Kennedy and Sloop (1968) combined a behavioral intervention with a trial of Methedrine for the treatment of nighttime incontinence with three retarded subjects. Results showed that all three subjects became dry throughout the night following the intervention. Unfortunately, the design of the study did not allow a separate analysis of the efficacy of Methedrine in controlling nighttime incontinence, nor did it look at the possibility that the medications could be faded.

Drew (1967) examined the use of imipramine and amitriptyline in the treatment of daytime incontinence. Although these medications are generally considered to be superior to the amphetamines in the treatment of incontinence, the use of these medications without a concurrent behavioral intervention was not found to be successful in reducing toileting accidents. Researchers need to examine the efficacy of combining medication and behavioral interventions in treating selected cases of incontinence in developmentally delayed individuals. A regimen of imipramine or amitriptyline may be useful during the early phases of treatment for individuals who are responding slowly to a behavioral intervention, or for some intractable cases of incontinence that present no apparent medical causes. These individuals may be experiencing bladder instability that results in difficulty in inhibiting urination. The anticholinergic effects of imipramine or amitriptyline may allow the individual to inhibit a void for a longer period of time, thus allowing him or her to access the toilet.

Finally, researchers have not examined the role of bladder or sphincter dysfunction in incontinence in developmentally delayed persons. There is a need for urodynamic studies of retarded individuals. Urodynamics are diagnostic procedures that measure bladder and sphincter responses to bladder filling and other events. It is assumed that many cases of incontinence in the mild to moderately retarded, particularly those who have previously acquired toileting skills, are due to bladder or sphincter dysfunction. Procedures similar to timed and regular toileting procedures have been shown to be effective in modifying or compensating for these dysfunctions in nonretarded populations (Clay, 1978; Frewen, 1978, 1979; Schnelle et al., 1983). A high success rate has also been reported with the use of biofeedback and self-management procedures for both bladder instability (Burgio, Whitehead, & Engel, 1985) and stress incontinence (Burgio, Robinson, & Engel, 1986). These procedures require active participation and compliance on the subject's part, but should be applicable to mild and perhaps moderately retarded individuals.

Behavioral procedures have proven to be extremely powerful tools in treating incontinence in the developmentally delayed population. The emphasis on environmental factors in incontinence is understandable given that most incontinence in this population is due to a deficit in toileting skills. The inclusion of physiological variables in our analysis of incontinence will improve our assessment of our clients and is likely to allow us to provide better incontinence treatments for them.

References

Ando, H. (1977). Training autistic children to urinate in the toilet through operant conditioning techniques. *Journal of Autism and Childhood Schizophrenia, 7*(2), 151–163.

Azrin, N.H., Bugle, C., & O'Brien, F. (1971). Behavioral engineering: Two apparatuses for toilet training retarded children. *Journal of Applied Behavior Analysis, 4,* 249–253.

Azrin, N.H., & Foxx, R.M. (1971). A rapid method of toilet training the institutionalized retarded. *Journal of Applied Behavior Analysis, 4,* 89–99.

Azrin, N.H., Sneed, T.J., & Foxx, R.M. (1973). Dry bed: A rapid method of eliminating bedwetting (enuresis) of the retarded. *Behavioral Research and Therapy, 11,* 427–434.

Bach, R., & Moylan, J.J. (1975). Parents administered behavior therapy for inappropriate urination and encopresis: A case study. *Journal of Behavior Therapy and Experimental Psychiatry, 5,* 239–241.

Barmann, B.C., Katz, R.C., O'Brien, F., & Beauchamp, K.L. (1981). Treating irregular enuresis in developmentally disabled persons. *Behavior Modification, 5*(3), 336–346.

Barton, E.S. (1975). Behavior modification in the hospital school for the severely subnormal. In C.C. Klernan & F.P. Woodford (Eds.), *Behavior modification with the severely retarded: IRMMH Study Group No. 8* (pp. 243–258). Amsterdam: Associated Scientific Publishers.

Baumeister, A., & Klosowski, R. (1965). An attempt to group toilet train severely retarded patients. *Mental Retardation, 3,* 24–26.

Bettison, S., Davison, D., Taylor, P., & Foxx, B. (1976). Long-term effects of a toilet training program for the retarded: A pilot study. *Australian Journal of Mental Retardation, 4,* 28–35.

Blechman, E.A. (1979). Short- and long-term results of positive home-based treatment of childhood chronic constipation and encopresis. *Child Behavior Therapy, 1,* 237–247.

Burgio, K.L., Robinson, J.C., & Engel, B.T. (1986). The role of biofeedback in Kegel exercise training for stress urinary incontinence. *American Journal of Obstetrics and Gynecology, 154,* 58–64.

Burgio, K.L., Whitehead, W.E., & Engel, B.T. (1985). Urinary incontinence in the elderly: Bladder-sphincter biofeedback and toileting skills training. *Annals of Internal Medicine, 103,* 507–515.

Clay, E.G. (1978). Incontinence of urine: A regime for retraining. *Nursing Mirror, 146,* 23–24.

Dayan, M. (1964). Toilet training retarded children in a state residential institution. *Mental Retardation, 2,* 116–117.

Dixon, J., & Smith, P.S. (1976). The use of a pants alarm in daytime toilet training. *British Journal of Mental Subnormality, 22*(2), 20–25.

Doleys, D.M. (1981). Encopresis. In M. Ferguson & B. Taylor (Eds.), *The Comprehensive Handbook of Behavioral Medicine* (pp. 145–157). New York: Spectrum Publications.

Drabman, R., Spitalnik, R., Hagamen, M.B., & Van Witsen, B. (1973). The five-two program: An integrated approach to treating severely disturbed children. *Hospital and Community Psychiatry, 34*(1), 33–36.

Drew, L.R. (1967). Drug control of incontinence in adult mental defectives. *The Medical Journal of Australia, 2*(5), 206–207.

Edelman, R.F. (1971). Operant conditioning treatment of encopresis. *Journal of Behavior Therapy and Experimental Psychiatry, 2,* 71–76.

Ellis, N. (1963). Toilet training the severely defective patient: An S-R reinforcement analysis. *American Journal of Mental Deficiency, 68,* 98–103.

Epstein, L.H., & McCoy, J.F. (1977). Bladder and bowel control in Hirschsprung's disease. *Journal of Behavior Therapy and Experimental Psychiatry, 8*, 97–99.

Foxx, R.M., & Azrin, N.H. (1973). *Toilet training the retarded*. Champaign, IL: Research Press.

Frewen, W.K. (1978). An objective assessment of the unstable bladder of psychosomatic origin. *British Journal of Urology, 50*, 246–249.

Frewen, W.K. (1979). Role of bladder training in the treatment of the unstable bladder in the female. *Urologic Clinics of North America, 6*, 273–277.

Giles, D.K., & Wolf, M.M. (1966). Toilet training institutionalized, severe retardates: An application of operant behavior modification techniques. *American Journal of Mental Deficiency, 70*, 766–780.

Hanson, R.H. (1981). Behavioral treatment of enuresis in institutionalized developmentally disabled youth: Five case studies. *Education and Treatment of Children, 4*(4), 349–356.

Hundziak, M., Maurer, R.A., & Watson, L.S. (1965). Operant conditioning in toilet training of severely mentally retarded boys. *American Journal of Mental Deficiency, 70*, 120–124.

International Continence Society. (1977). Standardization of terminology of lower urinary tract function. *Urology, 9*, 237–241.

Kennedy, W.A., & Sloop, E.W. (1968). Methedrine as an adjunct to conditioning treatment of nocturnal enuresis in normal and institutionalized retarded subjects. *Psychological Reports, 22*, 997–1000.

Kimbrell, D.L., Luckey, R.E., Barbuto, P.F., & Love, J.G. (1967). Operation dry pants: An intensive habit training program for severely and profoundly retarded. *Mental Retardation, 5*, 32–36.

Kohlenberg, R.J. (1973). Operant conditioning of human anal sphincter pressure. *Journal of Applied Behavior Analysis, 6*, 201–208.

Konarski, E.A., & Diorio, M.S. (1985). A quantitative review of self-help research with the severely and profoundly retarded. *Applied Research in Mental Retardation, 6*, 229–245.

Litrownik, A.J. (1974). A method for home-training an incontinent child. *Journal of Behavior Therapy and Experimental Psychiatry, 5*, 77–80.

Luiselli, J.K. (1977). Case report: An attendant-administered contingency management program for the treatment of a toileting phobia. *Journal of Mental Deficiency Research, 21*, 283–288.

Mahoney, K., Van Wagenen, K., & Meyerson, L. (1971). Toilet training of normal and retarded children. *Journal of Applied Behavior Analysis, 3*, 173–181.

Mowrer, O.H., & Mowrer, W.M. (1938). Enuresis—A method for its study and treatment. *American Journal of Orthopsychiatry, 8*, 436–459.

Ouslander, J.G., & Sier, H.C. (1986). Drug therapy for geriatric urinary incontinence. In J. Ouslander (Ed.), *Urinary incontinence: Clinics in geriatric medicine* (Vol. 2, No. 4, pp. 1–19). Philadelphia: W.B. Saunders.

Pedrini, B.C., & Pedrini, D.T. (1971). Reinforcement procedures in the control of encopresis: A case study. *Psychological Reports, 28*, 937–938.

Pfadt, A., & Sternlicht, K. (1980). *Clinical and administrative issues in the large scale implementation of the Azrin-Foxx self-initiation training program*. Paper presented at the AAMD Annual Meeting, San Francisco.

Phibbs, J., & Wells, M. (1982). The treatment of nocturnal enuresis in institutionalized retarded adults. *Journal of Behavior Therapy and Experimental Psychiatry, 13*(3), 245–249.

Richmond, G. (1983). Shaping bladder and bowel continence in developmentally retarded preschool children. *Journal of Autism and Developmental Disorders, 13*(2), 197–204.

Sadler, O.W., & Merkert, F. (1977). Evaluating Foxx and Azrin toilet training procedure for retarded children in a day training center. *Behavior Therapy, 8*, 499–500.

Schnelle, J.F., Traughber, B., Morgan, D.B., Embry, J.E., Binion, A.F., & Coleman, A. (1983). Management of geriatric incontinence in nursing homes. *Journal of Applied Behavior Analysis, 16*, 235–241.

Siegel, R.K. (1977). Stimulus selection and tracking during urination: Autoshaping directed behavior with toilet targets. *Journal of Applied Behavior Analysis, 10*, 255–265.

Singh, N.N. (1976). Toilet training of a severely retarded non-verbal child. *Australian Journal of Mental Retardation, 4*, 15–18.

Sloop, E.W., & Kennedy, W.A. (1973). Institutionalized retarded nocturnal enuretics treated by a conditioning technique. *American Journal of Mental Deficiency, 77*(6), 717–721.

Smith, P.S. (1983). A comparison of different methods of toilet training the mentally handicapped. *Behavioral Research and Therapy, 17*, 33–43.

Smith, P.S., Britton, P.G., Johnson, M., & Thomas, D.A. (1975). Problems involved in toilet training profoundly mentally retarded adults. *Behavioral Research and Therapy, 13*, 301–307.

Sternlicht, M. (1979). Fears of institutionalized mentally retarded adults. *Social Casework, 34*, 119–124.

Sugaya, K. (1967). Survey of the enuresis problem in an institution for the mentally retarded with emphasis on the clinical psychology aspects. *Japanese Journal of Child Psychiatry, 8*, 142–150.

Thompson, T., & Hanson, R. (1983). Overhydration: Precautions when treating urinary incontinence. *Mental Retardation, 21*(4), 139–143.

Tierney, A.J. (1973). Toilet training. *Nursing Times, 20*(27), 1740–1745.

Trott, M.C. (1977). Application of Foxx and Azrin toilet training for the retarded in a school program. *Education and Training of the Mentally Retarded, 12*, 336–338.

Van Wagenen, R.K., Meyerson, L., Kerr, N.J., & Mahoney, K. (1969). Field trials of a new procedure for toilet training. *Journal of Experimental Child Psychology, 8*, 147–159.

Wendland, C.J., & Ouslander, J.G. (1986). *A rehabilitative approach to urinary incontinence in long-term care: Monograph for nurses*. South Pasadena, CA: The Beverly Foundation.

Whitehead, W.E., Parker, L.H., Bosmajian, L.S., Morrill, E.D., Middaugh, S., Drescher, V.M., Cataldo, M.F., & Freeman J. (1982). Behavioral treatment of fecal incontinence secondary to spina bifida. *Gastroenterology, 82*, 1209 (Abstract).

Whitehead, W.E., & Schuster, M.M. (1985). *Gastrointestinal disorders: Behavioral and physiological basis for treatment*. New York: Academic Press.

Whitman, T.L., Sciback, J.W., & Reid, D.H. (1983). *Behavior modification with the severely and profoundly retarded: Research and application*. New York: Academic Press.

5
Obesity and Weight Regulation

ROBERT A. FOX, DONALD J. MEYER, AND
ANTHONY F. ROTATORI

Obesity is a prevalent condition among developmentally disabled (DD) children and adults (Rotatori & Fox, 1981). These obese individuals are likely to experience secondary medical and social problems as a result of this health-related condition. Obesity is not a unitary syndrome with a single causative factor. Rather, it reflects a complex interaction between an individual's biological and physical characteristics, past learning experiences, and present environmental circumstances. The short- and long-term health risks associated with obesity have stimulated an increased interest in this topic in the research literature as well as the popular press. Specific health risks include hypertension, hyperlipidemia, carbohydrate intolerance, coronary artery disease, diabetes mellitus, pulmonary and renal problems, complications during pregnancy, and higher perinatal mortality (Bray, 1976; Dawber, 1980; Kannel & Gorden, 1979; Van Itallie, 1979). Increased incidence of varicose veins, arthritis, gallstone and gallbladder disease, liver damage, and complications in surgery also have been linked to an obese condition (Agras & Werne, 1981). Moreover, obesity influences longevity. Overweight individuals, especially those who are overweight at younger ages, tend to die younger than average-weight individuals (Simopoulos & Van Itallie, 1984).

Relatively little is known about obesity in DD persons. In one of the first reviews to appear in the literature, Staugaitis (1978) cited only four sources specifically dealing with the DD population. Since that time, the literature has expanded (Burkhart, Fox, & Rotatori, 1985). Yet even today only a handful of researchers have been attracted to study this important area. This chapter reviews what we currently know about obesity and its management with DD individuals, and what we need to learn. References are made to the obese nondisabled population to provide a comparative context for this review.

Incidence of Obesity

Prevalence estimates for obesity among American adults range from 15% to 50% (Bray, 1976; Van Itallie, 1979). The National Center for Health Statistics (Abraham, 1983) estimates that 28% of women and 29% of men between the ages of

20 and 74 years, or a total of over 29 million Americans, are obese. The prevalence of obesity increases with membership in certain ethnic groups, age, and lower socioeconomic status (Stunkard, 1975). For example, black compared to white women and older compared to younger adults of both sexes are more likely to be obese.

Within the adult mentally retarded (MR) population, no similar, comprehensive epidemiological studies are available. However, a similar pattern of obesity to that which exists in the general population is likely. Kreze, Zelinda, Juhas, and Garbara (1974) compared the incidence of obesity between low-IQ (IQ up to 90), average-IQ (IQ between 91 and 110), and above-average-IQ groups (IQ 111 or more). They reported an inverse relationship between IQ and the prevalence of obesity. However, extending this conclusion to the MR population is unwarranted given that only eight subjects in their low-IQ category had IQs in the retarded range (less than 70). In a more recent study, Fox and Rotatori (1982) found that 16% of the males and 25% of the females, from a sample of 1,152 mentally retarded adults living in a variety of different environments (e.g., home with parents, public institution), were obese. Additionally, differences were found between levels of retardation and gender. From the sample of severe to profoundly retarded individuals (376 males, 272 females), 6.9% of the males and 13.6% of the females were obese. Among the mild to moderate retardation categories (258 males, 228 females), 27.9% of the males and 38.2% of the females were obese. In an institutional sample ($N = 149$ MR adults), Wallen and Roszkowski (1980) reported that 45% of the females and 26% of the males were overweight. Of interest in both of these studies was the finding that excess weight is more common in mild to moderate MR persons than in severe to profound MR individuals. Consequently, these data do not support extending the inverse relationship between IQ and obesity reported by Kreze et al. (1974) to the MR population. From their survey of 1,152 MR adults, Fox and Rotatori (1982) concluded that: 1) a higher proportion of women than men were obese, 2) a higher proportion of moderate/mild retarded persons were obese than were those in the severe/profound range, and 3) the incidence of obesity generally increased with age but not in a linear fashion.

The incidence of obesity among nonretarded and retarded children and adolescents has recently received attention. In one of the larger studies using a nonretarded, low-income sample of 1,830 children from 2 months to 18 years of age, DuRant, Martin, Linder, and Weston (1980) reported that 8% of black males and 10.3% of black females were obese; among whites, 10.8% of the males and 10.4% of the females were obese. These researchers used a weight-for-length index to determine the incidence of obesity in this sample. Using the same index, Fox, Hartney, Rotatori, and Kurpiers (1985) studied the incidence of obesity among retarded children ($N = 337$) between the ages of 5 and 15 years in a large, urban public school system. They found that 22.2% of the males and 22.9% of the females were obese. When dividing the sample into lower (moderate to profound) and higher (mild) MR levels, and younger (5.5 to 10.4 years) and older age groups (10.5 to 15.4 years), the incidence of obesity ranged from 12.5% in

TABLE 5.1. Incidence of obesity (%) based on the weight-for-length index by sex, age group, and mental retardation level for public school sample ($N = 337$)

	Males		Females	
	Higher MR[a]	Lower MR[a]	Higher MR[a]	Lower MR[a]
Younger[b]	12.5	30.8	20.0	35.7
Older[b]	26.0	21.2	20.3	23.5

[a] Higher MR = mild; Lower MR = moderate to profound.
[b] Younger = 5.5 to 10.4 years; Older = 10.5 to 15.4 years.

younger, higher functioning MR males to 35.7% in younger, lower functioning MR females (see Table 5.1).

In a study directly comparing nonretarded with institutionalized retarded children in Japan, Yokoyama (1983) reported that 7% to 17% of the MR boys ($N = 443$) and 11% to 31% of the MR girls ($N = 250$) were obese, based on standard weight tables from the Ministry of Education in Japan. In the nonretarded control sample ($N = 339$ boys, 302 girls), obesity ranged form 6% to 7% for both sexes. Given this limited data base, it would appear that obesity may be more common among retarded than nonretarded children. Using a restricted MR sample, Chumlea and Cronk (1981) evaluated data from three large growth studies of children with trisomy 21. They found that being overweight was characteristic of these children beginning as early as 2 to 3 years of age, and continuing up through the adolescent period.

Definition and Measurement

One common problem, evident across studies in the obesity area, is the variety of measures and formulae used to determine an individual's relative weight. The Task Force on Obesity (Bray, 1979) recognized the need to precisely define obesity in order to further understand its etiologies, to accurately identify obesity subcategories, and to develop differential treatment programs. Unfortunately, confusion between basic terminology has existed. As an example, the terms *overweight* and *obesity* are used interchangeably in clinical settings and in the research literature, yet they are not the same. Overweight refers to an excess in body weight relative to standards for height; obesity is defined as surplus body fat. It is important to maintain a distinction between these concepts because an overweight person may be underfat and an overfat individual may not be at all heavy (Seltzer & Mayer, 1965). In a study involving MR adults (40 males, 44 females) (Fox, Burkhart, & Rotatori, 1983a), 22.5% of the males and 13.7% of the females in the sample would be misclassified as nonobese using relative weight alone; 7.5% of the males and 2.3% of the females would be misclassified as nonobese using only a measure of obesity. In a comprehensive evaluation of any obese individual, both concepts and related measures of corpulence (obesity) and heaviness (overweight) should be included. A variety of clinical measures are available to determine relative weight and obesity status. Measures include gross body weight, relative body weight, and surplus body fat.

Gross Weight

Gross weight measures are perhaps the easiest to use, but have the major drawback of being an inexact measure of body fat. Since the entire body, including skeletal, musculature, and bodily fluids, as well as fat deposits, are included, gross body weight is affected by temporary bodily fluid retention and musculature development.

Relative Weight

ADULTS

One of the most popular forms of determining obesity is through comparison of an individual's gross weight with tables of desirable weight-for-height. The *Desirable Height and Weight Tables* (1977) developed by Metropolitan Life Insurance Company have generally been accepted as the best yardstick for normal weights (Craddock, 1978). The use of the Metropolitan tables has been criticized because: 1) subjects were self-selected and as such may not be representative of the population at large; 2) there is a lack of established criteria for body frame classification required to use the table; and 3) subjects were weighed with their shoes and clothes on, which may have added variability to the data. Additionally, when using the tables for clinical purposes, first the frame size of the individual must be determined (small, medium, or large), then the value (expressed in ranges) within the table to use for comparison with the person's present weight is obtained. For example, a woman 64 inches in height should weigh between 108 and 116 pounds if she has a "small frame," 113 and 126 pounds for a "medium frame," and 121 and 138 pounds for a "large frame." A 64-inch female of large frame size who weighs 151 pounds could be considered 20% or 9% overweight if the extremes of the desirable weight ranges were used.

In an attempt to develop solutions to the body frame problem inherent in using the tables, Harris (1976) developed a method for determining frame size in females. Measurements of wrist, ankle, and pelvic areas, plus subjective visual assessment of the body frame's silhouette are completed. Using the Harris method, Craddock (1978) reported that an individual's weight for height and build could be predicted within 3 pounds 90% of the time.

CHILDREN

DuRant and Linder (1981) evaluated five popular formulas for determining relative weight in children. They concluded that the weight-for-length index (WLI) was the most accurate. The WLI is calculated as follows:

$$\text{WLI} = A/B \times 100$$

where

$$A = \frac{\text{Actual weight (Kg)}}{\text{Actual height (cm)}}$$

$$B = \frac{\text{50th percentile expected weight (Kg) for age}}{\text{50th percentile expected height (cm) for age}}$$

The 50th percentile, expected height and weight for age data are derived from the National Center for Health Statistics Growth Charts (1976). Interpretation of WLI scores is straightforward: 90 to 109 represents the normal range with 100 the ideal score, 89 and below indicates the child is underweight, 110 to 119 is considered overweight, and obesity is defined as scoring 120 or more. DuRant et al. (1980) reported low correlations between the WLI and height and age for non-retarded children, adding support to the validity of this index. Fox, Hartney, Rotatori, and Litton (1986) also found low correlations between WLI and age and height for a MR sample. Further, this index was found to correlate significantly with MR subjects' triceps skinfold thickness, which provides a good measure of body fat. The advantages of the WLI include: 1) height and weight measures are easy to obtain, 2) the WLI is quickly computed, 3) the WLI includes national standards for height and weight, 4) the WLI is not related to the individuals age or height, 5) the WLI correlates well with more direct measures of obesity (skin-fold thickness), and 6) interpretation of WLI scores is straightforward.

Triceps Skinfold Thickness

Triceps skinfold thickness is one of the best indexes of the amount of fat in the body (Seltzer & Mayer, 1965). A skinfold caliper is used to obtain this measure. Normative tables derived from the Ten-State Nutrition Survey (1968–1970) for over 29,000 black and white participants between 1 and 80 years of age are available for triceps fatfold comparisons (Garn & Clark, 1976). Fox et al. (1983a) recommended that both relative weight measures and triceps skinfold thickness be used to ensure that an individual desiring or in need of treatment for obesity is accurately identified.

Etiology

Potential variables contributing to obesity include genetic factors (Bray, 1979; Withers, 1964), environmental factors (Cronk, Chumlea, & Roche, 1985), excessive caloric intake (Sims et al., 1968), and insufficient activity level (Chirico & Stunkard, 1960; Mayer, 1955). Although genetics were once generally believed to play a major role in the etiology of obesity, other evidence suggests that environmental factors may be more influential (Garn & Clark, 1976; Hartz, Rimm,

& Griefer, 1977; Schenker, Fisichelli, & Lang, 1974). Agras and Werne (1981) indicated that obesity is a complex condition with multiple precursors and subtypes. These factors make treating obesity a complicated process that should take into consideration the specific condition(s) contributing to the disorder and should tailor the treatment to the individual's unique needs.

Clinical Subtypes

The clinical subtypes of obesity are: 1) genetic, 2) endocrine, 3) hypothalamic, and 4) drug induced. Genetic obesity includes simple obesity, physical anomalies in fat distribution associated with lipomatosis and lipophilia, and the hereditary conditions of Alstrom, Prader-Willi, Down, Carpenter, Lawrence-Moon-Biedl, and Cohen syndromes. Endocrine forms of obesity include Von Gierke disease and hyperostosis frontalis inertia. Hypothalamic forms of obesity include Frohlich syndrome, Cushing syndrome, gynandrism, hypogonadism, hyperinsulinism, thyroid deficiency, and Stein-Leventhal syndrome. Drug-induced obesity generally is the result of side effects to the phenothiazines, estrogens, and tricyclic antidepressants.

GENETIC FACTORS

The genetic clinical subtypes of obesity account for only a small percentage of MR individuals. The majority of genetic syndromes are very rare. Prader-Willi children (Prader, Labhart, & Willi, 1956) are perhaps better known because of their unusual symptoms, which include indiscriminate eating (e.g., eating trash, pet food) and an insatiable hunger. Obesity, which may occur in the first or second year of life, if left untreated will result in significant obesity in adolescence and adulthood. Early attempts to treat this disorder were unsuccessful (Evans, 1964). More recently, behavioral interventions have shown some promise (Altman, Bundy, & Hirsch, 1978; Heiman, 1978; Thompson, Kodluboy, & Heston, 1980).

Cohen syndrome is another genetic disorder with both mental retardation and obesity as part of its clinical course. Truncal obesity associated with this disorder develops after 5 years of age (Doyard & Mattei, 1984). First reported by Cohen and colleagues (Cohen, Hall, Smith, Graham, & Kampert, 1973), this syndrome is also characterized by: delayed puberty onset, hypotonia, short stature (Goecke, Majewski, Kauther, & Sterzel, 1982; Kousseff, 1981), and in some cases, cardiovascular anomalies (Friedman & Sack, 1982). The clinical symptoms of mental retardation, obesity, and other anomalies (limb and ocular) link it to other well-documented conditions such as Prader-Willi syndrome (Hall & Smith, 1972) and Biedl-Bardet syndrome (Bauman & Hogan, 1973).

The prevalence of Down syndrome in the mentally retarded is greater than the other genetic anomalies associated with obesity. Mild to moderate obesity is found in Down syndrome children (Niesworth & Smith, 1978), adolescents, and adults (Robinson & Robinson, 1976). The specific mechanisms through which this syndrome influences the development of an obese condition are not well understood.

Laurence-Moon-Biedl syndrome is another rare condition that has obesity as one of its characteristics. Menolascino and Egger (1978) suggested that obesity associated with this disorder may be related to a brain defect rather than to over-eating or lack of exercise.

The genetic causes of retardation in which obesity is a clinical symptom explain only a small part of the total problem, since together the above syndromes are involved in a very limited percentage of the retarded population. Specific physical factors play a relatively small role in the majority of obesity cases for the retarded and nonretarded populations. However, more general physical factors such as body build, metabolic rate, and age of onset do contribute to an individual's tendencies towards obesity, and, consequently, may be important factors influencing treatment effectiveness.

Personality and Behavioral Factors

A number of personality and behavioral characteristics have been linked with obesity and overweight conditions, including anxiety, low self-esteem, neuroticism, and depression (Atkinson & Ringuette, 1967; Clancy, 1965; Held & Snow, 1972; Leckie & Withers, 1967; Levitt & Fellner, 1965; Werkman & Greenberg, 1967). Research results in this area have been contradictory and equivocal. For example, early studies on the psychological factors related to obesity suggested that anxiety contributed to overeating behavior (Bruch, 1973). Although some studies have supported increased eating patterns under stressful conditions in normal weight (Schachter, Goldman, & Gordon, 1968) and obese individuals (McKenna, 1972), the bulk of literature does not support the theory that food consumption reduces anxiety (Leon, 1974). Consistent with research in the general population, Fox, Burkhart, and Rotatori (1984) found no relationship between personality factors in mentally retarded adults, as measured by anxiety and self-concept scales, and an obese condition.

EATING STYLE

Faulty eating habits that lead to excessive food consumption may contribute to an obese condition (Stunkard & Kaplan, 1977; Wooley, Wooley, & Dyrenforth, 1979). The specific habits felt to play a part are rapid eating, insufficient chewing, taking large bites, and snacking. Obese children and adults have been found to eat more quickly and chew their food less than nonobese individuals (Adams, Ferguson, Stunkard, & Agras, 1978; Hill & McCutcheon, 1975). Obese individuals display a greater preference for and responsiveness toward food palatability (Haskin & Van Itallie, 1965; Nisbett, 1972; Wooley & Wooley, 1975; Wooley, Wooley, & Woods, 1975), suggesting that they may be more sensitive to and eat highly palatable foods. Obese individuals have also been found to be more sensitive to visually prominent food cues (Johnson, 1974; Ross, 1974). Schachter

(1968), interested in the effects of locus of control on eating behavior, postulated that eating behavior in obese individuals is under external stimulus control. This generated a number of well-controlled studies with conflicting results (Levitz, 1973). Other studies in this area have generally reported either no evidence of an obese eating style (Adams et al., 1978; Stunkard, Coll, Lindquist, & Meyers, 1980) or conflicting results (Stunkard & Kaplan, 1977).

Eating behavior has also been studied in MR persons (Fox, Burkhart, & Rotatori, 1983b). In this study, obese and nonobese MR adults individually were observed while eating in their natural environment (a sheltered workshop cafeteria). Measures were recorded for the first 15 minutes of the meal and included: number of individual bites of food or drinks of liquid, time spent actively eating (biting, chewing, drinking, or swallowing), pause time (cumulative time when the subject was not actively eating), and total calories consumed. The results indicated that there were no significant differences between the two groups on any of the measures. This relatively surprising finding has also been observed in similar studies with nonretarded subjects (Stunkard et al., 1980). However, in the Fox et al. (1983b) study with MR adults, high interindividual variability was observed within the obese and nonobese groups. For example, the total calories consumed by obese MR subjects ranged from 357 calories to 1,699 calories; caloric intake ranged from 380 to 1,232 calories for nonobese persons. Obese MR subjects took between 10 and 54 bites and drinks of food during the first 5 minutes of the meal; nonobese subjects ranged from 9 to 42 bites and drinks. Given this high variability between subjects, abandoning the study of eating style in obese MR subjects is premature. Although a distinct eating style may not be a characteristic common to all obese MR individuals, it may be an important variable contributing to an obese condition for a subset of this population.

ENVIRONMENTAL FACTORS AND PHYSICAL ACTIVITY

Environmental factors have also been associated with mental retardation and obesity. Although poor nutrition is prevalent in the MR population and has been most often cited as responsible for malnutrition (Crome & Stern, 1972), it may also play a significant role in obesity. For example, institutional diets, often high in starch and carbohydrates, may play a role in increased weights. Cronk et al. (1985) found increased weight levels of institutionalized Down syndrome children compared with those reared at home. They attributed weight differences to diet, activity, and general stimulation levels.

Although numerous studies have been conducted on the eating behavior of obese persons and its management (e.g., calorie-based diets), relatively little attention has been given to how obese persons expend energy through physical activity (Thompson, Jarvie, Lahey, & Cureton, 1982). A prominent issue in obesity and overweight conditions is addressed by the theory of energy imbalance. Briefly stated, when energy input exceeds energy expenditure over a period of time, overweight or obesity may result. This imbalance between food intake and energy expenditure has received increased research attention in recent years.

Preliminary research findings suggest that obese individuals exert less energy and are less active than nonobese individuals (Bullen, Reed, & Mayer, 1964; Dean & Garabedian, 1979; Meyers, Stunkard, Coll, & Cooke, 1980; Stefanik, Heald, & Mayer, 1959). Generally, males tend to be more active than females (Garfield, 1963), which may contribute to the greater prevalence of underweight in males than females in the retarded population (Wallen & Roszkowski, 1980). Further, hypotonia and hypoactivity may interact to contribute to an obese condition in several genetically related subgroups in the retarded population (e.g., Down, Cohen, Prader-Willi syndromes). Several researchers have suggested that inactivity may play a greater role in obesity than overeating (Johnson, Burke, & Mayer, 1956; Stefanik et al., 1959).

One way to study indirectly a person's physical activity is by assessing general physical fitness. The assumptions are that: 1) sedentary people are more likely to be in poorer physical condition than active individuals, and 2) obesity at least partly reflects an inactive life-style resulting in obese individuals being in relatively poor physical condition. A measure used to assess the physical condition of obese and nonobese MR subjects is the Ohio State University (OSU) Step Test, a submaximal measure of cardiovascular endurance (Mathews, 1978). The apparatus used includes a split-level bench with 15- and 20-inch steps, and an adjustable hand bar. The total test consists of 20 innings. Each inning includes a 30-second work period, during which subjects hold onto the hand bar with both hands and step up and down on the split-level bench, followed by a 20-second rest period. During the work period a tape-recorded cadence ("up-up-down-down") is played. The three different work loads on the OSU Step Test include: 1) six innings at a cadence of 24 steps per minute on the 15-inch bench, 2) six innings at a cadence of 30 steps per minute on the 15-inch bench, and 3) six innings at a cadence of 30 steps per minute on the 20-inch bench. During the 20-second rest period (between work periods), the subject's pulse rate is taken for 10 seconds beginning with Second 5 of the rest period and terminating at Second 15. The test is stopped when the pulse rate reaches 25 beats during the 20-second rest period (150 bpm) or when the subject finishes all 18 innings. The score for the test is the total number of innings completed. Unlike other measures of aerobic capacity (e.g., Cooper's 12-minute test, 1977), the OSU Step Test does not require maximum effort to obtain accurate results. This factor is particularly useful when the motivation of the individual may be in question. The OSU Step Test may also be used as a measure of change in physical conditioning by having individuals' perform the test prior to the initiation of an aerobic or other physical fitness program, and again after a number of weeks or months into the program. Adjustments in the fitness program may then be made to help individuals obtain maximum benefit from their efforts to improve conditioning and use up the calories necessary to lose weight.

Fox, Burkhart, et al. (1984) evaluated the OSU Step Test's ability to discriminate obese from nonobese retarded individuals. Thirty-eight subjects (19 obese and 19 nonobese) were evaluated using the OSU Step Test. Sixty-two percent of the sample successfully completed the OSU Step Test, 14 obese (7 males and 7 females) and 12 nonobese (2 males and 10 females). The remaining 16 were eliminated because they failed to maintain the cadence required by the test. The results indicated a significant difference between the obese and non-obese groups, with the obese subjects completing less innings than the nonobese. Also, significant sex differences were found with males completing more innings. As predicted, the obese retarded adults were in poorer physical fitness than nonobese retarded adults. The results suggest that physical inactivity may be important to our understanding of obesity. However, the picture at this point is far from being clear:

Obesity may be related over time to lowering levels of physical activity (which results in poor physical fitness), or, reduced levels of physical activity may be the result of an obese condition caused by other factors (e.g., caloric intake, physiological aspects), or by combinations of factors (Fox, Burkhart, et al., 1984, p. 66).

Treatment Strategies

A plethora of intervention approaches to obesity have surfaced over the years. They have included psychotherapy, group weight loss programs (such as "Take Off Pounds Sensibly"), innumerable diet regimes, exercise programs, medications, and even surgery. Although psychotherapy was once thought to be an effective treatment for obesity, there is little evidence to support this belief (Stunkard, 1976) and long-term follow-up data have been disappointing. Weight reduction groups have reported significant weight losses (Stunkard, Levine, & Fox, 1978). Group pressure for weight loss and strict diets have been important factors in their successes. Unfortunately, attrition of dieters has been a major problem for these support groups. Calorie-controlled and low-carbohydrate diets (Howard, 1975) have resulted in effective weight loss (Leon, 1974), yet the long-term effects of dieting alone for maintaining weight loss have been poor (Leon, 1976; Sohar & Sneh, 1973).

Exercise has increasingly become an important component of many weight loss programs. The potential benefits of regular physical activity (e.g., weight reduction, improved cardiopulmonary function, and stress reduction) are even greater for obese than nonobese individuals, since they are likely to be doing a greater amount of work exercising their larger and heavier bodies. Additionally, increased activity for inactive people may result in reduced caloric intake, since exercise acts as an appetite suppressant (Bakwin & Bakwin, 1972). Like caloric restrictions, many authors (Craddock, 1973; Stuart & Davis, 1972) believe exercise to be an important component in a weight reduction program. Unfortunately, Buskirk (1969) has suggested that obese individuals are not highly motivated for physical activity. Schurrer, Weltman, and Brammel (1985) recently demonstrated the benefits of exercise with MR persons. They found that subjects who attended exercise sessions on an average of three times per week and covered an average distance of 9.0 km per week, lost an average of 3.6 kg of weight and increased maximal oxygen consumption by 43% over the 23-week training program. Nardella, Sulzbacher, and Worthington-Roberts (1983) reported a study that assessed the impact of activity level on the weight of Prader-Willi subjects who were involved in a weight reduction program that combined exercise and a 1,000-calorie-per-day diet. Results revealed a significant correlation between activity level and weight loss.

Anorexiant medications also have been used to treat obesity. Unfortunately, the long-term effectiveness of prescription and nonprescription drugs for maintaining weight reduction has been poor (Feinstein, 1960; Leon, 1976; Stunkard & McLaren-Hume, 1959). The ideal anorectic medication which maintains reduced caloric intake but has no side effects, has yet to be discovered (Silverstone, 1975). Surgical procedures, such as intestinal bypass, stomach stapling, and removal of excessive fatty tissue, have been used with mixed results and have resulted in a number of postoperative complications (Bray & Benfield, 1977).

The majority of traditional treatment approaches described previously have not been applied in any systematic way to the obese DD/MR populations. Even in the general population these approaches have met with mixed results. In most cases, although initial and even substantial weight loss can be expected in most traditional treatment programs, long-term maintenance of weight loss is far less likely to occur.

Behavioral Approaches

For the general and DD/MR obese populations, behavioral approaches have made a significant impact in the obesity treatment field over the past 15 years. The inroads made by behavioral practitioners have been felt across the different professional disciplines dealing with obesity (e.g., psychology, medicine, nutrition, physical education). The influence of the behavioral orientation has spread in part due to its effectiveness. By the mid-1970s, when behavioral approaches to health-related disorders were still in their infancy, Abramson (1973, 1977) reported over 100 research and clinical reports in which behavioral techniques were used in the treatment of obesity. There are several elements common to programs employing behavioral strategies, including self-monitoring, reinforcement, stimulus control and eating style, and physical activity. Each of these components is briefly described below.

PROMOTING INCREASED AWARENESS

Self-monitoring techniques include having the dieter record: daily consumption of food, weight, and specific eating and physical activity patterns. The primary purpose is to help dieters become more aware of their eating behavior and the situations where eating takes place, and to associate the amount of food they eat with weight gain or loss. Self-monitoring alone has resulted in weight loss, especially when the recording is completed prior to eating, rather than after eating (Bellack, 1975). Through daily weigh-ins, dieters learn to associate weight change with changes in caloric intake. Finally, recording eating and activity patterns provides information pertaining to where change may be needed (e.g., reducing snacks, increasing amount of time walking). Self-recording techniques in general serve as a useful means of providing dieters feedback regarding their progress.

CHANGING EATING PATTERNS

Schachter (1971) suggested that the behavior of obese individuals is more influenced by external cues (i.e., the sight and smell of food), than by internal cues (i.e., actual hunger). Although this theory has been challenged, the purpose of stimulus control techniques is to reduce the potential influence of external cues on behavior. One strategy is to have the dieter make the eating situation as distinctive as possible, by using an entire place setting when eating and to limit the number of places where eating takes place (e.g., dining room, kitchen). A second technique is to have the dieter limit intake by instructing him or her to take only one average-size helping of each food served at a meal. A third technique is to lengthen the behavioral chain involved in overeating (e.g., putting down the eating utensil after each bite of food, and not picking it up again until the food in the mouth is completely chewed and swallowed). The final technique is to have the dieter substitute a pleasurable activity for eating, when the urge to overeat occurs. The substituted activity should be incompatible with eating, readily available, and physically separated from food areas (e.g., taking a walk, riding a bicycle, or going to a health club).

INCREASED PHYSICAL ACTIVITY

By increasing caloric energy expenditure through activity, dieters are working on using up energy and burning calories. When combined with reduced caloric intake, increased activity level enhances the effects of dieting, and results in greater weight loss in a shorter amount of time. Obese individuals are generally less active and may resist encouragement to increase their activity level. "Gradually introducing a highly reinforcing exercise program (e.g., aerobic dance) by small steps helps increase the dieter's likelihood of participation" (Fox, Switzky, Rotatori, & Vitkus, 1982, p. 240).

MAINTAINING BEHAVIORAL CHANGES

Positive reinforcement is used to enhance the development and use of techniques dieters are taught. Rotatori (1978) suggests that a combination of external and self-delivered rewards should be used. External rewards are used as incentives for learning and using the techniques for weight loss during the treatment period. After treatment, the dieter should have a fully developed self-reinforcement system, which promotes the continued use of dieting techniques.

Behavioral Intervention with Obese DD/MR Persons

The greatest success in weight loss for DD/MR children, adolescents, and adults is likely to be through a combination of behavioral techniques, weight control procedures, and increased activity levels. Table 5.2 summarizes a group of behavioral control studies and their outcome with mentally retarded individuals.

In a case study, Foxx (1972) used social reinforcement in a weight reduction program for an obese, mildly retarded, institutionalized, adolescent girl. As a reward for losing 1½ pounds per week, the researcher would accompany the girl to the facility canteen and share a diet soda with her. A weight reduction of 79 pounds (from 239 to 160 pounds) was reported over a 42-week period.

Gumaer and Simon (1979) involved parents and school staff (teachers and cafeteria workers) in an instructional program with 11 obese, trainable, mentally retarded students. Instruction was provided twice weekly on the use of a food intake chart, a nutritious diet, and the use of exercise to "burn off" calories. Contingent upon the loss of ½ pound per week, a variety of short-term reinforcers were used, including social recognition (through praise and display of a thermometer weight loss chart on a bulletin board) and admittance to a special activity. The long-term reinforcer involved a fashion show before the entire school, for those maintaining desired weight losses. Weight change by the end of the 14-month intervention period ranged from +13 to −30 pounds. An additional mean weight loss of 2.75 pounds was observed at a 3-month follow-up.

Buford (1975) developed a multicomponent treatment program with 15 moderately retarded students from 9 to 21 years of age. Parents and school staff were involved in establishing and providing individualized reinforcers for each participant. A public health nurse led this 8-month treatment program. The students lost an average of 8.3 pounds, with individual weight change ranging from +3 to −24 pounds.

A study by Altman et al. (1978) involved the treatment of two mentally retarded adolescents with Prader-Willi syndrome. A contingency contract was established between the dieters and their parents/caregivers, who agreed to provide reinforcers for compliance with program procedures and to withhold the reinforcers for noncompliance. The program components introduced sequentially were: 1) self-monitoring of caloric intake, daily morning weight, and exercise; 2) positive reinforcement for weekly weight loss and reduced caloric intake; and 3) positive reinforcement for weight loss only. The 18-year-old mildly retarded female lost 43 pounds (14% of her body weight) during the treatment phase, and an additional 22 pounds were lost during the maintenance phase. The second dieter, a 13-year-old moderately retarded female, lost 19 pounds during treatment and an additional 11 pounds during maintenance. An interesting finding was that the self-monitoring treatment condition did not produce significant weight loss for either subject. Contingent reinforcement did result in decreased caloric intake and weight reduction. Additionally, when reinforcement was given only for weight loss and removed for reduced caloric intake, weight losses continued.

TABLE 5.2. Behavioral weight studies with mentally retarded individuals

Author	N	Level of retardation	Active treatment period (weeks)	Average weight loss (pounds)	Research design
Foxx (1972)	1	Mild	42	79.0	Case study uncontrolled
Gumaer & Simon (1979)	11	Moderate	14	7.9	Single group outcome
Buford (1975)	15	Moderate	32	8.3	Single group outcome
Altman, Bundy, & Hirsch (1978)	2	Mild	33	31.0	Multiple baseline
Rotatori, Parrish, & Freagon (1979)	6	Moderate/mild	7	3.7	Single group outcome
Rotatori, Fox, & Switzky (1979)	6	Moderate	14	10.4	Single group outcome
Rotatori & Switzky (1979)	12	Moderate	14	9.7	Controlled group outcome
Rotatori & Fox (1980)	12	Moderate	14	10.3	Controlled group outcome
Jackson & Thorbecke (1982)	12	Moderate	14	9.2	Controlled group outcome
Fox, Haniotes, & Rotatori (1984)	16	Moderate	10	7.3	Controlled group outcome
Fox, Rosenberg, & Rotatori (1985)	15	Moderate	10	7.4	Controlled group outcome

A behaviorally based weight control program developed by Rotatori (1978) has been successfully used with retarded children (Rotatori, Parrish, & Freagon, 1979), adolescents (Rotatori & Switzky, 1979), and adults (Rotatori, 1978). This weight control program included 14 weeks of treatment, followed by 5 weeks of maintenance training. During the treatment phase, participants met three times weekly, where the following seven technique areas were systematically covered: 1) self-monitoring daily weight and food intake, 2) manipulating emotional responses to discourage urges to overeat, 3) eating only one average-size helping of each food present at a meal, 4) reducing eating rate, 5) performing food-cue elimination techniques, 6) increasing energy expenditure, and 7) eliminating or reducing snacking. Self-reinforcement was taught and incorporated into the program by having the participants grade themselves on their daily performance. Daily grades were exchanged for "activity-cards" and "self-reinforcer statement cards." Participants were weighed weekly and rewarded with an additional highly prized activity, contingent upon completing the recording forms and a 1-pound reduction in weight. During the 5-week maintenance phase, weight control techniques taught in the treatment phase were reviewed once or twice weekly and reinforcement procedures were continued. Follow-up weigh-ins were conducted to assess the program's long-term effects.

In a 7-week pilot study using this treatment package (Rotatori, Parrish, et al., 1979), six mild to moderately retarded children lost an average of 3.7 pounds. A second study with six moderately retarded Down syndrome adolescents (Rotatori, Fox, & Switzky, 1979), resulted in an average loss of 10.37 pounds during treatment, and 3.95 pounds during maintenance. A 26-week follow-up found no significant weight change from maintenance level weights. In both of these studies, parents and teachers were highly involved in the program. A third study (Rotatori & Switzky, 1979), designed to evaluate the effectiveness of a live versus videotaped presentation of the treatment package, was conducted with moderately retarded adolescents. A control group was also included. Live presentation members lost an average of 11 pounds during treatment, 2.96 pounds during maintenance, and 2.33 pounds during the 16-week follow-up. The videotaped presentation group members lost an average of 9.45 pounds during treatment, 2.58 pounds during maintenance, and 0.63 pounds during follow-up. No significant differences were found between the two treatment groups. Both treatment groups lost significantly more weight than the control group. The results of this study suggest that both live and videotaped presentations are equally as effective in applying this weight reduction program.

A fourth study (Rotatori & Fox, 1980) involved a comparison of the behavioral treatment package, with a nutrition-based weight control approach and a weight-list control group. The subjects were moderately retarded, public high school students. A school nurse led the nutrition group, which met four times weekly for 14 weeks. Emphasis was placed on good eating habits, the importance of weight loss, and other nutritional topics. While no significant differences were observed between the control group and the nutrition-based group, the behavior therapy group demonstrated significantly greater weight losses than either of the other groups.

In an attempt to determine if a shorter behavioral program could produce similar results, Fox, Haniotes, and Rotatori (1984) developed an abbreviated version of their behavioral weight loss program. The program was 10 weeks in length for the treatment phase, with meetings scheduled twice weekly. A 5-week maintenance phase immediately followed, with weekly meetings to review behavioral strategies, continue reinforcement procedures, and gradually fade out homework forms. A 1-year follow-up was conducted to obtain the body weights of all subjects. The subjects lost an average of 7.3 pounds, with a range of -1 to -16 pounds during treatment. Postmaintenance weigh-ins revealed an additional reduction of 2.1 pounds (range $= +2$ to -5 pounds). One-year follow-up weigh-ins revealed that they lost an additional 0.6 pounds (range $= +5$ to -8 pounds) from their original baseline weights. They concluded that the revised "treatment package was found to represent a more efficient approach to weight loss in the mentally retarded" (p. 77).

Fox, Rosenberg, and Rotatori (1985) studied the effects of parent and participant involvement in the abbreviated behavioral weight loss program. The parent involvement group lost significantly more weight ($M = 7.4$ pounds), with less intragroup variability ($SD = 2.26$ pounds) than the group with minimal parent involvement ($M = 2.4$ pounds; $SD = 4.38$ pounds). Using the number of daily homework forms completed as a measure of participant involvement, a strong correlation was found (r [13] $= 0.87, p < 0.01$) between this variable and weight loss.

Two major problems persist in treatment literature for both retarded and non-retarded persons: 1) high interindividual weight loss variability during a program's implementation, and 2) poor long-term maintenance of weight loss once treatment is concluded. Regarding the high interindividual variability, further investigations are needed to identify variables that contribute to the development and maintenance of obesity. Areas needing further research include: eating and activity patterns, caloric intake, metabolic factors, and biomedical correlates (Rotatori, Fox, et al., 1986). Because of poor long-term maintenance of weight loss, Rotatori, Zinkgraf, et al. (1986) investigated the effect of two weight loss maintenance strategies for 13 moderately/mildly retarded adults after they were first involved in a 12-week behavior therapy weight reduction program. One maintenance strategy involved posttreatment booster sessions (12 weeks) followed by weekly weigh-ins plus reinforcement for weight loss (40 weeks). The second maintenance strategy involved weekly weigh-ins and reinforcement for weight loss (52 weeks). Interestingly, subjects exposed to posttreatment booster sessions continued to lose weight, while those not exposed to booster sessions did not. However, a 12-month follow-up check revealed that treatment and maintenance successes were not well maintained.

Conclusions

Significant progress has been made in a relatively short time regarding our understanding, assessment, and treatment of an obese condition in DD/MR individuals. Much of what we have learned points to one conclusion, namely, that making analogies between obese nonretarded and retarded persons are warranted, with relatively rare exceptions (e.g., persons with syndromes such as Prader-Willi and Laurence-Moon-Biedl). Obesity is a prevalent condition in both groups from childhood through adulthood. Likewise, the etiology of an obese condition is similar across groups. That is, a person's unique physiological and biological makeup sets the parameters within which inappropriate eating and activity patterns may insidiously lead to an obese condition. Treatment of obesity remains a challenge for clinicians and researchers. Many of the treatment approaches that were found to be effective in the general obese population were found to be equally effective in the DD/MR population when tailored to the special characteristics of that group, (e.g., lower mental age).

Much yet needs to be learned. Disagreement continues on how obesity is best defined and measured, which makes comparing the findings of different research studies a difficult process. Also confounding the literature is the hypothesis that perhaps different nonphysiological subtypes of obesity exist. For example, in some individuals, limited physical activity may be more responsible for their condition than a problematic eating style. Such clinical subtypes require study to better delineate their characteristics and, ultimately, to arrive at the development of differential treatment strategies. This proposed differential treatment direction may help reduce the high variability in weight loss currently observed in programs for obese persons because treatment will be more tailored to the individual's unique characteristics. Long-term maintenance of weight loss after treatment has ended remains a major stumbling block for researchers. Current data imply that long-term success can only be achieved if relatively permanent changes in the general life-style of the obese person can be achieved. Treatment efforts falling short of this goal will likely have only a transient impact.

As in any important area concerning human health and behavior, more research is needed. This is particularly true for obesity, which is both prevalent and carries with it serious health consequences. Given the great difficulty in helping an obese individual attain a nonobese status, future research focusing on prevention of obesity in DD persons may be the most fruitful and rewarding direction to pursue.

References

Abraham, S. (1983). *Obese and overweight adults in the United States.* In *Vital and Health Statistics, National Center for Health Statistics* (Series 11, No. 230 DHHS Pub. No. 83–1650). Washington, DC: Public Health Service.

Abramson, E.E. (1973). A review of behavioral approaches to weight control. *Behavior Research and Therapy, 11,* 547–556.

Abramson, E.E. (1977). Behavioral approaches to weight control: An updated review. *Behavior Research and Therapy, 15,* 355–363.

Adams, N., Ferguson, J., Stunkard, A.J., & Agras, W.S. (1978). The eating behavior of obese and nonobese women. *Behaviour Research and Therapy, 16,* 225–232.

Agras, S., & Werne, J. (1981). Disorders or eating. In S.M. Turner, K.S. Calhoun, & H.E. Adams (Eds.), *Handbook of clinical behavior therapy* (pp. 214–239). New York: Wiley.

Altman, D., Bundy, A., & Hirsch, G. (1978). Behavioral treatment of obesity in patients with Prader-Willi syndrome. *Journal of Behavioral Medicine, 1,* 403–412.

Atkinson, R.M., & Ringuette, E.L. (1967). A survey of biographical and psychological features in extraordinary fatness. *Psychosomatic Medicine, 29,* 121–133.

Bakwin, H., & Bakwin, R.M. (1972). *Behavior disorders in children* (4th ed.). Philadelphia: W.B. Saunders.

Bauman, M.L., & Hogan, G.R. (1973). Laurence-Moon-Biedl syndrome. *American Journal of Diseases of Childhood, 126,* 119–123.

Bellack, A.S. (1975). A comparison of self-reinforcement and self-monitoring in a weight reduction program. *Behavior Therapy, 7,* 68–75.

Bray, G.A. (Ed.). (1976). *Obesity in America* (DHEW Publication 16, NIH 79–359). Washington, DC: U.S. Government Printing Office.

Bray, G.A. (Ed.). (1979). *Obesity in America* (NIH Publication No. 79–359). Washington, DC: U.S. Department of Health, Education and Welfare.

Bray, G.A., & Benfield, J.R. (1977). Intestinal bypass for obesity: A summary and perspective. *American Journal of Clinical Nutrition, 30,* 121–127.

Bruch, A. (1973). *Eating disorders: Obesity, anorexia nervosa, and the person within.* New York: Basic Books.

Buford, L.M. (1975). Group education to reduce overweight: Classes for mentally handicapped children. *American Journal of Nursing, 75,* 1994–1995.

Bullen, B.A., Reed, R.B., & Mayer, J. (1964). Physical activity of obese and nonobese adolescent girls appraised by motion picture sampling. *American Journal of Clinical Nutrition, 14,* 211.

Burkhart, J.E., Fox, R.A., & Rotatori, A.F. (1985). Obesity of mentally retarded individuals: Prevalence, characteristics, and intervention. *American Journal of Mental Deficiency, 90,* 303–313.

Buskirk, E.R. (1969). Increasing energy expenditure: The role of exercise. In N.L. Wilson (Ed.), *Obesity.* Philadelphia: F.A. Davis.

Chirico, A.M., & Stunkard, A.J. (1960). Physical activity and human obesity. *New England Journal of Medicine, 263,* 935–946.

Chumlea, W.C., & Cronk, C.E. (1981). Overweight among children with Trisomy 21. *Journal of Mental Deficiency Research, 25,* 275–280.

Clancy, J. (1965). Other aspects of depression. *Geriatrics, 20,* 92–98.

Cohen, M.M., Hall, B.D., Smith, D.W., Graham, C.B., & Kampert, K.J. (1973). A new syndrome with hypotonia, obesity, mental deficiency and facial, oral, ocular, and limb anomalies. *Journal of Pediatrics, 83,* 280–284.

Cooper, K.H. (1977). *The aerobics way.* New York: Bantam Books.

Craddock, D. (1973). *Obesity and its management* (2nd ed.). New York: Churchill Livingston.

Craddock, D. (1978). *Obesity and its management* (3rd ed.). New York: Churchill Livingston.

Crome, L., & Stern, J. (1972). *Pathology of mental retardation.* Baltimore: Williams & Wilkins.

Cronk, C.E., Chumlea, W.C., & Roche, A.F. (1985). Assessment of overweight children with Trisomy 21. *American Journal of Mental Deficiency, 90,* 34–39.

Dawber, T.R. (1980). *The Framingham study: The epidemiology of atherosclerotic disease.* Cambridge, MA: Harvard University Press.

Dean, R.S., & Garabedian, A.A. (1979). Obesity and level of activity. *Perceptual and Motor Skills, 49,* 690.

Doyard, P., & Mattei, J.F. (1984). Cohen's syndrome in two sisters. *Sem-Hospitals-Paris, 60,* 1143–1147.

DuRant, R.H., & Linder, C.W. (1981). An evaluation of five indexes of relative body weight for use with children. *Journal of the American Dietetic Association, 78,* 35–41.

DuRant, R.H., Martin, D.S., Linder, C.W., & Weston, W. (1980). The prevalence of obesity and thinness in children from a lower socioeconomic population receiving comprehensive health care. *American Journal of Clinical Nutrition, 33,* 2002–2007.

Evans, P.R. (1964). Hypogenitol dystrophy with diabetic tendency. *Guy's Hospital Report, 113,* 207.

Feinstein, A.R. (1960). The treatment of obesity: An analysis of methods, results, and factors which influence success. *Journal of Chronic Diseases, 11,* 349–393.

Fox, R.A., Burkhart, J.E., & Rotatori, A.F. (1983a). Appropriate classification of obesity of mentally retarded adults. *American Journal of Mental Deficiency, 88,* 112–114.

Fox, R.A., Burkhart, J.E., & Rotatori, A.F. (1983b). Eating behavior of obese and nonobese mentally retarded adults. *American Journal of Mental Deficiency, 5,* 570–574.

Fox, R.A., Burkhart, J.E., & Rotatori, A.F. (1984). Physical fitness and personality characteristics of obese and nonobese retarded adults. *International Journal of Obesity, 8*, 61–67.

Fox, R.A., Haniotes, H., & Rotatori, A. (1984). A streamlined weight loss program for moderately retarded adults in a sheltered workshop setting. *Applied Research in Mental Retardation, 5*, 69–79.

Fox, R.A., Hartney, C.W., Rotatori, A.F., & Kurpiers, E.M. (1985). Incidence of obesity among retarded children. *Education and Training of the Mentally Retarded, 20*, 175–181.

Fox, R.A., Hartney, C.W., Rotatori, A.F., & Litton, F. (March, 1986). *Assessing relative weight in mentally retarded children.* Paper presented at the regional meeting of the Southeastern Psychological Association, Orlando, FL.

Fox, R., Rosenberg, R., & Rotatori, A. (1985). Parent involvement in a treatment program for obese retarded adults. *Journal of Behavior Therapy & Experimental Psychiatry, 16* (1), 45–48.

Fox, R.A., & Rotatori, A.F. (1982). Prevalence of obesity in mentally retarded adults. *American Journal of Mental Deficiency, 87*, 228–230.

Fox, R.A., Switzky, H., Rotatori, A., & Vitkus, P. (1982). Successful weight loss techniques with mentally retarded children and youth. *Exceptional Children, 49*(3), 238–244.

Foxx, R.M. (1972). Social reinforcement of weight reduction: A case report on an obese retarded adolescent. *Mental Retardation, 10*, 21–23.

Friedman, E., & Sack, J. (1982). The Cohen syndrome: Report of five new cases and a review of the literature. *Journal of Craniological Genetics and Developmental Biology, 2*, 193–200.

Garfield, S.L. (1963). Abnormal behavior and mental deficiency. In N.R. Ellis (Eds.), *Handbook of mental deficiency: Psychology theory and research* (pp. 574–577). New York: McGraw-Hill.

Garn, S.M., & Clark, D.C. (1976). Trends in fatness and the origins of obesity. *Pediatrics, 57*, 443–456.

Goecke, T., Majewski, F., Kauther, K.D., & Sterzel, U. (1982). Mental retardation hypotonia, obesity, ocular, facial, dental, and limb abnormalities (Cohen syndrome): Report of three patients. *European Journal of Pediatrics, 138*(4), 334–338.

Gumaer, J., & Simon, R. (1979). Behavioral group counseling and schoolwide reinforcement program with obese trainable mentally retarded students. *Education and Training of the Mentally Retarded, 14*, 106–111.

Hall, B.D., & Smith, D.W. (1972). Prader-Willi syndrome. *Journal of Pediatrics, 81*, 286–293.

Harris, M.B. (1976). What is obesity. *World Medicine, 19*, 39.

Hartz, A., Rimm, A.A., & Griefer, E. (1977). *Relative importance of family environment and heredity on the etiology of childhood obesity.* Second International Congress on Obesity, Washington, DC.

Haskin, S.A., & Van Itallie, T.B. (1965). Studies in normal and obese subjects with a monitored food dispensing service. *Annals of the New York Sciences, 131*, 654–661.

Heiman, M.F. (1978). The management of obesity in the post-adolescent developmentally disabled client with Prader Willi syndrome. *Adolescence, 13*, 291–296.

Held, M.L., & Snow, D.L. (1972). MMPI, internal-external control, and problem checklist scores of obese adolescent females. *Journal of Clinical Psychology, 28*, 523–525.

Hill, S.W., & McCutcheon, N.B. (1975). Eating response of obese and nonobese humans during dinner meals. *Psychosomatic Medicine, 37,* 395–401.

Howard, A.N. (1975). Dietary treatment of obesity. In T. Silverstone (Ed.), *Obesity: Its pathogenesis and management.* Acton, MA: Publishing Sciences Group.

Jackson, H.J., & Thorbecke, P.J. (1982). Treating obesity of mentally retarded adolescents and adults: An exploratory program. *American Journal of Mental Deficiency, 87,* 302–308.

Johnson, M.I., Burke, B.S., & Mayer, J. (1956). Relative importance of inactivity and overeating on the energy balance of obese high school girls. *American Journal of Clinical Nutrition, 4,* 37.

Johnson, W.G. (1974). Effect of cue prominence and subject weight on human food directed performance. *Journal of Personality and Social Psychology, 29,* 843–848.

Kannel, W.B., & Gorden, T. (1979). Physiological and medical concomitants of obesity: The Framingham study. In G.A. Bray (Ed.), *Obesity in America* (NIH Publication No. 79–359, pp. 125–163). Washington, DC: U.S. Department of Health, Education and Welfare.

Kousseff, B.G. (1981). Cohen syndrome: Further delineation and inheritance. *American Journal of Medical Genetics, 17,* 317–319.

Kreze, A., Zelinda, M., Juhas, J., & Garbara, M. (1974). Relationship between intelligence and relative prevalence of obesity. *Human Biology, 46,* 109–113.

Leckie, E.V., & Withers, R.F.J. (1967). Obesity and depression. *Journal of Psychosomatic Research, 11,* 107–115.

Leon, G.R. (1974). Personality, body image, and eating pattern changes in overweight persons after weight loss. In A. Howard (Ed.), *Recent advances in obesity research.* London: Newman.

Leon, G.R. (1976). Current directions in the treatment of obesity. *Psychological Bulletin, 83*(4), 557–578.

Levitt, H., & Fellner, C. (1965). MMPI profiles of three obesity subgroups. *Journal of Consulting and Clinical Psychology, 29,* 91.

Levitz, L.S. (1973). *The susceptibility of human feeding behavior to external controls.* Paper presented at the Fogarty Internal Conferences on Obesity, Washington, DC.

Mathews, D. (1978). *Measurement in physical education.* Philadelphia: W.B. Saunders.

Mayer, J. (1955). The role of exercise and activity in weight control. In E.S. Eppright, A. Swanson, & A. Iverson (Eds.), *Weight control.* Ames, Iowa: Iowa State College Press.

McKenna, R.J. (1972). Some effects of anxiety level and food cues on eating behavior of obese and normal subjects: A comparison of the Schachterian and psychosomatic conception. *Journal of Personality and Social Psychology, 22,* 311–319.

Menolascino, F.J., & Egger, M.L. (1978). *Medical dimensions of mental retardation.* Lincoln: University of Nebraska Press.

Metropolitan Life Insurance Company. (1977). *Desirable height-weight tables.* New York: Author.

Meyers, A.W., Stunkard, A.J., Coll, M., & Cooke, C.J. (1980). Stairs, escalators, and obesity. *Behavior Modification, 4,* 355–359.

Nardella, M.T., Sulzbacher, S.I., & Worthington-Roberts, B.S. (1983). Activity levels of persons with Prader-Willi syndrome. *American Journal of Mental Deficiency, 87,* 498–505.

National Center for Health Statistics: NCHS Growth Charts. (1976). Monthly vital statistics report *25*(3), Dupp. (HRA) 76–1120. Rockville, MD.

Niesworth, J.T., & Smith, R.M. (1978). *Retardation: Issues, assessment, and intervention.* New York: McGraw-Hill.

Nisbett, R.E. (1972). Hunger, obesity and the ventromedial hypothalamus. *Psychological Review, 79,* 433–438.

Prader, A., Labhart, A., & Willi, H. (1956). Ein Syndrome von Adipositas Kleinwuchs, Kryptorchismus und Oligophrenie nach Myantonieartigem Zustand en Neugeboralter. *Schweizerische Medizinische Wochenschrift, 86,* 1260.

Robinson, M.M., & Robinson, H.B. (1976). *The mentally retarded child* (2nd ed.). New York: McGraw-Hill.

Ross, L. (1974). Effects of manipulating salience of food upon consumption of obese and normal eaters. In S. Schachter & J. Rodin (Eds.), *Obese humans and rats* (pp. 43–52). Potomac, MD: Lawrence Erlbaum.

Rotatori, A.F. (1978). The effect of different reinforcement schedules in the maintenance of weight loss with retarded overweight adults. *Dissertation Abstracts International, 38,* 4738-N.

Rotatori, A.F., & Fox, R. (1980). A comparison of two weight reduction programs for moderately retarded adolescents. *Behavior Therapy, 11,* 410–416.

Rotatori, A.F., & Fox, R. (1981). *Behavioral weight reduction program for mentally handicapped persons: A self-control approach.* Baltimore, MD: ProEd.

Rotatori, A.F., Fox, R.A., Matson, J., Metha, S., Baker, A., & Lopuch, W.R. (1986). Changes in biomedical and physical correlates in behavioral weight loss with retarded youths. *Journal of Obesity and Weight Regulation, 5,* 11–17.

Rotatori, A.F., Fox, R., & Switzky, H.N. (1979). Parent-teacher administered weight reduction program for obese Down's syndrome adolescents. *Journal of Behavior Therapy and Experimental Psychiatry, 10,* 339–341.

Rotatori, A.F., Parrish, P., & Freagon, S. (1979). Weight loss in retarded children: A pilot study. *Journal of Psychiatric Nursing, 17,* 33–34.

Rotatori, A.F., & Switzky, H. (1979). Successful behavioral weight loss with moderately mentally retarded individuals. *International Journal of Obesity, 3,* 223–228.

Rotatori, A.F., Zinkgraf, S., Matson, J., Fox, R., Sexton, D., & Wade, P. (1986). The effect of two weight reduction maintenance strategies for moderately/mildly retarded adults. *Journal of Obesity and Weight Regulation, 5,* 18–22.

Schachter, S. (1968). Obesity and eating. *Science, 161,* 751–756.

Schachter, S. (1971). Some extraordinary facts about obese humans and rats. *American Psychologist, 26,* 129–144.

Schachter, S., Goldman, R., & Gordon, A. (1968). Effects of fear, food deprivation and obesity on eating. *Journal of Personality and Social Psychology, 10,* 91–97.

Schenker, I.R., Fisichelli, U., & Lang, J. (1974). Weight difference between foster infants of overweight and nonoverweight foster mothers. *Journal of Personality and Social Psychology, 10,* 91–97.

Schurrer, O.R., Weltman, A., & Brammel, H. (1985). Effects of physical training on cardiovascular fitness and behavior patterns of mentally retarded adults. *American Journal of Mental Deficiency, 90*(2), 167–169.

Seltzer, C.C., & Mayer, J. (1965). A simple criterion of obesity. *Postgraduate Medicine, 38,* A101–A107.

Silverstone, T. (1975). Anorectic drugs. In T. Silverstone (Ed.), *Obesity: Its pathogenesis and management.* Acton, MA: Publishing Sciences Group.

Simopoulos, A.P., & Van Itallie, T.B. (1984). Body, weight, and longevity. *Annals of Internal Medicine, 100,* 285–295.

Sims, E.A., Goldman, R.F., Gluck, C.M., Horton, E.S., Kelleher, P.C., & Rowe, D.W. (1968). Experimental obesity in men. *Transactions of the Association of American Physicians, 81*, 153–170.

Sohar, E., & Sneh, E. (1973). Follow-up of obese patients: 14 years after a successful reducing diet. *American Journal of Clinical Nutrition, 26*, 845–848.

Staugaitis, S.D. (1978). New directions for effective weight control with mentally retarded people. *Mental Retardation, 16*, 157–163.

Stefanik, P.A., Heald, F.P., Jr., & Mayer, J. (1959). Caloric intake in relation to energy output of obese and nonobese adolescent boys. *American Journal of Clinical Nutrition, 7*, 55.

Stuart, R.B., & Davis, B. (1972). *Slim chance in a fat world: Changing health lifestyles.* Champaign, IL: Research Press.

Stunkard, A.J. (1975). From explanation to action in psychosomatic medicine: The case of obesity. *Psychosomatic Medicine, 37*, 195–236.

Stunkard, A.J. (1976). *The pain of obesity.* Palo Alto, CA: Bull Publishing.

Stunkard, A.J., Coll, M., Lindquist, S., & Meyers, A. (1980). Obesity and eating style. *Archives of General Psychiatry, 37*, 1127–1229.

Stunkard, A.J., & Kaplan, P. (1977). Eating in public places: A review of reports of the direct observations of eating behavior. *International Journal of Obesity, 1*, 89–101.

Stunkard, A., Levine, H., & Fox, S. (1978). The management of obesity. *Archives of Internal Medicine, 125*, 1067–1072.

Stunkard, A.J., & McLaren-Hume, M. (1959). The results of treatment for obesity. *Archives of Internal Medicine, 103*, 79–85.

Thompson, J.K., Jarvie, G.J., Lahey, B.B., & Cureton, K.J. (1982). Exercise and obesity: Etiology, physiology, and intervention. *Psychological Bulletin, 91*, 55–79.

Thompson, T., Kodluboy, S., & Heston, L. (1980). Behavioral treatment of obesity in Prader-Willi syndrome. *Behavior Therapy, 11*, 588–593.

Van Itallie, T.B. (1979). Adverse effects on health and longevity. *American Journal of Clinical Nutrition, 32*, 2723–2733.

Wallen, A., & Roszkowski, M. (1980). Patterns of weight disorders in institutionalized mentally retarded adults. *Nutrition Reports International, 21*, 469–477.

Werkman, S.L., & Greenberg. E.S. (1967). Personality and interest patterns on obese adolescent girls. *Psychosomatic Medicine, 29*, 72–80.

Withers, R.F.L. (1964). Problems in the genetics of human obesity. *Eugenics Review, 56*, 81–90.

Wooley, O.W., & Wooley, S.C. (1975). The experimental psychology of obesity. In T. Silverstone & J. Fincham (Eds.), *Obesity: Pathogenesis and management* (pp. 93–121). Lancaster, England: Technical and Medical Publishing Co.

Wooley, O.W., Wooley, S.C., & Woods, W.A. (1975). Effect of calories on appetite for palatable foods in obese and nonobese humans. *Journal of Comparative and Physiological Psychology, 89*, 619–625.

Wooley, S.C., Wooley, O.W., & Dyrenforth, S.R. (1979). Theoretical, practical and social issues in behavioral treatments of obesity. *Journal of Applied Behavior Analysis, 12*, 3–25.

Yokoyama, Y. (1983). The incidence of obesity in mentally retarded children. *Japanese Journal of Special Education, 21*, 27–35.

6
Health-Threatening Behaviors

JAMES K. LUISELLI

Health-threatening behaviors are those responses and life-style patterns that deleteriously affect physical well-being and establish risk for subsequent medical illness. Problems of this type are common within contemporary society: cigarette smoking, alcohol consumption, poor exercise habits, and high-cholesterol diets. Intervention to reduce these and similar risk factors is a primary therapeutic goal within behavioral medicine. Such efforts are classified as secondary prevention (Luiselli, 1987; Masek, Epstein, & Russo, 1981).

Many developmentally disabled persons engage in health-threatening behaviors. Typically, these consist of responses that are functionally controlled by organismic and operant variables. Responding of this type usually occurs at extremely high frequencies and persists for prolonged periods unless systematic treatment is introduced. In some cases, the resulting conditions can actually be life terminating. Oftentimes, multiple behaviors occur concurrently.

This chapter addresses the assessment and treatment of health-threatening behaviors in developmentally disabled individuals. It begins with a discussion of the crucial role of applied behavior analysis in determining the variables that maintain problematic responding and how this information is used to select an appropriate method of intervention. The major portion of the chapter consists of a review of treatment methodology for several health-threatening behaviors frequently encountered among handicapped populations. For each dysfunction, incidence rates are reported, treatment techniques are defined, and critical procedural guidelines are highlighted. A concluding section briefly summarizes several issues of relevant concern.

Functional Assessment Within Applied Behavior Analysis

The topic of behavioral assessment has been considered at length in the professional literature (Barlow, Hayes, & Nelson, 1984; Hersen & Bellack, 1981) and emphasized throughout chapters in this book. Proper behavioral assessment requires the operational definition of target responses, the design of a recording protocol, repeated measurement within clinically relevant settings, and accurate determination of reliability and validity. Adherence to these guidelines is essential to identify empirically the incidence of behavior before, during, and following intervention. In this way, the effects of treatment can be discerned objectively.

Another goal of behavioral assessment is to identify the variables that control and maintain the responses targeted for intervention. This process entails observing the client within varied setting conditions while focusing on events that precede and follow his or her behavior. By functionally analyzing sources of control, treatment programs can be formulated accordingly. There are several influences that can affect maladaptive responding.

Organismic

This category includes neuromuscular, anatomical, and biochemical influences, namely a person's physiology. As an example, problems in self-feeding, chewing, and swallowing food among many individuals with cerebral palsy can be linked directly to deficits of the motor response system. Similarly, a child with cleft palate may experience feeding difficulties due to associated structural abnormalities. The severe behavioral pathology of self-injury is, at times, an outcome of organismic dysfunctions such as biochemical deficiencies in Lesch-Nyhan disease and increased pain thresholds in Riley-Day syndrome (Cataldo & Harris, 1982).

Anxiety-Provoking Antecedents

When environmental stimuli become paired with aversive experiences, those stimuli develop conditioned properties such that exposure to them can provoke anxious responding. Fears and phobias represent primary clinical disorders stemming from such conditioning. A phobia is manifested by increased physiological arousal when confronted with conditioned stimuli, followed by avoidance of these antecedents. Such "two-factor" learning (Wilson & O'Leary, 1980) is common in patients subjected to invasive, painful, or noxious medical procedures. The distress associated with such diagnostic and therapeutic approaches may result in problems such as avoidance of services (e.g., dental care), anticipatory discomfort (Redd & Andrykowski, 1982), and agitated behavior (Varni, 1983), to name a few.

Sensory Reinforcement

Some behavior disorders, most typically stereotypy, can be sustained by the sensory consequences they produce. Research by Rincover and associates (Rincover, 1978; Rincover, Cook, Peoples, & Packard, 1979), for example, has demonstrated that various forms of self-stimulation displayed by developmentally disabled children can be reduced dramatically by blocking or masking response-elicited sensory events. In one case, a child's object spinning that appeared to be reinforced by auditory stimulation was decreased by carpeting a table top such that accompanying sound was prevented. In another study, the visually reinforced finger and hand manipulation of two children was reduced to low levels when they wore blindfolds. Sensory reinforcing effects are also implicated in the occurrence of rumination and some forms of self-injury as discussed in subsequent sections of the chapter.

Attention-Eliciting Consequences

Many maladaptive behaviors are maintained by contingent adult and peer attention. Research has demonstrated that when disorders such as aggression, self-injury, and tantrums are followed by social responses (eye contact, verbalizations), these behaviors can increase dramatically (Carr & McDowell, 1980; Lovaas, Freitag, Gold, & Kassorla, 1965; Martin & Foxx, 1973). In such situations, the social consequences function as a form of positive reinforcement. Within medicine, the concept of "secondary gain" refers to the persistence of a patient's "sick-role" behavior due to the frequent attention usually delivered by significant others. Problems of hospital malingering and repeated requests for medical services (Munchausen syndrome) are often sustained by the solicitous caring and regard from professional staff. In cases such as chronic pain, various physical dimensions of the dysfunction are highly responsive to socioenvironmental influences (Varni, Bessman, Russo, & Cataldo, 1980).

Escape and Avoidance

The removal of an aversive stimulus or termination of an undesired event contingent upon a response is defined as negative reinforcement. The escape or avoidance function of negative reinforcement results in an increase in behavior. The occurrence of negatively reinforced behavior disorders was demonstrated by Carr, Newsom, and Binkoff (1980) in a study with retarded children. Under conditions where instructional demands were delivered to the children, high rates of aggression were displayed; in the absence of demands, aggressive behavior was virtually absent. Similarly, Weeks and Gaylord-Ross (1981) found that the management problems of developmentally disabled children occurred at higher rates when presented with difficult discrimination tasks in contrast to easy tasks. The findings from these studies suggest that for some handicapped individuals, demands and difficult response requirements serve as aversive stimuli that provoke escape and avoidance in the form of behavior problems.

Additional Considerations

Pertinent to the preceding discussion is the fact that the variable(s) that originally "caused" a behavior disorder may no longer be maintaining the expression of that problem. Thus, a child's rumination may have stemmed initially from gastrointestinal distress, but continues because it produces termination of meals that he or she finds unpleasant. It is also important to note that many behaviors are multiply determined. A child who displays self-injurious eye pressing during "free-play" situations may do so because such responding is sensory pleasurable;

during interaction with adults, the behavior may occur because it is reinforced by contingent attention (e.g., statements such as, "Stop that—you shouldn't hurt yourself!"). And finally, one typography of behavior, (e.g., pica) may be maintained by one set of controlling variables while a second behavior, (e.g., self-stimulation) is controlled by another.

To isolate functionally controlling variables, behavioral observations should be performed within environmental and interpersonal contexts that approximate different sources of control. To illustrate, Iwata, Dorsey, Slifer, Bauman, and Richman (1982) assessed the self-injurious responding of nine developmentally handicapped children under four stimulus conditions. Eight observational sessions (two per condition) were carried out each day using a multi-element design (Barlow & Hayes, 1979). In the *Social Disapproval* condition, each occurrence of self-injury resulted in a verbal statement (e.g., "Don't do that!") from a supervising adult. This condition was intended to approximate an attention-eliciting contingency. In the *Academic Demand* condition, different and non-mastered manipulatable tasks were presented to the children at a predetermined rate. When self-injury was displayed, the experimenter terminated task presentation for a brief period, a consequence designed to evaluate an escape/avoidance function. The third condition, *Unstructured Play*, allowed each child to engage in isolate or cooperative play with contingent attention for non-self-injury delivered intermittently. In the final condition *(Alone)*, the children were observed in a therapy room without access to toys or the presence of an attending adult. This context was intended to approximate an "impoverished" physical and interpersonal environment in order to evaluate the self-stimulatory motivation of self-injury.

The results of Iwata et al. (1982) revealed that for three of the children, self-injury was greater in the *Alone* condition, for two it occurred at higher levels in the *Academic Demand* condition, and with one child, it was more frequent within the condition of *Social Disapproval*. Thus, for six of the nine children studied, rates of self-injury were correlated with specific stimulus conditions, thereby suggesting that their responding was maintained differentially. Higher rates in the *Alone* condition indicate that the self-injurious behavior was most probably reinforced by sensory stimulation. Where frequencies were greater in the *Academic Demand* condition, it suggests that escape/avoidance was the controlling variable. Increased responding during the *Social Disapproval* phase implicates an attention-eliciting function.

The procedures described by Iwata et al. (1982) represent an operant assessment methodology that can be instituted within an analogue situation or adapted to an actual clinical context. The information acquired from such assessment should be used to plan and design treatment strategies. Behaviors that appear to be maintained by social reinforcement contingencies would require the contingent withholding of attention combined with the reinforcement of incompatible responses. The brief interruption in reinforcement via time-out could also be included as a method of intervention. For behaviors that are escape/avoidance motivated, several treatment options are available. One approach is to increase the density of reinforcement within the environment in an effort to reduce the motivation to escape or avoid. Other strategies include "working through" incidents of behavior to prevent negative reinforcement from operating ("escape extinction") (Carr et al., 1980) or training functionally equivalent but behaviorally appropriate escape responses (Carr & Durand, 1985). In cases of sensory reinforced behaviors, the application of sensory extinction procedures (Rincover et al., 1979) or programming the preferred sensory stimuli to reinforce alternative responses are possible treatment methods. When the behavior disorder appears to be provoked by fear or increased anxiety, desensitization approaches based on graduated exposure, participant modeling, or similar counter-conditioning techniques should be implemented (Kratochwill & Morris, 1983).

Finally, the initial phase of treating health-threatening behaviors should include a comprehensive medical screening. Such evaluation is essential in order to identify possible organic pathology as an underlying cause of the presenting disorder. Problems that are clearly linked to a physical etiology would then be treated accordingly in an interdisciplinary fashion. As an example, encopretic children with anal muscle dysfunction might be trained to increase rectosphincteric pressure via biofeedback combined with a contingency reward program for appropriate bowel elimination (Whitehead, Parker, Masek, Cataldo & Freeman, 1981).

Treatment Techniques

This section is a review of treatment techniques for several types of health-threatening behavior. The review samples a wide range of behavioral intervention strategies but is not intended to be an exhaustive coverage of the vast extant literature. The techniques selected for review are those that have undergone substantive research evaluation and have been shown to be clinically efficacious. Also, an effort has been made to concentrate on relatively recent developments in treatment technology, namely research within the past 8 years (1980 to 1988).

Self-Injury

Self-injurious behavior (SIB) represents any repetitive, self-inflicted motor response that produces physical harm. Such behavior can occur in many forms: eye gouging, face/body punching, head banging, hand biting, rectal digging, and skin picking. There are numerous ill effects caused by SIB. Lacerations, contusions, bruises, and internal bleeding may result from blows inflicted on the body. Biting, scratching, and picking the skin produce dermal abrasion, open wounds, and the potential for infection. In some cases of SIB, sensory organs can be impaired as with children who blind themselves stemming from abuse to the eyes.

Data on the prevalence of SIB among developmentally disabled populations have been gathered almost exclusively from incidence surveys of institutionalized mentally retarded persons. Singh (1981a) summarized this information and reported rates ranging from 5.3% to 37.1%. In a more recent report, Griffin, Williams, Stark, Altmeyer, and Mason (1986) documented SIB in 13.6% of 10,000 mentally retarded residents within 13 state institutions. All surveys show consistently that SIB is most prevalent in persons classified as severely to profoundly retarded. Frequently, these individuals exhibit multiple topographies of self-injury as well as other types of maladaptive behavior (e.g., aggression, noncompliance, property destruction).

POSITIVE REINFORCEMENT

The implementation of positive reinforcement procedures to shape alternative behaviors and/or reward the absence of problem responding should be a component of any formalized management program. One method to deliver reinforcement is via a time-based schedule in which a reinforcing stimulus is presented following nonoccurrence of the target behavior during a predefined interval (DRO: Differential Reinforcement of Other Behavior). Another strategy is to reinforce behaviors that are topographically incompatible with the problem response (DRI: Differential Reinforcement of Incompatible Behavior).

Several studies have documented the successful treatment of self-injury through the application of DRO and DRI programs. In an early study, Peterson and Peterson (1968) reduced head slapping and head banging in an 8-year-old mentally retarded child by rewarding periods without self-injury (using edibles and praise) and briefly withdrawing these reinforcers when SIB occurred. A time-out contingency was subsequently added to the program and this produced a further decrease in responding. Luiselli and colleagues conducted two studies in which control over SIB was established using DRO procedures without the addition of other response-deceleration techniques. One project (Luiselli, Helfen, Colozzi, Donellon, & Pemberton, 1978) treated the hand biting of a 10-year-old moderately retarded boy within three classroom instructional settings. The DRO contingency consisted of providing edible reinforcers to the child when SIB did not occur during timed intervals beginning at 1 minute and increasing gradually to 15 to 21 minutes. The program, as evaluated in a multiple-baseline design, produced virtual elimination of the hand-biting response. In the second study (Luiselli, Myles, Evans, & Boyce, 1985, Study 2), self-injurious eye pressing of a 10-year-old blind, hearing-impaired girl was targeted for intervention. Following an initial baseline phase, a DRO program was introduced in the context of a multielement design. This entailed applying DRO during select periods of the day while maintaining baseline conditions during other periods so as to functionally analyze the effects of treatment. The DRO program specified the presentation of a highly preferred reinforcing stimulus (stuffed animal toy) for a 1-minute period contingent upon gradually increasing intervals without SIB. The result was a reduction in eye pressing to near-zero levels with the DRO program in effect;

without DRO, self-injurious responding persisted at high rates. Reduced levels of SIB were maintained when the program was extended throughout the day and at 1- and 3-month follow-up assessments.

One of the limitations associated with a DRO schedule is that the contingency does not specify an actual response to be reinforced, but rather, the *absence* of the maladaptive behavior. It may be that with seriously behaviorally deficient individuals it would by therapeutically advantageous to reinforce directly alternative responses through a DRI schedule as opposed to periods of nonresponding. Tarpley and Schroeder (1979) compared the reductive effects from DRO and DRI contingencies with three profoundly retarded, institutionalized residents displaying self-injurious head banging. Both contingencies reduced SIB from baseline (no treatment) conditions, but DRI was consistently superior to DRO in the rapidity and magnitude of behavior change. These findings suggest that, whenever possible, the reinforcement of physically incompatible behaviors should be the method of choice when programming reinforcers with self-injurious clients.

Favell, McGimsey, and Schell (1982) described an interesting approach to the reinforcement control of SIB that appeared to be maintained by pleasurable sensory stimulation. Working with six profoundly retarded, multiply handicapped persons, they attempted to reduce three topographies of self-injury by providing each client with alternative play activities that elicited sensory feedback similar to that produced by the SIB. For example, the eye-poking behavior of two clients decreased substantially when they were allowed to play with toys having highly visual properties (colored beads, mirrors, a prism). In several cases, further reductions in SIB were achieved when toy-play was reinforced directly. As a strategy to treat sensory reinforced SIB, the procedures designed by these investigators represent an economical, easily manipulated, and nonaversive method of behavioral control. A topic for future research on this is whether the sensory effects from toy-play must be *matched* to those produced by SIB or whether any alternative form of stimulation will suffice.

Although the preceding discussion highlights some clinical successes from reinforcement-oriented treatment programs, the effective management of SIB through reinforcement, in and of itself, is typically the exception rather than the rule. In fact, many of the intervention techniques described in later sections were designed and evaluated because of the numerous situations in which reinforcement did not work. How to utilize reinforcement efficaciously remains a crucial programmatic concern since, as stated previously, any attempt to reduce SIB (or other health-threatening behaviors) should seek to increase adaptive responses through positive means. The majority of behavioral treatments for SIB, however, generally are comprised of reinforcement procedures *combined with* response-contingent interventions.

SENSORY EXTINCTION

The concept of sensory extinction is described briefly in an earlier section. To reiterate, this strategy posits that some maladaptive behaviors may be reinforced by their own response-elicited stimulation and that by blocking or otherwise attenuating such sensory events, reductions in undesired responding can be achieved. Sensory extinction was evaluated originally as a treatment for stereotypic behaviors (Rincover, 1978; Rincover et al., 1979) and in recent years has been extended to the management of SIB.

In order to mask response-produced stimulatory effects when applying sensory extinction, the self-injurer is required to wear some form of protective equipment noncontingently throughout the day or during selected setting conditions. The usual approach to treat head banging, for example, is to have the client wear headgear, usually a football helmet or similar device. Two studies have demonstrated that this form of sensory extinction produced meaningful reductions in head hitting (striking head with fists, banging head against fixed surfaces) displayed by mentally retarded adolescents (Dorsey, Iwata, Reid, & Davis, 1982; Parrish, Aguerrevere, Dorsey, & Iwata, 1980). Rincover and Devany (1982) eliminated face scratching in a 4-year-old developmentally disabled girl by having her wear thin rubber (dishwashing) gloves to prevent skin damage from fingernails. And Luiselli (1988) compared two methods of sensory extinction to control arm biting of a 6-year-old boy with multiple congenital handicaps. The child's SIB was restricted to the area around his wrists. Therefore, one approach entailed the wearing of tennis wrist bands to block teeth-to-skin contact. When this method proved to be ineffective, the child was fitted with removable, Orthoplas,® wrist/ forearm cuffs. Arm biting was reduced substantially with this program.

As a strategy to treat sensory-reinforced SIB, sensory extinction represents a promising method of intervention. It is important to note that although protective equipment is required, the application of such devices is not intended to physically restrict movement in the manner characteristic of mechanical restraint. Rather, the approach is predicated on the manipulation of sensory consequences that reinforce SIB. Therefore, when wearing a protective device, the client is free to perform the self-injurious response (and other behaviors), but without experiencing the reinforcing effect. It is also important to distinguish the *assessment* and *treatment* functions associated with sensory extinction. That is, the purported visually reinforced eye poking of a child could be assessed by having him or her wear a blindfold and showing that self-injury is eliminated or greatly reduced when it is in place but occurs frequently when it is removed. However, as a treatment for this typography of SIB, the wearing of a blindfold would be contraindicated for obvious reasons. Thus, in some cases, the methods and devices to identify sensory reinforcement and to ultimately establish clinical control will be different.

Finally, since sensory extinction requires the conspicuous appearance of equipment and materials, it would be desirable to fade-out such stimuli gradually while maintaining therapeutic effects. One approach in this regard is to have the client spend increasingly longer periods out of the equipment, again provided that response rates do not increase (Rincover & Devany, 1982). Another procedure is to change slowly the physical features of the equipment, for example, progressively cutting back a stocking cap for the treatment of self-injurious hair pulling. The analysis of such stimulus fading techniques awaits experimental evaluation.

MECHANICAL RESTRAINT, ADAPTIVE CLOTHING, AND RESTRAINT FADING

Like sensory extinction, programs incorporating mechanical restraint require the self-injurer to wear protective, and sometimes specially adapted, equipment. Mechanical restraint differs from sensory extinction in that the equipment is intended to prevent or impede responding as opposed to rearranging reinforcement contingencies. Although clinical experiences would indicate that mechanical restraint is utilized with some regularity (particularly with extremely intractable cases of SIB), this method has not received extensive research evaluation. Where data are available, they show that when successful behavioral control is achieved, it may be compromised by decreases in social interaction between clients and caregivers (Rojahn, Schroeder, & Mulick, 1980). Other disadvantages associated with mechanical restraint include restricted range of motion and the possibility of muscle atrophy or bone decalcification. Also, since restraint methods simply prevent SIB, responding is likely to reoccur upon removal of the protective equipment.

Mechanical restraint can be applied as a functional treatment for SIB by providing immediate suppression of high-rate responses, allowing the clinician to reinforce alternative behaviors, and then gradually eliminating the physical equipment through "restraint fading." Pace, Iwata, Edwards, and McCosh (1986) evaluated such a methodology with a mentally retarded adolescent exhibiting self-injurious hand, arm, and shoulder biting. Restraint was applied with Orthoplas® tubes that extended from shoulders to hands of each arm. The tubes, initially measuring 47 cm in length, were reduced in successive steps to a size of 5 cm and eventually were replaced with tennis wrist bands. The restraint fading procedure, coupled with reinforcement for alternative behaviors, reduced SIB to manageable levels.

Ball, Campbell, and Barkemeyer (1980) reported an innovative application of mechanical restraint and restraint fading in a treatment program for self-injurious finger sucking of a 22-year-old mentally retarded woman. Restraint was established by placing the client in inflatable air splints around the arms. The splints permitted appropriate range of motion but prevented her from placing fingers into mouth. They were set initially at maximum inflation on flexion, an effect that produced elimination of the target behavior. Over time, the pressure was reduced gradually and low levels of SIB were maintained. Subsequently, a DRO procedure was introduced to reinforce the reduced finger sucking that had been achieved following faded restraint.

Control over SIB in clients who engage in "self-restraint" has been produced through adaptive clothing (Rojahn, Mulick, McCoy, & Schroeder, 1978). Self-restraint refers to the purposeful restriction of self-abusive responses (e.g., inserting fingers into belt loops, sitting on hands). Favell, McGimsey, and Jones (1978) showed that restraint functioned as positive reinforcement among several self-injurious, mentally retarded clients. In a study with a 13-year-old profoundly retarded boy, Silverman, Wantanabe, Marshall, and Baer (1984) found that the reduction in self-injury achieved through noncontingent protective equipment was correlated with decreases in self-restraint. These findings suggest that one approach to modify SIB in persons who self-restrain might be to provide adaptive clothing that permits appropriate immobilization. In the study by Rojahn et al. (1978), the wearing of a jacket with large pockets allowed for acceptable self-restraint and greatly reduced head and shoulder hitting of a 30-year-old profoundly retarded adult. The authors pointed out that since restraint with the jacket (placing hands in pockets) occurred at an increased rate, the implementation of procedures to release hands and arms should be the next therapeutic goal.

To summarize, mechanical restraint and adaptive clothing have a place in the treatment of SIB as methods of response prevention to be combined with stimulus control fading techniques. The ultimate goal of such programming should be to free the client from restraint and to develop compensatory skills. The use of restraint for prolonged periods or without a predefined fading sequence should be avoided.

GROSS MOTOR ACTIVITY

The integration of gross motor activities such as physical exercise and aerobic conditioning is a recent development in treatment programming for severe behavior disorders. Such intervention has been designed, in part, in an effort to establish more simplified and easily managed therapy programs. Although only two such programs for SIB have been reported in the literature, both reveal positive findings and, therefore, warrant a brief description.

Baumeister and MacLean (1984) examined the effects of a daily, 1-hour jogging program on SIB (face slapping, head hitting) of 23-year-old and 19-year-old mentally retarded males. The clients were observed from 9:00 to 10:00 a.m. and 3:00 to 4:00 p.m. each day. The jogging activity was scheduled from 1:00 to 2:00 p.m. daily, beginning with 1 mile each period for 2 weeks, then 2 miles per period for 2 weeks, and finally 3 miles for 2 weeks. Evaluation was performed using a reversal design and demonstrated that, for both individuals, SIB decreased dramatically in the afternoon observation immediately following the jogging period. Responding during the morning observation was less affected but also decreased relative to baseline phases.

Positive effects from regularly scheduled gross motor activities on the self-injurious tantrums of three, multihandicapped youngsters were reported by Lancioni, Smeets, Ceccarani, Capodaglio, and Campanari (1984). During baseline phases of an ABAB reversal design, the participants performed routine activities that required minimal exertion. Treatment consisted of noncontingently scheduled gross motor activities that demanded increased physical effort but were not intended to produce excessive fatigue. Examples included transporting materials, performing household tasks, and walking obstacle courses. For each participant, reduced frequencies of SIB were associated with treatment; in two cases, a decrease in tantrum duration was also recorded.

It is difficult to determine precisely the variables responsible for therapeutic change observed in the preceding studies. Possibly, the gross motor activities induced sufficient fatigue to minimize the participants' level of arousal. It is also possible that the motor responses provided sensory consequences similar to those produced by the aberrant behaviors. Indeed, the activities designed by Lancioni et al. (1984) were intended to provoke a wide variety of pleasurable sensory events without tiring the participants. Or, as stated by Baumeister and MacLean (1984), regular physical exertion may have produced neurochemical changes that affected outward behavior. Interactions among these and other influences, of course, cannot be ruled out. It is apparent that much more research is required on the role of physical exercise in the control of SIB, although, to date, the results appear promising. Obvious restrictions governing this approach include physically resistant clients, those who are motorically impaired, and persons with medical contraindications.

CONTINGENT EFFORT

Intervention based on contingent effort includes several procedures that require a client to perform an extended series of motor responses following occurrences of maladaptive behavior. These procedures are usually applied by having the practitioner guide the client through the response requirements, using the minimal degree of physical assistance necessary to sustain continuous movement. Each treatment application is instituted for a predefined time period (e.g., 3 to 5 minutes). Ultimately, the goal is to have the client engage in the effort procedures without assisted guidance.

Overcorrection is one form of contingent effort that has been evaluated extensively as a treatment for SIB and other severe behavior disorders (Marholin, Luiselli, & Townsend, 1980). As designed by Foxx and Azrin (1973), the rationale for the procedure is to have the client correct the environmental effects of his or her behavior (termed *restitution*) and then to practice alternative ways of responding (termed *positive practice*). The earliest reports of overcorrection by this research team suggested that both the restitutional and positive practice components should be implemented in combination to achieve the maximum therapeutic outcome. However, subsequent studies have revealed consistently that either component applied by itself can be equally effective (Foxx & Bechtel, 1982).

One method of overcorrection consists of instructing a client to move a body part (usually the one involved in the maladaptive behavior) in a repetitive sequence. This form of "practice" at other motor responses and instruction following is intended to represent alternative, topographically appropriate behaviors. An early example of this technique is that of Azrin, Gottlieb, Hughart, Wesolowski, and Rahn (1975). They worked with 11 developmentally handicapped persons with chronic histories of SIB such as face slapping, head banging, and finger biting. Treatment included positive reinforcement, required relaxation, and pertinent to this discussion, a "hand control" positive practice overcorrection procedure. Each episode of overcorrection required a client to extend his arms up, down, and to the side, every 10 seconds, following instructions from an individual trainer. The duration of each overcorrection episode lasted 20 minutes. As evaluated in an AB design, treatment was associated with a 99% decrease in SIB at the end of 3 months. Other studies have shown that similar overcorrection formats can reduce various topographies of self-injury without the addition of other treatment components (Halpern & Andrasik, 1986; Luiselli, Suskin, & McPhee, 1981; Zehr & Theobald, 1978).

Another method of overcorrection is to have the client correct the physically damaging effects of his or her SIB. Thus, mentally retarded children who display hand banging have been required to apply first aid or ice packs to the afflicted areas (Barnard, Christophersen, & Wolf, 1976). Luiselli & Michaud (1983) treated the arm biting of a 19-year-old blind, severely retarded male with a multi-component management program based upon the principle of "hygiene training" (Foxx & Azrin, 1973). It consisted of instructing and guiding the client to cleanse his arm with an antiseptic solution whenever he bit himself. Matson, Stephens, and Smith (1978) had a 57-year-old profoundly retarded woman practice brushing her hair contingent on self-injurious hair pulling.

A second type of contingent effort is forced body movement. Essentially, this represents a variant of overcorrection in which graduated guidance is applied but *without* accompanying instructions. In a study with a 3-year-old blind child, Kelly and Drabman (1977) reduced eye poking by prompting him to raise and lower his arm 12 times contingent on the target SIB. Interestingly, intervention in this case generalized to a different setting where treatment contingencies were not in effect. Harris and Romanczyk (1976) evaluated a similar methodology with an 8-year-old mentally, retarded, sensory impaired boy who banged his head and chin. Each occurrence of SIB produced 10 minutes of guidance in the form of hand and arm movements (hands up/down and left/right; arms to side, in front, and overhead). The procedure was implemented within the child's home and school and it produced rapid suppression of both topographies of self-injury. Finally, Luiselli (1986b, Study 2) reported the effective use of contingent arm raising in combination with differential reinforcement to eliminate multiple topographies of SIB (hand biting, body striking, head banging, hair pulling) in a 10-year-old mentally retarded boy.

Contingent exercise is a third category of effort procedures. Unlike the previous description of physical exercise and gross motor activity as an *antecedent control* strategy, contingent exercise is applied as a decelerating consequence within an operant treatment format. Following a designated problem behavior, a client is prompted to perform one or a series of exercise movements such as sit-ups or knee-bends. To date, only one published study has described this technique in the treatment of SIB (Borreson, 1980). In it, the self-biting of a profoundly retarded boy was eliminated with a contingent forced running consequence.

Contingent effort is one of the most extensively researched behavioral treatment methodologies. The variations of this procedure have been extremely effective with numerous forms of SIB encountered with diverse clinical populations. Various parameters of contingent effort have also been investigated and have led to several practical refinements. Whereas early research suggested that extended durations of treatment should be implemented (e.g., 20 minutes per overcorrection episode), it is now apparent that extremely brief periods of application (e.g., 30 seconds to 2 minutes) can be efficacious (Carey & Bucher, 1983; Luiselli, 1984). Other research findings have shown that the motor requirements comprising a contingent effort program do not have to be matched topographically to the target problem. Therefore, it is possible to reduce head banging against objects with an effort procedure that involves the hands. This means that multiple forms of SIB can be treated with a single intervention technique, a factor that should reduce the time required to design and implement management programs. Related to the issue of practicality is the finding that, in some cases, reductive effects from effort procedures are possible with intermittent versus continuous application (Luiselli et al., 1981). The utilization of effort techniques would be contraindicated for clients who are seriously motorically impaired or extremely physically resistant.

RESPONSE INTERRUPTION AND IMMOBILIZATION

This procedure is another physical intervention technique that has been applied successfully with varied behavior disorders (aggression, tantrums, stereotypy). It is comprised of two components. First, contingent upon the maladaptive behavior, the client's responding is stopped by the practitioner (interruption). Next, the body part involved in the response is restrained briefly in a stationary position (immobilization). A child who strikes out with his hands, for example, would have his hands placed by the sides of his body and maintained there for a predefined duration. For an individual displaying stereotypic body rocking, his or her movement would be stopped and shoulders held against the back of the chair. When immobilization is applied, the implementor uses the minimal degree of physical force required to sustain a stationary position.

   The application of contingent immobilization combined with differential reinforcement has been evaluated in several studies with self-injurious, developmentally disabled children (Luiselli, 1986b, Study 1; Luiselli, Evans, & Boyce, 1986; Slifer, Iwata, & Dorsey, 1984). The general methodology in these cases was to reinforce intervals of no SIB with stimuli such as social attention (Luiselli et al., 1986), consumables (Luiselli, 1986b, Study 1), or increased stimulation (Slifer et al., 1984). When self-injury was emitted, the children's hands were restrained manually against their body, lap, or sides of chair for durations ranging from 10 seconds to 2 minutes. SIB in these cases was virtually eliminated with application of the treatment programs. Contingent interruption-immobilization has also been highly effective when implemented by itself without explicit attempts to reinforce other behaviors (Rapoff, Altman, & Christophersen, 1980; Singh, Dawson, & Manning, 1981). However, as with other response-contingent deceleration techniques, it is advisable to always include a reinforcement component in combination with immobilization.

   The study by Singh et al. (1981) is noteworthy in that it evaluated two methods of physical immobilization and two durations of treatment administration. This study was actually comprised of two separate experiments. The participant in each was a 16-year-old, deaf-blind, profoundly retarded girl whose SIB involved face slapping and punching. In Experiment I, a reversal design was used to compare an immobilization procedure applied for either 1 minute or 3 minutes following each instance of SIB. To implement immobilization, the girl was placed in a soft jacket that physically restrained arm movements. The second experiment used an alternating treatments design, again comparing 1-minute versus 3-minute durations. This time immobilization consisted of holding the girl's hands by her sides. Both experiments found immobilization to be an effective treatment relative to baseline phases and, in each case, the 1-minute application was more efficacious than the 3-minute duration. Parametric analyses of this type serve a useful purpose by identifying adaptations of treatment strategies that can lead to enhanced practicality and cost efficiency.

Like contingent effort procedures, the method of response interruption and immobilization has been subjected to sufficient empirical validation to recommend it as a functional treatment for SIB. On the negative side, it is subject to the same physical contraindications associated with effort techniques. Furthermore, immobilization would not be clinically desirable for self-injurious clients who are reinforced by restraint. The advantage of interruption-immobilization is that it is not as procedurally complex as other physical intervention approaches (e.g., overcorrection) so that it is easily taught to practitioners and relatively simple to implement.

VISUAL OCCLUSION

In 1974, Lutzker and Spencer described a then novel procedure for the management of SIB. It consisted of a client wearing a large terrycloth bib fastened around the neck with a soft cloth tie. When SIB occurred, the bib was "flipped up" over the client's face and held there for a brief duration. The bib obstructed vision but was maintained loosely so as to not to impede breathing. This procedure was eventually termed facial screening and it has since been evaluated in a number of self-injurious treatment studies. Two methods related to facial screening include: 1) placing a blindfold over the eyes, and 2) placing one hand over the eyes while supporting the head with the other hand (vision screening). Facial screening, blindfold, and vision screening are classified as visual occlusion techniques (Lutzker & Wesch, 1983).

The study by Lutzker and Spencer (1974) was carried out with two severely retarded males, a 20-year-old and a 9-year-old, each displaying hand-to-head striking. In a multiple-baseline design across subjects, they were treated with facial screening lasting either 3 or 15 seconds. Each application of facial screening was preceded by a firm, "No!" One of the participants was also exposed to several additional phases comprised of baseline conditions, stating, "No" without using the screening technique, and wearing the bib but not applying it contingently. Results indicated that facial screening reduced SIB in both individuals. Neither stating the reprimand by itself nor wearing the bib without application was effective.

The analyses performed by Lutzker and Spencer (1974) occurred within a controlled laboratory setting. As always, one of the crucial questions regarding the design of behavior-change interventions is whether they can be transferred properly to naturalistic settings. Lutzker (1978) demonstrated that for one of the participants studied previously, facial screening suppressed SIB across three classroom settings. Significantly, a different teacher implemented the procedure within each location. Barmann and Vitali (1982) trained parents and home-care providers to institute facial screening as a treatment for chronic hair pulling (trichotillomania) in three developmentally disabled youngsters. Self-injury was reduced after approximately 11 days of intervention with each child and maintained at zero levels up to a 7-month follow-up assessment. Singh (1980) also showed that parents could be instructed in the use of facial screening, in this case to eliminate severe thumb biting of an 11-month severely retarded boy. Complete suppression of thumb biting was achieved within 3 weeks and remained absent 1 year later. Thus, it appears that facial screening can be imparted to natural behavior-change agents and that its proper use by these individuals can support long-term therapeutic effects.

An important feature of recent facial screening research with SIB has been the investigation of several treatment parameters and procedural variations. In a single-case analysis with a 14-year-old severely retarded boy, Demetral and Lutzker (1980) found that the procedure was significantly more effective when employed in a contingent versus noncontingent fashion. Other studies have compared the use of opaque and translucent screening materials (Demetral & Lutzker, 1980; Winton, Singh, & Dawson, 1984). In each of three separate cases, this research found that control over SIB was established only with an opaque bib. Therefore, visual blocking appears to be the crucial component of the facial screening procedure. Another study examined the effects from 3-second, 1-minute, and 3-minute durations of facial screening on face striking of an 18-year-old severely retarded girl (Singh, Beale, & Dawson, 1981). The 1-minute duration produced the largest and most immediate response reduction. Finally, two studies have compared different methods of visual occlusion. Winton et al. (1984) treated face hitting of a 12-year-old profoundly retarded boy in the context of an alternating treatments design that compared a standard facial screening procedure with contingent application of a blindfold. Both techniques were equally successful. The second study (Watson, Singh, & Winton, 1986) also utilized an alternating treatments design to compare facial screening with vision screening on self-injurious finger sucking of two profoundly retarded adolescents. Both procedures reduced SIB from baseline levels and for one participant, vision screening produced more complete suppression.

Many practitioners who are informed of visual occlusion procedures or witness them being implemented express concerns regarding the conspicuousness and unusual appearance of this method of intervention. Indeed, programs of this type may seem highly intrusive to some. The choice of such treatment, as any other, should follow a careful behavior analysis of the presenting disorder. For example, if a time-out procedure was ineffective as a treatment strategy because it appeared that the client enjoyed visual stimulation during the time-out interval, the addition of a vision occlusion method might be considered. Conversely, for individuals who are blind or severely visually impaired, it is unlikely that such a strategy would be effective. Similar to other punishment approaches, visual occlusion procedures should work quickly (within four to five treatment sessions) or else be abandoned (Lutzker & Wesch, 1983). It might also be noted that the majority of research on visual occlusion with SIB and other behavior disorders has been performed by a small group of clinical investigators. Systematic replications and extensions by other research teams would strengthen the generality of these findings.

CONTINGENT PROTECTIVE EQUIPMENT

Previous sections describe the application of protective equipment in programs of sensory extinction and mechanical restraint. A third option is to place the self-injurer in protective equipment *contingent upon* targeted behaviors. The equipment remains in place for a brief, predetermined duration and is then removed. While wearing the equipment, the client has free range of motion and can continue to perform the self-injurious responses since his or her movement is not restricted. However, the protection afforded by the equipment prevents physical harm from occurring.

The clinical application of contingent protective equipment for SIB was reported initially by Dorsey et al. (1982). Three institutionalized, severely to profoundly retarded adolescents were observed during two 10-minute sessions each day. The types of SIB recorded included head hitting, hand biting, and eye gouging. During baseline and DRO phases, self-injury remained high for each participant. Next, they were exposed to a condition during which they wore foam-padded gloves and a football helmet throughout treatment sessions. Lastly, the procedure of continuous protective equipment was compared with a program of contingent application. It entailed placing the protective devices on the participants for a 2-minute period following self-injurious responses. Both the continuous and contingent wearing procedures greatly reduced SIB. Subsequently, the contingently applied program was extended to the participant's living units where clinical control over SIB was also achieved.

Three additional reports, each single-case studies, have documented further the successful management of SIB in applied settings through contingent wearing of protective equipment. Clients and settings included a 9-year-old moderately retarded, autistic girl in a community-based group home (Neufeld & Fantuzzo, 1984), a 17-year-old severely retarded male in an institution (Parrish, Iwata, Dorsey, Bunck, & Slifer, 1985), and a 16½-year-old deaf-blind boy in a residential school (Luiselli, 1986a). These studies featured brief applications of protective equipment (30 seconds to 2 minutes) combined with reinforcement for alternative behaviors and, in each case, all forms of SIB were eliminated or reduced to manageable levels. It appears, then, that this relatively novel procedure is receiving strong empirical validation. Furthermore, in at least one study

(Luiselli, 1986a), a social validity questionnaire revealed that the procedure was rated highly in terms of practitioner acceptability and satisfaction.

The therapeutic control exerted by contingently applied protective equipment may occur because the procedure functions as a method of time-out from positive reinforcement (both social and sensory), response interruption, negative reinforcement of nonagitation, aversive stimulation, or perhaps, some combination of these variables. Like physical immobilization techniques, the procedure provides a means of contingently withdrawing sources of reinforcement while preventing further instances of SIB. Unlike restraint methods, it does not require physical holding and, therefore, avoids problems of active resistance, struggling, and the like. Essential for the implementation of this approach is the careful design and adaptation of equipment, namely that it fits properly, ensures protection, and cannot be removed by the client following application.

AVERSIVE STIMULATION

Treatment by aversive stimulation has been and remains an area of considerable controversy. Aversive conditioning procedures entail the presentation of a noxious stimulus contingent upon targeted problem behaviors. The most intense form of aversive stimulation is punishment by electric shock (Carr & Lovaas, 1983). The shock stimulus is typically applied to a fleshy area of the body (arm, thigh) for a brief duration (1 to 2 seconds), delivered via either a hand-held inductorium or remote-controlled body unit worn by the client. The result is a localized sensation that terminates when the stimulation is discontinued. Subjectively, this sensation resembles the pain experienced when being struck by a strap or having drilling performed on an unanesthetized tooth.

Shock programs for SIB have been reported frequently in the behavioral literature (Corte, Wolf, & Locke, 1971; Lovaas, Schaeffer, & Simmons, 1965; Lovaas & Simmons, 1969; Romanczyk & Goren, 1975; Young & Wincze, 1974). These studies described effective control over severe, chronic, and, at times, life-threatening forms of self-injury. The suggestion by some was that contingent electric shock should be considered as a viable treatment option for particularly intractable typographies of SIB or when other interventions have failed. However, certain limitations must be noted. First, a common finding from this research was that the therapeutic effects from shock were extremely situation specific. Control over SIB was established in the treatment environment and in the presence of program staff but did not generalize beyond these conditions. Although a lack of generalization is typically associated with a variety of treatment strategies (Marholin & Luiselli, 1978; Marholin, Siegal, & Phillips, 1976), it is a crucial consideration given the intensity of shock as a punishing stimulus. That is, to facilitate generalization, intervention must be extended to multiple settings and personnel, thereby exposing the client to more frequent aversive stimulation. It should also be pointed out that very few behavioral clinicians are trained sufficiently or have the necessary "hands-on" experience to design and implement a program incorporating contingent electric shock. Therefore, the cost to hire such expert consultants may be prohibitive. Perhaps the greatest impediment to the development of shock programs is the emergence of state regulatory guidelines for the use of aversive and deprivation procedures (Accreditation Council for Services for Mentally Retarded and Other Developmentally Disabled Persons, 1981; Foxx, Plaska, & Bittle, 1986). Given the philosophy of *least restrictive treatment*, stringent restrictions have been placed on the utilization of electric shock. In some settings, the procedure is simply not allowed. This may account for the fact that since approximately 1975, clinical research and publications on shock have all but disappeared.

The limitations associated with electric shock have been addressed by identifying stimuli that are more easily applied, "less intrusive," and likely to find greater acceptance by practitioners and the lay public. One alternative, aromatic ammonia, consists of holding a crushed vial of this substance under the client's nose contingent on SIB. The vial is either held in place for several seconds or until self-injurious responding terminates. At least four studies have reported the successful treatment of SIB in mentally retarded children, adolescents, and adults using this approach (Altman, Haavik, & Cook, 1978; Baumeister & Baumeister, 1978; Singh, Dawson, & Gregory, 1980a; Tanner & Zeiler, 1975). A second recently investigated noxious stimulus is lemon juice. Mayhew and Harris (1979) reduced multiple self-injurious responses in a 19-year-old mentally retarded male by squirting a small amount of diluted, food-grade citric acid into his mouth on a contingent basis. Similarly, Gross, Wright, and Drabman (1980) decreased finger gnawing of a 5-year-old handicapped boy by touching his lips with lemon juice delivered from a plastic bottle with a sponge applicator. On a positive note, this body of research documents empirically alternatives to electric shock. Once again, though, several precautions are worth noting. Aromatic ammonia, for instance, can cause damage to the nasal mucosa or skin irritation from prolonged contact. Other persons in the immediate environment may also be affected since the odor does not dissipate totally following application. Problems with lemon juice include the possibility of mouth irritations, aspiration into the lungs, and erosion of tooth enamel. Clearly, rigorous physical monitoring should be a mandatory feature of any program based on aversive conditioning with these stimuli.

Another aversive stimulus recently evaluated as a treatment for SIB is water mist spray. In a multiple-baseline-across-persons design, Dorsey, Iwata, Ong, and McSween (1980) treated seven profoundly retarded residents who performed hand biting, skin tearing, and head banging responses. During intervention, each occurrence of self-injury resulted in a fine mist of water being sprayed at the client's face. Tap water maintained at room temperature was dispensed from a plastic plant sprayer held no closer than 0.3 m from the face. For each client, the spray mist punishment produced rapid and complete suppression of SIB. A second experiment by the same investigators compared the procedure with two less intrusive interventions: differential reinforcement of no SIB (DRO) and a contingent reprimand (shouting, "No!"). Neither procedure was successful in reducing SIB of two mentally retarded clients. A combined treatment package of water spray, reprimand, and DRO quickly suppressed responding. Further support for the clinical efficacy of water spray as an aversive stimulus in SIB treatment is provided by Murphey, Ruprecht, Baggio, and Nunes (1979) and Jenson, Rovner, Cameron, Petersen, and Kesler (1985).

Given the preceding discussion, what conclusions can be drawn regarding the aversive treatment of SIB? The various precautions notwithstanding, it is evident that such intervention does work. For many clients with chronic and severe SIB, aversive procedures were the only methods that established long-lasting clinical control. Perhaps a better question is not does aversive conditioning have a place in the management of SIB but rather, under what conditions should it, or should it not, be utilized? In effect, a compromise is presented: is it more beneficial to expose the client to a brief and controlled period of discomfort as compared to the years of self-imposed physical harm that will persist in the absence of treatment? If the answer in a particular case is affirmative, then several guidelines should be followed. First, aversive treatment should always be considered the method of last resort and should only be instituted following the demonstrated ineffectiveness of less invasive procedures. Such intervention must be applied simultaneously with efforts to shape and reinforce alternative behaviors. The conditions of treatment should be tightly controlled, publicly verifiable, and supervised by an experienced clinician. It is also essential that the treatment program is designed in accordance with prevailing regulatory protocol and is only implemented subsequent to informed, written consent from parents, guardians, and relevant third parties. And last, it must be emphasized that aversive conditioning techniques are intended to produce rapid response deceleration. If a client's behavior has not decreased substantially following several treatment sessions, the program should be abandoned. Subjecting an individual to prolonged aversive treatment is contrary to the goal of ensuring that intervention does not increase the pain and distress already posed by the presenting clinical disorder.

Rumination

Rumination is the deliberate regurgitation or bringing up of previously ingested food into the mouth, followed by reconsumption of the vomitus. Frequently, the behavior is induced by rapid, thrusting tongue movements or inserting fingers into the mouth or throat. The disorder is different from *involuntary* regurgitation often associated with infections, central nervous system disease, or nonobstructive organic problems (Singh, 1981b), a condition that usually remits following appropriate medical treatment. Chronic rumination can produce serious ill effects such as dehydration, lowered resistance to disease, malnutrition, electrolyte imbalance, and weight loss. Mortality rates among ruminating infants have ranged from 12% to 20% (Gaddini & Gaddini, 1959; Kanner, 1957; Sajwaj, Libet, & Agras, 1974). Some theorists view rumination as a subclassification of self-injurious behavior (Singh, 1981b).

There are no published reports of the prevalence of rumination among developmentally disabled persons. In an unpublished survey, Singh and Dawson (1980) reviewed the entire inpatient population of an institution for mentally retarded persons. Out of 349 residents, 21 (6.02%) were identified as ruminators. Of these individuals, 8 were profoundly retarded and 13 were severely retarded. Overall, 22.2% of the profoundly retarded and 8.5% of the severely retarded residents at the institution displayed rumination. Although based on a small sample size, these data reflect a common observation that within mentally retarded populations, ruminating behavior is most often encountered among those persons with a severe to profound classification.

FOOD SATIATION

A reinforcing stimulus or event loses its controlling effects when delivered in excessive amounts (Kazdin, 1984). When previously steady-state responding decreases following prolonged presentation of reinforcement, the outcome is said to occur due to *satiation*. One way to conceptualize the etiology and maintenance of rumination is that emesis occurs due to reconsumption of vomitus. In effect, ingestion of the vomitus reinforces the preceding ruminative behavior. Food satiation approaches are intended to lessen this reinforcing response by providing large, and sometimes unlimited, quantities of food intake.

Jackson, Johnson, Ackron, and Crowley (1975) first described this strategy in a treatment program with two profoundly retarded males. Each individual was allowed to consume additional portions of their regular meals plus supplemental items such as ice cream and milkshakes. Vomiting was reduced by 94% for one client and 50% for the second. Libby and Phillips (1978) reported the elimination of rumination in a profoundly retarded boy using food satiation, although conclusive interpretations of treatment are difficult due to methodological design limitations. Employing a multiple-baseline design, Foxx, Snyder, and Schroeder (1979) observed reductions in ruminative vomiting following introduction of a satiation program with two profoundly retarded adults. Further decreases in rumination were recorded when an oral hygiene overcorrection procedure was combined with satiation.

Some of the procedural parameters associated with food satiation treatment of rumination have been investigated in an interesting series of studies by Rast and associates. In one study (Rast, Johnston, Drum, & Conrin, 1981), the postmeal vomiting of three severely to profoundly retarded males (ages 19 to 24) was recorded under three conditions within a reversal design: 1) baseline (no intervention), 2) providing larger portions at meals, and 3) providing larger portions *plus* all the potatoes, unflavored instant grits, cream of wheat, and/or bread each client would consume freely. For all three cases, the frequency and duration of vomiting incidents remained high during baseline and increased portion conditions but decreased rapidly during satiation phases. Rast, Johnston, and Drum (1984) measured ruminative vomiting of 22-year-old, 32-year-old, and 34-year-old profoundly retarded, institutionalized residents. Following initial baseline assessment, phases were introduced during which starches were added to daily meals in gradual 10-ounce increments. For each client, rumination decreased to near-zero levels only when satiation quantities at meals were achieved. A return-to-baseline condition resulted in a recovery of rumination to preintervention rates. And finally, Rast, Ellinger-Allen, and Johnston (1985) evaluated several variations of food satiation in a study with four profoundly retarded males, ages 17 to 22. Three of the clients received increased portions at meals (15 to 20 ounces of starch, 28.5 ounces of starch, or all extra starch consumed freely), while the fourth client was presented with either small or double-size portions alternated at daily lunch and supper meals. For this latter client, the larger quantity meals actually resulted in more frequent rumination. However, for the other three clients who received greater increases in supplemental starches, ruminating decreased substantially.

The research by Rast and associates reveals some essential features of food satiation as a rumination treatment strategy. It appears that the procedure will not be effective if meal size is increased *gradually*. Rather, satiation quantities should be presented initially to ensure positive results. However, the actual controlling mechanisms involved in food satiation have not been adequately determined. For example, does it matter what types of food, particle size, or nutritional content are consumed? Or, as demonstrated in a recent study (Rast, Johnston, Ellinger-Allen, & Drum, 1985), the caloric value of satiation diets or possible oropharyngeal and esophageal stimulation may be influential variables. It is also common that clients who receive food satiation treatment invariably gain weight. Initially, this is a desirable outcome for ruminators since they are usually underweight and malnourished. Conversely, such treatment could not be recommended on a prolonged basis since clients would become excessively overweight. Therefore, changing satiation diets to more normalized meal quantities while maintaining treatment effects is an essential programmatic concern to be addressed in future research.

POSITIVE REINFORCEMENT

As with other health-threatening behaviors, there are few examples of treatment programs for rumination that have relied exclusively on the use of positive reinforcement procedures. Because the response decrements from reinforcement methods tend to be very gradual, there is a reluctance to institute such treatment for behaviors that are physically harmful to the client. Instead, more immediate suppression of responding is desired.

Where reinforcement techniques have been investigated, equivocal findings have resulted. O'Neil, White, King, and Carek (1979) successfully treated a 26-month-old developmentally delayed child through a DRO procedure. After rumination remained unresponsive to an aversive stimulation punishment program, DRO was added in the form of a honey-water solution delivered whenever 15 to 30 seconds elapsed without a ruminating response. Rumination was reduced to near-zero levels with this intervention and remained low during the withdrawal of the punishment component. Mulick, Schroeder, and Rojahn (1980) found that reinforcing a specific alternative behavior (toy-play) while concurrently ignoring rumination was an effective treatment for a 15-year-old profoundly retarded boy.

Reinforcement for the absence of vomiting without a specific alternative response (DRO) was less successful.

Barmann (1980) also attained a reduction in rumination displayed by a 6-year-old profoundly retarded male through reinforcement of an alternative response. Because the child's vomiting was frequently preceded by hand-in-mouth behavior, reinforcement consisted of contingent vibration (a pleasant stimulus for the child) for responses such as hands on lap or playing with toys. This intervention produced rapid decreases in hand-mouthing and rumination. At a 1-year follow-up, the program had been eliminated and both behaviors remained virtually absent.

As discussed in the review of SIB, these studies provide examples of how to design and program reinforcement strategies for severe maladaptive behaviors. Again, given the serious medical concerns posed by ruminative disorders, efforts at clinical intervention will most probably continue to emphasize the application of reinforcement procedures combined with response deceleration methods.

OVERCORRECTION

Overcorrection treatment of rumination has consisted primarily of contingencies that require the client to clean up the environmental effects of the behavior or hygienically cleanse the oral cavity. At times, both procedures are implemented concurrently.

Azrin and Wesolowski (1975) used a combination of self-correction and positive practice for the management of ruminative vomiting in a 36-year-old profoundly retarded woman. Self-correction required the woman to clean up her vomitus and change her soiled clothing or bed sheets. The positive practice component included rehearsal of proper vomiting responses (entering a bathroom and vomiting into a toilet). This combination of procedures, evaluated in a case-study (AB) design, resulted in complete suppression of vomiting within 2 weeks and therapeutic maintenance 1 year later. A similar restitutional overcorrection procedure was applied by Duker and Seys (1977) with a 19-year-old profoundly retarded ruminator. Contingent on a vomiting response, she was prompted to wash her face, clean up the physical surroundings, and change into new clothing. Rumination was brought quickly under control with this program as revealed in a reversal design. In another methodologically sound study, Singh, Manning, and Angell (1982) examined the effects of oral hygiene overcorrection on rumination displayed by 17-year-old profoundly retarded twins. Overcorrection consisted of the participants cleansing their teeth for 2 minutes with a toothbrush that had been soaked in oral antiseptic, followed by wiping of the lips with a face cloth. A multiple-baseline design across participants and daily meals showed that treatment produced a reduction in rumination to near-zero levels. Interestingly, as rumination decreased, stereotypic behaviors such as body rocking and object manipulation increased in frequency. This outcome indicates negative covariation among responses and, as suggested by the authors, could be addressed by positively reinforcing alternative, incompatible behaviors.

The attractiveness of overcorrection as a treatment for rumination is that it enables the practitioner to respond to the problem in an educative fashion. For example, when oral hygiene overcorrection is used, it allows for the antiseptic cleansing of the teeth and gums (Singh et al., 1982). Restitutional overcorrection strategies teach the client how to respond properly when one's physical surroundings are affected. Unfortunately, there are still too few studies with sufficient methodological rigor to warrant conclusive interpretations as to treatment efficacy and generalizability. Also, as noted by others (Marholin, Luiselli, & Townsend, 1980; Singh, 1981b), overcorrection is comprised of several procedures including response interruption, time-out, physical immobilization, negative reinforcement, and compliance training. As such, it is difficult to determine with certainty which procedure, or combination of procedures, is responsible for therapeutic control. Overcorrection, therefore, should be considered as a potentially useful management strategy but one that must be evaluated more extensively.

AVERSIVE STIMULATION

The general format for applying aversive stimulation has been specified previously. Two categories of aversive stimuli have been examined in the treatment of rumination: electric shock and distasteful solutions. Operationally, one strategy entails presenting the stimulus contingent upon emesis. A second variation consists of intervening following occurrences of a behavioral precursor to the vomiting response such as stomach contractions or reverse peristalsis.

Among mentally retarded children and adults, several publications have reported substantial decreases or suppression of rumination through contingent electric shock (Kohlenberg, 1970; Luckey, Watson, & Musick, 1968; Watkins, 1972; White & Taylor, 1967). However, it is noteworthy that each of these studies includes one or more experimental shortcomings, for example, an absence of quantitative data, no estimates of interobserver reliability, and lack of controlled research design (Singh, 1981b). Such limitations mean that these results can only be suggestive at best. Furthermore, the procedural and ethical problems with shock already indicated for SIB apply here as well.

One of the earliest examples of aversive control over rumination with a distasteful solution as the noxious stimulus was provided by Sajwaj et al. (1974). Treatment was instituted with a 6-month-old normal infant and consisted of squirting 5 to 10 ml of lemon juice into her mouth contingent on rumination or antecedent behaviors. As a result of this intervention, the child's rumination was suppressed while other positive effects in the forms of weight gain and increased social behaviors occurred. These findings have been replicated subsequently with a variety of developmentally handicapped persons. Becker, Turner, and Sajwaj (1978) used contingent lemon juice to reduce ruminative vomiting of a 36-month-old retarded child. The same procedure was employed by Marholin, Luiselli, Robinson, and Lott (1980, Study 1) to eliminate chronic rumination exhibited by a 16-year-old profoundly retarded youngster. A very recent study by Glasscock, Friman, O'Brien, and Christophersen (1986) documented further the reduction of rumination via contingent citrus application and also reported an interesting procedural variation. Using contingent squirts of lemon juice, the ruminative gagging of a 13-year-old girl with Batten's disease decreased substantially. When responding exceeded a preset criterion, lime juice was substituted and reduced rates were achieved once again. Following a second increase in rumination, lemon juice was reintroduced, producing an immediate decrement in responding that was maintained for the remainder of the study. The authors suggested that this alteration of aversives may be a useful tactic to overcome habituation that sometimes occurs with punishment programs incorporating noxious stimuli.

Of significant note is the finding that, in some cases, taste aversion punishment with ruminators has proven ineffective when lemon juice was the aversive stimulus but has been successful subsequently when another stimulus was applied. Singh (1979, Study 1) implemented a lemon juice punishment procedure similar to that of Sajwaj et al. (1974) with a 4.8-year-old profoundly retarded boy contingent on several rumination responses (actual emesis, tongue thrusting, reconsumption of vomitus). This treatment was not effective in reducing rumination until Tabasco-brand pepper sauce was substituted for the lemon juice. With this stimulus, response suppression was obtained quickly and maintained 1 year later. The same findings were reported in a second study by Marholin, Luiselli, Robinson, et al. (1980, Study 2). In it, the ruminative vomiting of an 11-year-old profoundly retarded boy with tuberous sclerosis was unaffected by lemon juice treatment but was eliminated with Tabasco sauce as the punisher. These results underscore the fact that a punishing stimulus can only be determined by empirically verifying its controlling effects on behavior and not by its purported aversive properties.

It bears repeating that the aversive treatment of rumination, like other health-threatening behaviors, requires careful consideration, by experienced clinicians, and usually occurs as the method of last resort. For the most part, programs incorporating electric shock are seldom utilized in contemporary treatment. Punishment by distasteful solutions, on the other hand, is receiving more extensive evaluation. This may be due to the fact that, compared to electric shock, such stimuli are more readily acceptable to practitioners. Other positive characteristics are that the stimuli can be applied quickly following rumination or antecedent behaviors and that they are topographically related to the target response. This form of intervention, of course, demands extensive and systematic monitoring to ensure proper implementation and the prevention of possible physical side effects.

Pica

Pica is an appetitive disorder observed most frequently in mentally retarded populations. It consists of the ingestion of nonnutritive or inedible substances such as string, garbage, plaster, paper products, and paint chips. Some of the serious ill effects from this behavior include lead poisoning, anemia, and intestinal obstruction (Kanner, 1957; Milar & Schroeder, 1983). If fecal matter is ingested (coprophagy), gastrointestinal parasites may result.

In a survey of 598 institutionalized, mentally retarded persons, Singh and Winton (1982) identified pica in 8.4% of their sample. Danford and Huber (1982) also recorded incidence rates in an institutionalized setting for the mentally retarded and found that among 991 residents, 25.8% engaged in pica. Additional data from this survey revealed that frequency of pica increased with the severity of retardation and that various other behavior and food-related problems were associated with the disorder.

Positive Reinforcement

Efforts to reduce pica through positive reinforcement procedures have been evaluated in young children with lead poisioning (Finney, Russo, & Cataldo, 1982; Madden, Russo, & Cataldo, 1980). One method of reinforcement, discrimination training, was based upon the assumption that children should first know the difference between edible and nonedible objects. Discrimination training sessions were conducted, during which food items (raisins, candy) and paint chips (real and simulated) were presented to the children followed by the questions, "Is this something you should put in your mouth?" Correct responses were reinforced with praise and food treats. An incorrect response produced corrective feedback, for example, "No, this is paint—it will make you sick if you eat it." A second method of reinforcement consisted of a standard DRO schedule that specified reinforcers to be presented to the children if they did not engage in pica responses during timed intervals. Both the discrimination training and DRO procedures were implemented and evaluated within an inpatient hospital setting.

Out of a total of seven children studied by Finney et al. (1982) and Madden et al. (1980), two were classified as mildly retarded based upon standardized IQ testing. One, a 3-year-old male, was unaffected by the discrimination training program but did evince significant reductions in pica during DRO treatment sessions. The other child, a 5.8-year-old female, demonstrated high, average rates of pica following exposure to both reinforcement strategies. Pica was reduced to near-zero levels when an overcorrection procedure was combined with DRO.

Due to the very limited research conducted in general, and with developmentally disabled persons in particular, it is not possible to evaluate the clinical efficacy of reinforcement-control strategies for pica. It would appear that in the case of DRO, treatment would have to be extended into the client's natural environment (home, school) to be maximally effective. The discrimination training procedures may only apply to persons with mild to moderate intellectual and language impairments. As a form of least restrictive treatment, both methods warrant further scrutiny, particularly as components of multimethod intervention packages.

OVERCORRECTION

Overcorrection programs for pica are similar to those employed in treating rumination. Usually, the individual engaging in pica is required to cleanse his or her mouth, hands, and the environment. To illustrate, Foxx and Martin (1975) applied the following procedures with three profoundly retarded women contingent upon their ingestion of feces or upon detection of fecal matter on the hands or mouth: 1) walk to the toilet and expectorate the ingested material; 2) brush mouth, teeth, and gums with a soft toothbrush that had been soaked in oral antiseptic; 3) wash hands and scrub fingernails in warm, soapy water; 4) cleanse the anal area with a soapy cloth; and 5) mop up the area where feces eating or handling had been observed, using a disinfectant. In all three cases, pica was essentially eliminated within one week of treatment. Also, biweekly stool specimens taken during the study revealed an absence of previous parasite infestation. Mulick, Barbour, Schroeder, and Rojahn (1980) reduced pica (ingestion of bits of clothing, string, small metal objects) in two profoundly retarded adults using a similar methodology. In the study by Finney et al. (1982) cited previously, brief overcorrection that consisted of brushing mouth and teeth with an antiseptic-soaked toothbrush for 1 minute was combined with DRO to decrease pica in a mildly retarded, 5.8-year-old child with lead poisoning.

A component analysis of the typical overcorrection package for pica was carried out by Singh and Winton (1985) in a study with two profoundly retarded women. Both participants had long-standing histories of pica behavior that included the ingestion of cigarette butts, buttons from clothing, and food remains. The differential effects from three separate components were assessed. The *oral hygiene* component required the women to spit out or throw away any object that was mouthed, followed by 5 minutes of toothbrushing with an oral antiseptic. *Personal hygiene* consisted of 5 minutes of washing hands and scrubbing fingernails. The third component, *tidying*, required a 5-minute period of picking up inedible objects and depositing them in a trash can. Each overcorrection component was programmed randomly within one of three environmental settings in the form of an alternating treatments design. All three procedures reduced pica of both participants, but the oral hygiene component produced the most substantial decrease in responding. These findings provide further evidence that short durations of overcorrection can be programmed successfully, thereby lessening the burden on treatment personnel. The results are particularly encouraging given the seriousness of pica as a health-threatening behavior.

PHYSICAL IMMOBILIZATION

Bucher, Reykdal, and Albin (1976) first reported the use of physical immobilization to control pica in a developmentally disabled population. Two mentally retarded children were treated with a reprimand ("No!") and 30 seconds of contingent hand restraint. While reduced levels of responding were obtained with both children, the study suffers from the fact that reprimand and immobilization procedures were applied concurrently. Therefore, it is difficult to separate the differential control exerted by each technique.

Research by Singh and associates has examined the efficacy of physical immobilization without an accompanying reprimand. These investigations also included several procedural comparisons and data on collateral behavior change. Winton and Singh (1983) programmed two durations of contingent immobilization for pica in 19-year-old and 12-year-old profoundly retarded boys. Durations of 10 seconds and 30 seconds were compared with one participant and 10 seconds and 3 seconds with the other. To apply immobilization, a trainer removed any object the children placed in their mouths and then restrained arms at the sides of the body for the specified duration. The comparison of durations was accomplished using an alternating treatments design and showed that 10 seconds was the most effective duration for each child. During intervention, gradual increases in pica were noted in nontreated settings. The behavior was suppressed rapidly, however, when immobilization was introduced into these locations. Collateral behaviors such as picking and handling inedible objects changed variably over the course of treatment.

A comparison of physical immobilization and overcorrection was performed by Singh and Bakker (1984). Two profoundly retarded, institutionalized young adults (20 and 21 years old) who ingested stones, cigarette butts, bits of string, and other similar substances served as participants. Following baseline conditions in an alternating treatments design, the immobilization and overcorrection interventions were programmed daily with each resident, in each of two settings. When overcorrection was in effect, the occurrence of pica resulted in 15 minutes of cleansing the mouth, washing hands, and picking up and depositing trash. With physical immobilization, the participants were required to expectorate ingested items, whereafter their hands were restrained manually for 10 seconds. While both treatments reduced pica, immobilization was the most effective method. Picking and handling materials, which were precursors to pica, decreased under both treatments. Stereotypic behaviors and desirable social responses (smiling, laughter, peer interaction) appeared to be unaffected by either intervention.

The results from physical immobilization treatment of pica, although limited to only a few studies, are promising. When applied for brief durations, the procedure is certainly an economical one for most practitioners. In fact, social validity responses by treatment personnel in the Singh and Bakker (1984) study revealed a uniform preference for immobilization when compared to overcorrection, most probably because the procedure required less time for implementation and staff training.

Additional Disorders

In addition to the substantive research conducted on self-injury, rumination, and pica, recent studies, although fewer in number, have been carried out with other health-threatening behaviors. This section provides a brief review of these disorders, specifically bruxism, respiratory problems, and liquid avoidance.

Bruxism

Bruxism is the repetitive clenching or grinding of the teeth and may occur during the day (diurnal bruxism) or evening (nocturnal bruxism). This disorder can produce myofacial pain, erosion of tooth enamel, damage to the soft tissue surrounding the teeth, and hypertrophy of masticatory muscles (Glaros & Rao, 1977). Richmond, Rugh, Dolfi, and Wasilewsky (1984) surveyed 433 residents of a state institution for mentally retarded persons and found that bruxism was identified in 41% of this population based upon caregiver reports. Tooth-wear examinations performed by dental staff placed the incidence rate at 58%. Informal survey data collected by Blount, Drabman, Wilson, and Stewart (1982) revealed that 21.5% of 65 profoundly retarded residents engaged in nocturnal tooth-grinding habits.

The treatment of bruxism in developmentally disabled persons has been reported in two publications. Gross and Isaac (1983) evaluated a management program that combined differential reinforcement of nonbruxing behavior and contingent forced-arm exercise with two 4-year-old mentally retarded boys. The exercise component required 2 minutes of repetitive arm movements each time bruxism was detected. A multiple-baseline design across participants demonstrated that intervention successfully eliminated bruxism of both children. In the second study, Blount et al. (1982) treated diurnal bruxism of 16-year-old and 32-year-old profoundly retarded women. Treatment consisted of contingent "icing," a procedure that entails application of an ice cube to the cheeks or chin for several seconds. Bruxism was greatly reduced in both women during treatment sessions and also decreased during generalization (no-treatment) assessments.

Respiratory Problems

Singh et al. (1980b) implemented a punishment procedure to suppress chronic hyperventilation in a 17.5-year-old profoundly retarded female. As a respiratory problem, hyperventilation is associated with numbness in the extremities, palpitations, carpopedal spasm, and fainting. In this case, the client's hyperventilation was recorded during 30-minute assessment sessions in four settings within a state institution. Treatment was introduced sequentially across the four settings in the form of a multiple-baseline design. Each time the client hyperventilated, a vial of aromatic ammonia was placed under her nose for 3 seconds. This program produced immediate and complete suppression of the behavior as soon as it was introduced into each setting. It was subsequently extended on an 8-hour-per-day basis and, again, total elimination of responding was established.

Air swallowing (aerophagia) is a condition that can lead to abdominal distension, a compressed diaphragm, and gastrointestinal distress (Guaderer, Halpin, & Izart, 1981). Holburn and Dougher (1985) worked with two mentally retarded air swallowers in an institutional setting. One client was a 19-year-old profoundly retarded female whose 10-year history of air swallowing had doubled the size of her stomach. She was treated initially with an overcorrection procedure that entailed the placement of one hand over the mouth for a 5-second duration contingent upon air-swallowing responses. When overcorrection failed to decrease responding, various forms of time-out (e.g., placement in isolation, removal of a preferred activity) were programmed. However, rates of air swallowing remained at baseline levels. For the second client, a 22-year-old profoundly retarded male, intervention was more positive. It consisted of the previously described overcorrection procedure, first applied for 5 seconds and then increased to 10 seconds and 15 seconds. As treatment duration increased, frequency of air swallowing declined steadily and stabilized at near-zero levels. Unfortunately, the client displayed intense oppositional behavior during treatment, resulting in termination of the overcorrection program. Following discontinuation of the treatment, air swallowing increased once again.

Liquid Avoidance

Adipsia refers to a lack of thirst or chronic avoidance of fluid consumption. Failure to ingest liquids over an extended period of time produces a state of dehydration. In its most extreme form, a prolonged absence of liquid consumption may be fatal. Friedin, Borakove, and Fox (1982) reported a case study in which behavioral shaping procedures were used to treat a 14-year-old profoundly retarded boy who failed to swallow liquids from a glass and was periodically dehydrated. Milk was initially presented to him on a small teaspoon, followed by a small amount of applesauce (a preferred substance) when the milk was swallowed. Gradually, the stimulus for presenting milk was changed to a tablespoon, a partially filled cup, and, finally, a regular glass. After 9 weeks of programming, the boy was able to drink freely from a glass, an outcome that was maintained at a 1-year follow-up assessment. At that time, he was also ingesting other liquids and dehydration was no longer a problem.

Summary and Conclusions

This chapter focuses on the assessment and treatment of health-threatening behaviors in persons with developmental disabilities. Its primary purpose is to review therapeutic procedures as applied to specific disorders. In doing so, an effort is made to present research findings while discussing the particular benefits and disadvantages of the various techniques. With some disorders, for example, self-injury, a large variety of methods have been successfully employed. Certain techniques have been therapeutically effective with a number of disorders (e.g., overcorrection and physical immobilization). Overall, it may be concluded that behavioral technology has much to offer in the area of secondary prevention with developmentally handicapped individuals. As research and clinical practice evolve, many issues and concerns will present themselves.

The continued refinement of assessment methodology and its integration with standard medical practices remains a primary goal. In an earlier section, it is emphasized that the role of behavioral assessment is not only to obtain objective data, but also to functionally identify those variables that control the occurrence of the presenting disorder(s). Analytic assessment, such as the system developed by Iwata et al. (1982), represents an exemplary model in this regard. Although increasing, the incorporation of this approach with severe behavior disorders is still in its infancy (cf. Mace, Page, Ivancic, & O'Brien, 1986). Of course, such analyses may not be required in all cases or may be too lengthy relevant to certain medical conditions. However, through systematic research and design of functional assessment methodologies, behavior analysts can contribute greatly to the development of empirically based treatment choices.

For the majority of studies described in this chapter, treatment procedures were implemented by natural change-agents. Many programs were instituted by direct-care staff (aides, nursing assistants) within residential facilities. Other personnel have included parents, clinical specialists, and, at times, educators. The essential role of these individuals as practitioners demands continued development of cost-efficient and easily managed intervention strategies. In some cases, treatment failures can be linked to poorly designed protocols that are either too complex, cumbersome, or time consuming. It is encouraging to find that many contemporary researchers within behavioral medicine are conducting comparative analyses between various methods and components in an attempt to isolate optimum parameters. The evaluation of practitioner acceptability and satisfaction through social validity assessment is another meaningful step toward enhancing procedural methodology (Kazdin & Matson, 1981; Luiselli, Chapter 1, this volume).

When one considers the severity of many health-threatening behaviors, the ideal measure of clinical success is total suppression of responding. Although many studies in fact achieved this goal, many others did not. The experiences of most behavioral clinicians include clients who demonstrated significant reductions in maladaptive behaviors but not elimination. And in some instances, only moderate changes are obtained, or possibly no change (cf. Holburn & Dougher, 1985). Such results argue for better predictors of therapeutic effectiveness. The bias in professional publications, of course, is toward positive findings and success. However, reports of treatment failures may provide useful information to assist in the selection of therapy techniques and the design of multifaceted interventions.

Finally, it should be stressed that the effective treatment of health-threatening behaviors rests with a reciprocal and interdisciplinary approach between psychologists, physicians, and medical specialists. Behavior therapy, as elucidated in this chapter, represents one approach that may serve a primary, complimentary, or secondary function in any given clinical case. The proper focus of behavioral medicine on health-threatening conditions of developmentally disabled persons is one that combines multiple disciplines in a comprehensive diagnostic, assessment, and treatment orientation.

References

Accreditation Council for Services for Mentally Retarded and Other Developmentally Disabled Persons. (1981). *Standards for services for developmentally disabled individuals.* 5101 Wisconsin Avenue, N.W., Washington DC.

Altman, K., Haavik, S., & Cook, J.W. (1978). Punishment of self-injurious behavior in natural settings using contingent aromatic ammonia. *Behaviour Research and Therapy, 16,* 85–96.

Azrin, N.H., Gottlieb, L., Hughart, L., Wesolowski, M.D., & Rahn, T. (1975). Eliminating self-injurious behavior by educative procedures. *Behaviour Research and Therapy, 13,* 101–111.

Azrin, N.H., & Wesolowski, M.D. (1975). Eliminating habitual vomiting in a retarded adult by positive practice and self-correction. *Journal of Behavior Therapy and Experimental Psychiatry, 6,* 145–148.

Ball, T.S., Campbell, R., & Barkemeyer, R. (1980). Air splints applied to control self-injurious finger sucking in profoundly retarded individuals. *Journal of Behavior Therapy and Experimental Psychiatry, 11,* 267–271.

Barlow, D.H., & Hayes, S.C. (1979). The alternating treatments design: One strategy for comparing the effects of two treatments in a single subject. *Journal of Applied Behavior Analysis, 12,* 199–210.

Barlow, D.H., Hayes, S.C., & Nelson, R.O. (1984). *The scientist practitioner: Research and accountability in clinical and educational settings.* New York: Pergamon Press.

Barmann, B.C. (1980). Use of contingent vibration in the treatment of self-stimulatory hand-mouthing and ruminative vomiting behavior. *Journal of Behavior Therapy and Experimental Psychiatry, 11,* 307–312.

Barmann, B.C., & Vitali, D.L. (1982). Facial screening to eliminate trichotillomania in developmentally disabled persons. *Behavior Therapy, 13,* 735–742.

Barnard, J.D., Christophersen, E.R., & Wolf, M.M. (1976). Parent-mediated treatment of children's self-injurious behavior using overcorrection. *Journal of Pediatric Psychology, 1,* 56–61.

Baumeister, A.A., & Baumeister, A.A. (1978). Suppression of repetitive self-injurious behavior by contingent inhalation of aromatic ammonia. *Journal of Autism and Childhood Schizophrenia, 8,* 71–77.

Baumeister, A.A., & MacLean, W.E. (1984). Deceleration of self-injurious and stereotypic responding by exercise. *Applied Research in Mental Retardation, 5,* 385–393.

Becker, J.V., Turner, S.M., & Sajwaj, T.E. (1978). Multiple behavioral effects of the use of lemon juice with a ruminating toddler-age child. *Behavior Modification, 2,* 267–278.

Blount, R.L., Drabman, R.S., Wilson, N., & Stewart, D. (1982). Reducing severe diurnal bruxism in two profoundly retarded females. *Journal of Applied Behavior Analysis, 15,* 565–571.

Borreson, P.M. (1980). The elimination of a self-injurious avoidance response through a forced running sequence. *Mental Retardation, 18,* 73–76.

Bucher, B.B., Reykdal, R., & Albin, J. (1976). Brief restraint to control pica in retarded children. *Journal of Behavior Therapy and Experimental Psychiatry, 7,* 137–140.

Carey, R.G., & Bucher, B.B. (1983). Positive practice overcorrection: The effects of duration of positive practice on acquisition and response reduction. *Journal of Applied Behavior Analysis, 16,* 101–110.

Carr, E.G., & Durand, V.M. (1985). Reducing problem behaviors through functional communication training. *Journal of Applied Behavior Analysis, 18,* 111–126.

Carr, E.G., & Lovaas, O.I. (1983). Contingent electric shock as a treatment for severe behavior problems. In S. Axelrod & J. Apsche (Eds.), *The effects of punishment on human behavior* (pp. 245–269). New York: Academic Press.

Carr, E.G., & McDowell, J.J. (1980). Social control of self-injurious behavior of organic etiology. *Behavior Therapy, 11,* 402–409.

Carr, E.G., Newsom, C.D., & Binkoff, J.A. (1980). Escape as a factor in the aggressive behavior of two retarded children. *Journal of Applied Behavior Analysis, 13,* 101–117.

Cataldo, M.F., & Harris, J. (1982). The biological basis of self-injury in the mentally retarded. *Analysis and Intervention in Developmental Disabilities, 2,* 21–39.

Corte, H.E., Wolf, M.M., & Locke, B.J. (1971). A comparison of procedures for eliminating self-injurious behavior of retarded adolescents. *Journal of Applied Behavior Analysis, 4,* 201–213.

Danford, D.E., & Huber, A.M. (1982). Pica among mentally retarded adults. *American Journal of Mental Deficiency, 87,* 141–146.

Demetral, G.D., & Lutzker, J.R. (1980). The parameters of facial screening in treating self-injurious behavior. *Behavior Research of Severe Developmental Disabilities, 1,* 261–277.

Dorsey, M.F., Iwata, B.A., Ong, P., & McSween, T.E. (1980). Treatment of self-injurious behavior using a water mist : Initial response suppression and generalization. *Journal of Applied Behavior Analysis, 13,* 343–353.

Dorsey, M.F., Iwata, B.A., Reid, D.H., & Davis, P.A. (1982). Protective equipment: Continuous and contingent application in the treatment of self-injurious behavior. *Journal of Applied Behavior Analysis, 15,* 217–230.

Duker, P.C., & Seys, D.M. (1977). Elimination of vomiting in a retarded female using restitutional overcorrection. *Behavior Therapy, 8,* 255–257.

Favell, J.E., McGimsey, J.F., & Jones, M.L. (1978). The use of physical restraint in the treatment of self-injurious behavior and positive reinforcement. *Journal of Applied Behavior Analysis, 11,* 225–241.

Favell, J.E., McGimsey, J.F., & Schell, R.M. (1982). Treatment of self-injury by providing alternate sensory activities. *Analysis and Intervention in Developmental Disabilities, 2,* 83–104.

Finney, J.W., Russo, D.C., & Cataldo, M.F. (1982). Reduction of pica in young children with lead poisoning. *Journal of Pediatric Psychology, 7,* 197–207.

Foxx, R.M., & Azrin, N.H. (1973). The elimination of autistic self-stimulatory behavior by overcorrection. *Journal of Applied Behavior Analysis, 6,* 1–14.

Foxx, R.M., & Bechtel, D.R. (1982). Overcorrection. In M. Hersen, R.M. Eisler, & P.M. Miller (Eds.), *Progress in behavior modification* (Vol. 13). New York: Academic Press.

Foxx, R.M., & Martin, E.D. (1975). Treatment of scavenging behavior (coprophagy and pica) by overcorrection. *Behaviour Research and Therapy, 13,* 153–162.

Foxx, R.M., Plaska, T.G., & Bittle, R.G. (1986). Guidelines for the use of contingent electric shock to treat aberrant behavior. In M. Hersen, R.M. Eisler, & P.M. Miller (Eds.,), *Progress in behavior modification* (Vol. 20, pp. 1–34). New York: Academic Press.

Foxx, R.M., Snyder, N.S., & Schroeder, F. (1979). A food satiation and oral hygiene punishment program to suppress chronic rumination by retarded persons. *Journal of Autism and Developmental Disorders, 9,* 399–412.

Friedin, B.D., Borakove, L.S., & Fox, K.T. (1982). Treatment of abnormal avoidance of liquid consumption. *Journal of Behavior Therapy and Experimental Psychiatry, 13,* 85–88.

Gaddini, R.D.B., & Gaddini, E. (1959). Rumination in infancy. In L. Jessner & E. Pavenstadt (Eds.), *Dynamic psychopathology in childhood*. New York: Grune & Stratton.

Glaros, A.G., & Rao, S.M. (1977). Bruxism: A critical review. *Psychology Bulletin, 84*, 767–781.

Glasscock, S.G., Friman, P.C., O'Brien, S., & Christophersen, E.R. (1986). Varied citrus treatment of ruminant gagging in a teenager with Batten's disease. *Journal of Behavior Therapy and Experimental Psychiatry, 17*, 129–133.

Griffin, J.C., Williams, D.E., Stark, M.T., Altmeyer, B.K., & Mason, M. (1986). Self-injurious behavior: A state-wide prevalence survey of the extent and circumstances. *Applied Research in Mental Retardation, 7*, 105–116.

Gross, A.M., & Isaac, L. (1983). Forced arm exercise and DRO in the treatment of bruxism in cerebral palsied children. *Child and Family Behavior Therapy, 4*, 175–181.

Gross, A.M., Wright, B., & Drabman, R.S. (1980). The empirical selection of a punisher for a retarded child's self-injurious behavior: A case study. *Child Behavior Therapy, 2*, 59–65.

Guaderer, M.W., Halpin, T.C., & Izart, R.J. (1981). Pathologic childhood aerophagia: A recognizable clinical entity. *Journal of Pediatric Surgery, 16*, 301–305.

Halpern, L.F., & Andrasik, F. (1986). The immediate and long-term effectiveness of overcorrection in treating self-injurious behavior in a mentally retarded adult. *Applied Research in Mental Retardation, 7*, 59–66.

Harris, S.L., & Romanczyk, R.G. (1976). Treating self-injurious behavior of a retarded child by overcorrection. *Behavior Therapy, 7*, 235–239.

Hersen, M., & Bellack, A.S. (1981). *Behavioral assessment*. New York: Pergamon Press.

Holburn, C.S., & Dougher, M.J. (1985). Behavioral attempts to eliminate air-swallowing in two profoundly mentally retarded adults. *American Journal of Mental Deficiency, 89*, 524–536.

Iwata, B.A., Dorsey, M.F., Slifer, K.J., Bauman, K.E., & Richman, G.S. (1982). Towards a functional analysis of self-injury. *Analysis and Intervention in Developmental Disabilities, 2*, 3–20.

Jackson, G.M., Johnson, C.R., Ackron, G.S., & Crowley, R. (1975). Food satiation as a procedure to decelerate vomiting. *American Journal of Mental Deficiency, 80*, 223–227.

Jenson, W.R., Rovner, L., Cameron, S., Petersen, B.P., & Kesler, J. (1985). Reduction of self-injurious behavior in an autistic girl using a multifaceted treatment program. *Journal of Behavior Therapy and Experimental Psychiatry, 16*, 77–80.

Kanner, L. (1957). *Child psychiatry*. Springfield, IL: Thomas.

Kazdin, A.E. (1984). *Behavior modification in applied settings*. Homewood, IL: Dorsey Press.

Kazdin, A.E., & Matson, J.L. (1981). Social validation in mental retardation. *Applied Research in Mental Retardation, 2*, 39–54.

Kelly, J.A., & Drabman, R.S. (1977). Generalizing response suppression of self-injurious behavior through an overcorrection punishment procedure: A case study. *Behavior Therapy, 8*, 468–472.

Kohlenberg, R.J. (1970). The punishment of persistent vomiting: A case study. *Journal of Applied Behavior Analysis, 3*, 241–245.

Kratochwill, T.R., & Morris, R.J. (1983). *Treating children's fears and phobias: A behavioral approach*. New York: Pergamon Press.

Lancioni, G.G., Smeets, P.M., Ceccarani, P.S., Capodaglio, L., & Campanari, G. (1984). Effects of gross-motor activities on the severe self-injurious tantrums of multihandicapped individuals. *Applied Research in Mental Retardation, 5*, 471–482.

Libby, D.G., & Phillips, E. (1978). Eliminating rumination in a profoundly retarded adolescent: An exploratory study. *Mental Retardation, 16,* 57.

Lovaas, O.I., Freitag, G., Gold, V.J., & Kassorla, I. (1965). Experimental studies in childhood schizophrenia: I. Analysis of self-destructive behavior. *Journal of Experimental Child Psychology, 26,* 67–84.

Lovaas, O.I., Schaeffer, B.B., & Simmons, J.Q. (1965). Experimental studies in childhood schizophrenia: Building social behavior in autistic children by use of electric shock. *Journal of Experimental Research in Personality, 1,* 99–109.

Lovaas, O.I., & Simmons, J.Q. (1969). Manipulation of self-destruction in three retarded children. *Journal of Applied Behavior Analysis, 2,* 142–157.

Luckey, R.E., Watson, C.M., & Musick, J.K. (1968). Aversive conditioning as a means of inhibiting vomiting and rumination. *American Journal of Mental Deficiency, 73,* 139–142.

Luiselli, J.K. (1984). Effects of brief overcorrection on stereotypic behaviors of mentally retarded students. *Education and Treatment of Children, 7,* 125–138.

Luiselli, J.K. (1986a). Modification of self-injurious behavior: An analysis of the use of contingently applied protective equipment. *Behavior Modification, 10,* 191–204.

Luiselli, J.K. (1986b). Behavior analysis of pharmacological and contingency management interventions for self-injury. *Journal of Behavior Therapy and Experimental Psychiatry, 17,* 275–284.

Luiselli, J.K. (1987). Behavioral medicine research and treatment in developmental disabilities. In R.P. Barrett & J.L. Matson (Eds.), *Advances in developmental disorders* (pp. 1–39). Greenwich, CT: JAI Press.

Luiselli, J.K. (1988). Comparative analysis of sensory extinction treatments for self-injury. *Education and Treatment of Children, 11,* 149–156.

Luiselli, J.K., Evans, T.E., & Boyce, D.A. (1986). Pharmacological assessment and comprehensive behavioral intervention in a case of pediatric self-injury. *Journal of Clinical Child Psychology, 15,* 323–326.

Luiselli, J.K., Helfen, C.S., Colozzi, G., Donellon, S., & Pemberton, B.W. (1978). Controlling self-inflicted biting of a retarded child by the differential reinforcement of other behavior. *Psychological Reports, 42,* 435–438.

Luiselli, J.K., & Michaud, R.L. (1983). Behavioral treatment of aggression and self-injury in developmentally disabled, visually impaired students. *Journal of Visual Impairment and Blindness, 77,* 388–391.

Luiselli, J.K., Myles, E., Evans, T.E., & Boyce, D.A. (1985). Reinforcement control of severe dysfunctional behavior of blind, multihandicapped students. *American Journal of Mental Deficiency, 90,* 328–334.

Luiselli, J.K., Suskin, L., & McPhee, D.F. (1981). Continuous and intermittent application of overcorrection with a self-injurious autistic child: Alternating treatments design analysis. *Journal of Behavior Therapy and Experimental Psychiatry, 12,* 355–358.

Lutzker, J.R. (1978). Reducing self-injurious behavior by facial screening. *American Journal of Mental Deficiency, 82,* 510–513.

Lutzker, J.R., & Spencer, T. (1974). *Punishment of self-injurious behavior in retardates by brief application of a harmless face cover.* Paper presented at Annual Convention, American Psychological Association, New Orleans, LA.

Lutzker, J.R., & Wesch, D. (1983). Facial screening: History and critical review. *Australia and New Zealand Journal of Developmental Disabilities, 9,* 209–223.

Mace, F.C., Page, T.J., Ivancic, M.T., & O'Brien, S. (1986). Analysis of environmental determinants of aggression and disruption in mentally retarded children. *Applied Research in Mental Retardation, 7,* 203–221.

Madden, N.A., Russo, D.C., & Cataldo, M.F. (1980). Behavioral treatment of pica in children with lead poisoning. *Child Behavior Therapy, 2,* 67-81.

Marholin, D., II, & Luiselli, J.K. (1978). Children's problems. In R.P. Liberman (Ed.), *Psychiatric clinics of North America: Symposium on behavior therapy in psychiatry* (pp. 202-225). Philadelphia: W.B. Saunders.

Marholin, D., II, Luiselli, J.K., Robinson, M., & Lott, I.T. (1980). Response-contingent taste aversion in treating chronic ruminative vomiting of institutionalized, profoundly retarded children. *Journal of Mental Deficiency Research, 24,* 47-56.

Marholin, D., II, Luiselli, J.K., & Townsend, N.M. (1980). Overcorrection: An examination of its rationale and treatment effectiveness. In M. Hersen, R.M. Eisler, & P.M. Miller (Eds.), *Progress in behavior modification,* (Vol. 9, pp. 49-80). New York: Academic Press.

Marholin, D., II, Siegel, L., & Phillips, D. (1976). Treatment and transfer: A search for empirical procedures. In M. Hersen, R.M. Eisler, & P.M. Miller (Eds.), *Progress in behavior modification* (Vol. 3, pp. 293-342). New York: Academic Press.

Martin, P.L., & Foxx, R.M. (1973). Victim control of the aggression of an institutionalized retardate. *Journal of Behavior Therapy and Experimental Psychiatry, 4,* 161-165.

Masek, B.J., Epstein, L.H., & Russo, D.C. (1981). Behavioral perspectives in preventive medicine. In S.M. Turner, K.S. Calhoun, & H.E. Adams (Eds.), *Handbook of clinical behavior therapy* (pp. 475-499). New York: Wiley.

Matson, J.L., Stephens, R.M., & Smith, C. (1978). Treatment of self-injurious behavior with overcorrection. *Journal of Mental Deficiency Research, 22,* 175-178.

Mayhew, G., & Harris, F. (1979). Decreasing self-injurious behavior: Punishment with citric acid and reinforcement of alternative behavior. *Behavior Modification, 3,* 322-336.

Milar, C.R., & Schroeder, S.R. (1983). The effects of lead on retardation of cognitive and adaptive behavior. In J.L. Matson & F. Andrasik (Eds.), *Treatment issues and innovations in mental retardation* (pp. 129-158). New York: Plenum Press.

Mulick, J.A., Barbour, R., Schroeder, S.R., & Rojahn, J. (1980). Overcorrection of pica in two profoundly retarded adults: Analysis of setting events stimulus, and response generalization. *Applied Research in Mental Retardation, 1,* 241-252.

Mulick, J.A., Schroeder, S.R., & Rojahn, J. (1980). Chronic ruminative vomiting: A comparison of four treatment procedures. *Journal of Autism and Developmental Disorders, 10,* 203-213.

Murphey, R.J., Ruprecht, M.J., Baggio, P., & Nunes, D.L. (1979). The use of mild punishment in combination with reinforcement of alternative behaviors to reduce the self-injurious behavior of a profoundly retarded individual. *AAESPH Review, 4,* 187-195.

Neufeld, A., & Fantuzzo, J.W. (1984). Contingent application of a protective device to treat severe self-biting behaviors of a disturbed autistic child. *Journal of Behavior Therapy and Experimental Psychiatry, 15,* 79-83.

O'Neil, P.M., White, J.L., King, C.R., & Carek, D.J. (1979). Controlling childhood rumination through differential reinforcement of other behavior. *Behavior Modification, 3,* 355-372.

Pace, G.M., Iwata, B.A, Edwards, G.L., & McCosh, K.C. (1986). Stimulus fading and transfer in treatment of self-restraint and self-injurious behavior. *Journal of Applied Behavior Analysis, 19,* 381-389.

Parrish, J.M., Aguerrevere, L., Dorsey, M.F., & Iwata, B.A. (1980). The effects of protective equipment on self-injurious behavior. *The Behavior Therapist, 3,* 28-29.

Parrish, J.M., Iwata, B.A., Dorsey, M.F., Bunck, T.J., & Slifer, K.J. (1985). Behavior analysis, program development, and transfer of control in the treatment of self-injury. *Journal of Behavior Therapy and Experimental Psychiatry, 16*, 159–168.

Peterson, R.F., & Peterson, L.R. (1968). The use of positive reinforcement in the control of self-destructive behavior in a retarded boy. *Journal of Experimental Child Psychology, 6*, 351–361.

Rapoff, M.A., Altman, K., & Christophersen, E.R. (1980). Elimination of a retarded child's self-hitting by response-contingent brief restraint. *Education and Treatment of Children, 3*, 231–236.

Rast, J., Ellinger-Allen, J.A., & Johnston, J.M. (1985). Dietary management of rumination: Four case studies. *The American Journal of Clinical Nutrition, 42*, 95–101.

Rast, J., Johnston, J.M., & Drum, C. (1984). A parametric analysis of the relationship between food quantity and rumination. *Journal of the Experimental Analysis of Behavior, 41*, 125–134.

Rast, J., Johnston, J.M., Drum, C., & Conrin, J. (1981). The relation of food quantity to rumination behavior. *Journal of Applied Behavior Analysis, 14*, 121–130.

Rast, J., Johnston, J.M., Ellinger-Allen, J., & Drum, C. (1985). Effects of nutritional and mechanical properties of food on ruminative behavior. *Journal of the Experimental Analysis of Behavior, 44*, 195–206.

Redd, W.H., & Andrykowski, M.A. (1982). Behavioral intervention in cancer treatment: Controlling aversion reactions to chemotherapy. *Journal of Consulting and Clinical Psychology, 50*, 1018–1029.

Richmond, G., Rugh, J.D., Dolfi, G., & Wasilewsky, J.W. (1984). Survey of bruxism in an institutionalized mentally retarded population. *American Journal of Mental Deficiency, 88*, 418–421.

Rincover, A. (1978). Sensory extinction: A procedure for eliminating self-stimulatory behavior in developmentally disabled children. *Journal of Abnormal Child Psychology, 6*, 299–310.

Rincover, A., Cook, A.R., Peoples, A., & Packard, D. (1979). Sensory extinction and sensory reinforcement principles for programming multiple adaptive behavior change. *Journal of Applied Behavior Analysis, 12*, 221–233.

Rincover, A., & Devany, J. (1982). The application of sensory extinction to self-injury. *Analysis and Intervention in Developmental Disabilities, 2*, 67–82.

Rojahn, J., Mulick, J.A., McCoy, D., & Schroeder, S.R. (1978). Setting effects, adaptive clothing, and the modification of head-banging and self-restraint in two, profoundly retarded adults. *Behavior Analysis and Modification, 2*, 185–196.

Rojahn, J., Schroeder, S.R., & Mulick, J.A. (1980). Ecological assessment of self-protective devices in three profoundly retarded adults. *Journal of Autism and Developmental Disorders, 10*, 59–66.

Romanczyk, R.G., & Goren, E.R. (1975). Severe self-injurious behavior: The problem of clinical control. *Journal of Consulting and Clinical Psychology, 43*, 730–739.

Sajwaj, T.E., Libet, J., & Agras, W.S. (1974). Lemon-juice therapy: The control of life-threatening rumination in a six-month-old infant. *Journal of Applied Behavior Analysis, 7*, 557–563.

Silverman, K., Wantanabe, K., Marshall, A.M., & Baer, D.M. (1984). Reducing self-injury and corresponding self-restraint through the strategic use of protective clothing. *Journal of Applied Behavior Analysis, 17*, 545–552.

Singh, N.N. (1979). Aversive control of rumination in the mentally retarded. *Journal of Practical Applications to Developmental Handicap, 3*, 2–6.

Singh, N.N. (1980). The effects of facial screening on infant self-injury. *Journal of Behavior Therapy and Experimental Psychiatry, 11*, 131–134.

Singh, N.N. (1981a). Current trends in the treatment of self-injurious behavior. In L.A. Barness (Ed.), *Advances in pediatrics* (Vol. 28 pp. 377–440). Chicago: Year Book.

Singh, N.N. (1981b). Rumination. In N.R. Ellis (Ed.), *International review of research in mental retardation* (Vol. 10, pp. 139–181). New York: Academic Press.

Singh, N.N., & Bakker, L.W. (1984). Suppression of pica by overcorrection and physical restraint: A comparative analysis. *Journal of Autism and Developmental Disorders, 14*, 331–341.

Singh, N.N., Beale, I.L., & Dawson, M.J. (1981). Duration of facial screening and suppression of self-injurious behavior: Analysis using an alternating treatments design. *Behavioral Assessment, 3*, 411–420.

Singh, N.N., & Dawson, M.J. (1980). *The prevalence of rumination in institutionalized mentally retarded children*. Unpublished data, Mangere Hospital and Training School, Auckland, New Zealand.

Singh, N.N., Dawson, M.J., & Gregory, P.R. (1980a). Self-injury in the profoundly retarded: Clinically significant versus therapeutic control. *Journal of Mental Deficiency Research, 24*, 87–97.

Singh, N.N., Dawson, J.J., & Gregory, P.R. (1980b). Suppression of chronic hyperventilation using response-contingent aromatic ammonia. *Behavior Therapy, 11*, 561–566.

Singh, N.N., Dawson, M.J., & Manning, P.J. (1981). The effects of physical restraint on self-injurious behavior. *Journal of Mental Deficiency Research, 25*, 207–216.

Singh, N.N., Manning, P.J., & Angell, M.J. (1982). Effects of an oral hygiene punishment procedure on chronic rumination and collateral behaviors in monozygous twins. *Journal of Applied Behavior Analysis, 15*, 309–314.

Singh, N.N., & Winton, A.S.W. (1982). *Pica in institutionalized mentally retarded persons*. Unpublished data, University of Canterbury.

Singh, N.N., & Winton, A.S.W. (1985). Controlling pica by components of an overcorrection procedure. *American Journal of Mental Deficiency, 90*, 40–45.

Slifer, K.J., Iwata, B.A., & Dorsey, M.F. (1984). Reduction of eye gouging using a response interruption procedure. *Journal of Behavior Therapy and Experimental Psychiatry, 15*, 369–375.

Tanner, B.A., & Zeiler, M. (1975). Punishment of self-injurious behavior using aromatic ammonia as the aversive stimulus. *Journal of Applied Behavior Analysis, 5*, 163–175.

Tarpley, H.D., & Schroeder, S.R. (1979). Comparison of DRO and DRI on rate of suppression of self-injurious behavior. *American Journal of Mental Deficiency, 84*, 188–194.

Varni, J.W. (1983). *Clinical behavioral pediatrics*. New York: Pergamon Press.

Varni, J.W., Bessman, C.A., Russo, D.C., & Cataldo, M.F. (1980). Behavioral treatment of chronic pain in children: Case study. *Archives of Physical Medicine and Rehabilitation, 61*, 375–379.

Watkins, J.T. (1972). Treatment of chronic vomiting and extreme emaciation by an aversive stimulus: A case study. *Psychological Reports, 31*, 803–805.

Watson, J., Singh, N.N., & Winton, A.S.W. (1986). Suppressive effects of visual and facial screening on self-injurious finger-sucking. *American Journal of Mental Deficiency, 90*, 526–534.

Weeks, M., & Gaylord-Ross, R. (1981). Task difficulty and aberrant behavior in severely handicapped students. *Journal of Applied Behavior Analysis, 14*, 449–463.

White, J.C., & Taylor, D.J. (1967). Noxious conditioning as a treatment for rumination. *Mental Retardation, 5*, 30–33.

Whitehead, W.E., Parker, L.H., Masek, B.J., Cataldo, M.F., & Freeman, J.M. (1981). Biofeedback treatment of fecal incontinence in patients with myelomeningocele. *Developmental Medicine and Child Neurology, 23,* 313–322.

Wilson, G.T., & O'Leary, K.D. (1980). *Principles of behavior therapy.* Englewood Cliffs, NJ: Prentice-Hall.

Winton, A.S.W., & Singh, N.N. (1983). Suppression of pica using brief-duration physical restraint. *Journal of Mental Deficiency Research, 27,* 93–103.

Winton, A.S.W., Singh, N.N., & Dawson, M.J. (1984). Effects of facial screening and blindfold on self-injurious behavior. *Applied Research in Mental Retardation, 5,* 29–42.

Young, J.A., & Wincze, J.P. (1974). The effects of the reinforcement of compatible and incompatible alternative behaviors on the self-injurious and related behaviors of a profoundly retarded female adult. *Behavior Therapy, 5,* 619–623.

Zehr, M.P., & Theobald, D.E. (1978). Manual guidance used in a punishment procedure: The active ingredient in overcorrection. *Journal of Mental Deficiency Research, 22,* 263–272.

7
Behavioral Pharmacology

Nirbhay N. Singh and Alan S.W. Winton

A view held by professionals working with mentally retarded persons is that, of all people who are in need of educational, social, or medical services, their clients represent the single most medicated group. If current prevalence figures for psychotropic drug prescriptions are taken as an indication, then this view may well be true. Thus, it is imperative that nonmedical professionals working with mentally retarded persons have some knowledge of behavioral pharmacology, the field of study that investigates how pharmacological agents affect behavior.

This chapter reviews how drug therapy is used to ameliorate behavior problems of mentally retarded persons, with a special emphasis on recent research. The following topics are covered: prevalence and patterns of drug use; issues in evaluating the effects of pharmacotherapy; research involving the five major drug classes (neuroleptics, antidepressants and antimanics, anxiolytics, stimulants, and antiepileptics), with novel psychoactive agents, and with minerals, diets, and vitamins; and, an analysis of current issues in the field. Where appropriate, readers are referred to previous reviews for information not covered in this chapter.

Prevalence and Patterns of Drug Use

Since the first study by Lipman (1970), there have been several surveys of psychotropic use by institutionalized and noninstitutionalized mentally retarded persons. As these studies have been reviewed recently by Gadow (1986) and Aman and Singh (1988a), only a brief summary of the findings is presented here.

Institutions

Reported use of psychotropic drugs in institutions for mentally retarded individuals range from a low of 19% to a high of 86%, with most surveys reporting between about 30% and 50%. Antiepileptic medication use ranges from a low of 24% to a high of 56%, although it is typically between 25% and 45%. Overall, the institutional use of psychotropic and antiepileptic medication ranges from 50% to 70%, with some residents being prescribed both types simultaneously.

Individuals in the Community

Few studies have surveyed the medication of mentally retarded persons residing in the community. For children, the reported use of psychotropic drugs ranges from 2% to 7%, while for adults, the range is 14% to 36% (see Aman & Singh, 1988a). The prevalence of antiepileptic medication is between 12% and 31% for children and 18% and 24% for adults. Combined, the prevalence of psychotropic and antiepileptic medication is between 18% and 33% for children and 36% and 48% for adults.

In a recent study, Fox and Westling (1986) reported on the drugs used by 92 profoundly mentally handicapped children and young adults in one school district. They found that 54% were on medication; 45% on antiepileptics, 3% on major tranquilizers, 5% on minor tranquilizers, and 9% on other medication, with some being on more than one drug. Of note was the high percentage of subjects on antiepileptics compared to that reported in other studies. In particular, Gadow and Kalachnik (1981) reported a figure of only 12% with moderately mentally retarded children. However, it is likely that the difference was due to the level of retardation of the subjects in the two studies, since the probability of seizures tends to increase with the degree of retardation.

Factors Influencing Drug Use

A number of factors have been found to influence drug use by mentally retarded persons. Gender has been implicated in two studies (Tu & Smith, 1979, 1983), where drug prevalence was higher among institutionalized females. However, this finding was not reported in other surveys (Aman, Field, & Bridgman, 1985; Hill, Balow, & Bruininks, 1985; Intagliata & Rinck, 1985). The amount of medication has been found to correlate highly with increasing age and intellectual impairment (Aman et al., 1985; Hill et al., 1985). A strong relationship has also been reported between the type of residential facility and the use of psychotropic medication (Aman et al., 1985; Martin & Agran, 1985). More medication was prescribed in larger facilities and in those where the residents had very restrictive environments. Finally, as would be expected, several studies have reported a strong positive correlation between the amount and the degree of the subjects' behavioral and psychiatric problems and the use of medication (Intagliata & Rinck, 1985; Tu & Smith, 1983; Zimmerman & Heistad, 1981). The problems most frequently treated with drugs included aggression, hyperactivity, self-injury, excitability, screaming, and anxiety.

Since treatment in residential facilities is governed largely by medical staff (physicians and senior nurses), it is not surprising that behavior problems are often treated with medication (Aman, Singh, & Fitzpatrick, 1987; Aman, Singh, & White, 1987). Whether such treatment is appropriate or is applied appropriately is questionable. In the only study investigating this problem throughout an institution, Bates, Smeltzer, and Arnoczky (1986) examined the medication prescribed for the psychiatric problems of 242 residents whose psychiatric diagnosis had been assigned unanimously by a multidisciplinary team. Bates et al. reported that only 45% of the diagnosis-medication combination was found to be appropriate. This suggests that for a substantial number of residents in many institutions the prescribed medication may be inappropriate for their diagnosis.

In a single-subject study, Singh and Winton (1984) carried out detailed observations of the self-injurious behavior of a profoundly mentally retarded boy who was given pharmacological treatment. The clinical effectiveness of various doses of carbamazepine, thioridazine, and chlorpromazine prescribed by the boy's ward physician was assessed. Their data showed that decisions to change drug prescriptions were often not based on related changes in the target behavior. Although this is the only study to examine clinical decision making in terms of pharmacological intervention with the mentally retarded population, it does suggest that some residents may be on inappropriate medication for behavior problems.

Reducing the Use of Medication

The high prevalence figures and the reported side effects of drugs have resulted in calls to use less medication with mentally retarded persons. Several programs in which active steps were taken to reduce the general use of psychotropic drugs have been reported in the literature (e.g., Berchou, 1982; Briggs, Hamad, Garrard, & Wills, 1985; Inoue, 1982; James, 1983; LaMendola, Zaharia, & Carver, 1980). Other studies have reported reductions in the use of certain classes of drugs (e.g., neuroleptics), ranging from 18% (Ellenor & Frisk, 1977) to 57% (Fielding, Murphy, Reagan, & Peterson, 1980). Prevalence rates substantially declined to between 21% and 33% in institutions where such drug reduction programs were instituted (Inoue, 1982; LaMendola et al., 1980). These figures are well below the 50% to 70% discussed above.

Evaluating the Effects of Pharmacotherapy

There are several basic requirements for a drug study to be scientifically valid. Sprague and Werry (1971) proposed six minimal requirements, namely: having appropriate control groups, randomly assigning subjects to treatments, providing placebo and double-blind evaluations to minimize rater bias, standardizing measures of drug effects, doing adequate statistical analyses, and using standardized doses. Reviews of the drug literature show that few studies prior to 1980 included all or even most of these controls (Aman & Singh, 1980, 1983).

Additional requirements have been suggested by other investigators. Marholin and Phillips (1976) suggested that a drug's effects on appropriate social and adaptive behaviors should also be assessed since a targeted inappropriate behavior may be reduced due to behavior being generally suppressed rather than due to any specific therapeutic effect. We concur with this recommendation but suggest monitoring several collateral behaviors, both positive and negative, since a drug may affect untargeted maladaptive behaviors as well as prosocial and adaptive behaviors. Sprague and Baxley (1978) have suggested that drug treatment should regularly be compared with some alternative type of therapy. This takes into account the fact that most drugs are prescribed for behavior disorders for which proven alternative therapies are available. Aman and Singh (1980) have suggested that during any drug evaluation other contemporaneous drug treatments be discontinued so that the effects of the different drugs are not confounded. In reviewing research on the effects of thioridazine on childhood disorders, they found that in several studies patients had been receiving other medication simultaneously.

Singh and Beale (1986) have described behavioral assessment procedures that are suitable for use in psychopharmacological research with individual subjects. They noted that the basic principles of behavioral assessment used in applied behavior analysis generally hold for single-subject drug studies (e.g., data collection, interobserver agreement). They also discussed considerations that particularly pertain to drug studies, including phase lengths, the timing of observations, and single- and double-blind control conditions.

Barlow and Hersen (1984) and Singh and Beale (1986) have discussed a number of experimental designs that are appropriate for use in single-subject drug studies. These include several variants of the withdrawal (A-B-A-B) design, the multiple-baseline design, and the alternating treatments design. Both withdrawal and multiple-baseline designs can be used to assess the effects of a single drug relative to either a placebo or baseline (Ayllon, Layman, & Kandel, 1975; Wulbert & Dries, 1977), the relative effects of two different drugs or two doses of the same drug (e.g., Shafto & Sulzbacher, 1977), or the differential effects of pharmacotherapy and alternative therapies, such as behavior therapy (e.g., Rapport, Murphy, & Bailey, 1982; Wells, Conners, Imber, & Delamater, 1981). In addition, the multiple-baseline design can be used to measure the relative effects of different doses of the same drug. For example, Millichamp and Singh (1987) used a multiple-baseline-across-subjects design to assess the effects of intermittent drug therapy on the behavior of profoundly mentally retarded persons.

The alternating treatments design allows comparison of the effects of either two fast-acting drugs (e.g., stimulants), or a fast-acting drug versus a nondrug procedure. This design cannot be used with two drugs that have long-lasting effects (e.g., antipsychotics, antiepileptics) because of a possible carryover of the effects. However, the effects of behavior modification and a drug of this sort combined can be compared with those of the drug alone. For example, Singh and Falconer (1986) used an alternating treatments design to test the relative effects of a neuroleptic (thioridazine) alone and in combination with a visual screening procedure.

As is usual in applied behavior analysis studies, data from single-subject drug studies may be analyzed visually. This is acceptable if the differences in behavior between phases (conditions) are clear and unobscured by variability within each phase. If there are trends across phases or great variability within phases, visual analysis may need to be supported by inferential statistical analysis. With A-B-A-B designs, a time-series analysis can be used if there are a sufficient number of data points available (Hartmann et al., 1980; Tryon, 1982). With multiple-baseline designs that have four or more levels, the R_n statistic (Revusky, 1967) can be used. For alternating treatments designs, treatment effects can be assessed using randomization tests (Kratochwill & Levin, 1980).

Effects of Drugs on Behavior

Over the last 15 years a great deal has been published on the use of drugs with developmentally disabled individuals, particularly with persons with mental retardation. Most studies carried out before 1980 were methodologically flawed to such an extent that their results are scientifically uninterpretable. Several excellent reviews of this earlier work are already available (e.g., Aman, 1983; Aman & Singh, 1983, 1988; Sprague & Baxley, 1978; Sprague & Werry, 1971), so the following section reviews only recent research. The older material is referred to only to illustrate a particular point.

Neuroleptics

In the authors' view, there is no compelling rationale for using neuroleptics with mentally retarded persons. Its current use appears to be based on an apparent similarity between the behavior of persons who are mentally ill and those who are mentally retarded. Problem behaviors common to both groups include motor and verbal stereotypy, self-stimulation, self-injury, isolation, and a lack of self-care. Neuroleptics, in particular chlorpromazine (Thorazine), have been reasonably effective with many of these behaviors in schizophrenic or other psychotic individuals. However, topographically similar behaviors in both populations are not necessarily controlled by the same factors or affected by a given treatment in the same way. Until proven otherwise, it is prudent to question whether the etiologies of the behaviors are the same in the two populations or, even if they are, whether the model of drug action in one population is equally applicable to the other.

   The continued use of neuroleptics with mentally retarded individuals, particularly those in institutions or other residential care facilities, may be based on their presumed efficacy or folklore (see Aman & Singh, 1980) or their nonselective sedative effects. This is not to say that neuroleptics do not have a beneficial effect on some mentally retarded persons, but rather that, at present, no adequate biochemical explanation of the beneficial actions of these drugs with this population has been postulated.

PREVALENCE

Earlier surveys showed that about 40% to 50% of institutionalized mentally retarded residents received neuroleptic drugs. Recent trends to decrease the use of medication have produced a considerable decline in these figures. For example, in a national study of prescribed drugs in institutions and community residential facilities (Hill et al., 1985), it was found that only 30% of institutionalized retarded persons were on neuroleptics. In community residential facilities, the prevalence of neuroleptic use is typically lower (e.g., 29% [Intagliata & Rinck, 1985], 21% [Hill et al., 1985], and 11% in adults and 2% in school children [Aman et al., 1985]).

THERAPEUTIC EFFECTS

Schroeder (1988) has stated, "the modern era of pharmacotherapy was ushered in by Aman and Singh's (1980) review of the effectiveness of thioridazine, the most frequently used neuroleptic in mental retardation" (p. 88). Aman and Singh (1980) had noted that there were few methodologically rigorous studies that shed light on how thioridazine affects behavior of mentally retarded children. Since then there have been a number of studies on the effects of neuroleptic drugs with this population. Many of these were conducted by Stephen Breuning and his colleagues, but these will not be discussed since allegations of scientific fraud have been made regarding these studies (see Holden, 1987), and the data reported in them may not be accurate (see Ferguson, Cullari, & Gadow, 1987; Gadow, 1987; Gualtieri, 1987; Sprague, 1987). For a critique of some of these studies, the interested reader is referred to a paper by Aman and Singh (1986).

The three main neuroleptics used with mentally retarded persons are thioridazine (Mellaril), chlorpromazine (Thorazine), and haloperidol (Haldol).

THIORIDAZINE

While the early studies suggested that the behavior of mentally retarded children generally improved while on this drug, no clear drug-related changes were documented. Studies that attempted to measure specific changes in behavior reported improvements in hyperactivity, aggression, eating, and stereotypy (see Aman & Singh, 1980).

Two drug-withdrawal studies (Heistad, Zimmerman, & Doebler, 1982; Schroeder & Gualtieri, 1985) and three prospective studies (Jakab, 1984; Menolascino, Ruedrich, Golden, & Wilson, 1985; Singh & Aman, 1981) have been reported over the last 5 years. Heistad et al. (1982) conducted a short (4 to 5 weeks) double-blind, crossover, placebo-controlled study of thioridazine in 106 residents. Although there was a nonsignificant reduction in positive behaviors under the placebo condition, the main effect was an 18% increase in self-stimulation when the residents were taken off thioridazine. No neuroleptic withdrawal symptoms (e.g., involuntary movements) were reported, although the authors suggested that this may have been due to the inexperience of the raters.

Schroeder and Gualtieri (1985) withdrew the drugs of 23 profoundly retarded patients (2 on haloperidol and 21 on thioridazine) either abruptly or gradually in a placebo-controlled, double-blind, crossover design. This produced complex interactive effects on the subjects' behaviors, depending on such variables as setting, staff reactions to the subjects, and the presence of tardive dyskinesia. Overall, the subjects displayed quite individual responses ranging from improvement to serious deterioration of target behaviors.

Singh and Aman (1981) carried out a dose-response study of thioridazine on 19 severely or profoundly retarded residents. All subjects received a mean titrated dose that they had previously been on (5.23 mg/kg), a standardized dose of 2.5 mg/kg, and a placebo in a double-blind crossover design. Hyperactivity, bizarre and stereotyped behavior decreased under both dosages, but cognitive behaviors were not affected. No differential effects of the two doses occurred.

In another prospective study, Jakab (1984) compared the short-term effects of thioridazine tablets versus thioridazine in suspension on a range of behaviors of emotionally disturbed, mentally retarded children. Observations were taken in two settings (structured activity and free play) in the classroom before and after medication was administered. A placebo condition was not included. Results showed that both forms of thioridazine were effective in reducing aggression, tantrums, self-injury, pica, and stereotyped self-stimulation.

Finally, in a methodologically weak study (no placebo or double-blind conditions, no interrater reliability), Menolascino et al. (1985) evaluated the comparative effects of thiothixene and thioridazine on 61 retarded and nonretarded schizophrenics. The subjects showed considerable improvement under both drugs on the Brief Psychiatric Rating Scale but not on a number of other rating scales. It is difficult to fully interpret the findings of this study due to the methodological problems.

CHLORPROMAZINE

Uncontrolled studies of chlorpromazine suggest that it may be effective in reducing maladaptive behaviors in mentally retarded children. However, as shown in a recent review (Aman, 1984), well-controlled studies suggest that chlorpromazine may actually reduce some appropriate behaviors. In the only controlled study published in the last 5 years, Aman, White, and Field (1984) evaluated the effects of chlorpromazine on the stereotyped and adaptive behaviors of six profoundly retarded residents in a placebo-controlled, crossover study. Stereotypy (body rocking) was reduced in the wards, but no other behavioral changes were observed. Chlorpromazine also impaired the performance of most subjects on an operant lever-pulling task. The authors suggested that chlorpromazine may have a selective effect on stereotypy in the mentally retarded population.

HALOPERIDOL

With the exception of a study by Aman, Teehan, White, Turbott, and Vaithiana-than (in press), no recent study of haloperidol has been conducted with mentally retarded individuals. Uncontrolled studies suggest that haloperidol may be effective in controlling hyperactive, aggressive, hostile, and impulsive behaviors (Sprague & Baxley, 1978). However, no data are available from methodologically sound studies to support this view.

Aman, Teehan, et al. (in press) conducted a double-blind, placebo-controlled, crossover dose-response (0.025 mg/kg, 0.05 mg/kg/day) study of haloperidol with 20 mentally retarded residents. Reinforced instruction improved under the drug conditions and gross motor activity increased at the high dosage. Stereotypy was significantly reduced at the high dose, especially in subjects with initially high rates.

In summary, it is clear that most of the recent research on neuroleptics has been directed at thioridazine, a drug that shows the most promise in the treatment of certain behavioral problems of mentally retarded persons. Other than the work of Aman and his colleagues, virtually nothing has been done with the other two major neuroleptics. Obviously, much more research with neuroleptics is needed before their effects on this population can be established. As has been pointed out elsewhere (Aman & Singh, 1983), neuroleptics have a role to play in the management of severe behavior problems of mentally retarded persons. However, our current attempts at neuroleptic treatment with this population are based more on trial and error than established knowledge.

SIDE EFFECTS

The antipsychotics have a number of serious side effects, including: 1) anticholinergic effects—dry mouth, constipation, urinary retention, blurred vision, meiosis, reduced gastric motility, mental confusion, and tachycardia; 2)alpha adrenergic blockade—postural hypotension, mydriasis, and flushing of the skin; and 3) dopaminergic—acute dystonia, akathesia, and tardive dyskinesia. For further discussion see Werry (1982).

Antidepressants and Antimanic Drugs

The two major subgroups of antidepressants are the monoamine oxidase inhibitors (MAOI) and the tri- and quadricyclics. The MAOIs are not considered proven treatments for any childhood psychiatric illness (Rapoport & Mikkelsen, 1978) and are seldom, if ever, used in pediatric pharmacotherapy. They appear to be of some use for treating narcolepsy and hypertension and there is some suggestion that they may be useful in treating severe phobic disturbances in children. There is no indication for their use with mentally retarded children. The main rationale for the use of tri- and quadricyclics is to treat severe depression in adults. Since there are indications that mentally retarded children also suffer from severe and chronic depression (see Matson & Barrett, 1982), it is likely that the same rationale is used for prescribing antidepressants in this population.

Of the antimanics, lithium is the only drug that is important in the treatment of childhood disorders. It is used mainly for affective disorders although it is purported to reduce aggression, hyperactivity, and conduct disorders in mentally retarded children (Aman & Singh, 1983).

PREVALENCE

Antidepressants are not widely used with mentally retarded persons. About 1% to 4% of institutionalized mentally retarded persons are prescribed antidepressants (Hill et al., 1985; Lipman, 1970), although it is not always clear whether these are given to treat depression or some other disorder (e.g., enuresis, conduct problems). The figures for community samples range from about 1% to 6% (Aman et al., 1985; Hill et al., 1985; Intagliata & Rinck, 1985; Martin & Agran, 1985).

The antimanics are not widely used in either residential or community settings. For both settings the figures are less than 1% (Hill et al., 1985; Intagliata & Rinck, 1985), except for the 8% reported in one community-based setting (Martin & Agran, 1985).

THERAPEUTIC EFFECTS

According to Gualtieri and Hawk (1982), "the only unequivocal indication for the use of tricyclic antidepressants in the mentally retarded is unipolar depression" (p. 231). With the exception of two recent studies (Aman, White, Vaithianathan, & Teehan, 1986; Field, Aman, White, & Vaithianathan, 1986), all other studies of antidepressant treatment with mentally retarded persons were carried out prior to 1967 (see Aman & Singh, 1983 for a review). These studies were methodologically weak and no general conclusions can be drawn from them.

Antidepressants have been used to control a number of behavior disorders in mentally retarded children, such as hyperkinetic and aggressive behaviors, but there are no empirical data from well-controlled studies to show that they are indeed effective. In nonretarded children, antidepressants have been used to treat enuresis and, while these drugs do not provide a cure, they certainly suppress bed wetting to some degree in most children (Blackwell & Currah, 1973). The evidence for such an effect in mentally retarded persons is mixed, although there is no obvious reason why their reaction should be any different from that of their nonretarded peers.

It is likely that antidepressants are underutilized with mentally retarded individuals because of problems associated with the diagnosis of affective disorders in this population. Certainly, as Sovner and Hurley (1983) have reported, mentally retarded persons appear to suffer the full range of affective disorders and, in the absence of other proven treatments, especially with severely and profoundly retarded individuals, it is imperative that the effects of antidepressants be evaluated.

Of the antimanics, lithium appears to be the drug of choice for mentally retarded persons who have bipolar or recurrent unipolar depression and whose aggressive, assaultive, and destructive behaviors cannot be controlled by other means. The empirical literature on the effects of lithium is not as robust as one would hope, since the majority of the data are derived from clinical case studies or uncontrolled investigations.

Several case studies have been reported that suggest that manic-depressive mentally retarded persons who do not respond to neuroleptics may in fact show a good response to lithium (Hasan & Mooney, 1979; Kelly, Koch, & Buegel, 1976; Reid & Leonard, 1977). In a partially controlled study, Rivinus and Harmataz (1979) reported a substantial reduction in manic-depressive symptoms in five patients given lithium. Finally, in a placebo-controlled study Naylor, Donald, Le Poidevin, and Reid (1974) reported a study of 14 mentally retarded patients who had mood swings or recurrent behavioral changes. Their results indicated that these symptoms decreased while the patients were on lithium.

A number of case studies indicate that lithium may reduce aggressive, assaultive, and destructive behaviors in mentally retarded persons (e.g., Cooper & Fowlie, 1973; Dostal & Zvolsky, 1970; Goetze, Grunberg, & Berkowitz, 1977; Lion, Hill, & Madden, 1975; Micev & Lynch, 1974; Mullerova, Novotna, Rehan, & Skula, 1974). In the only controlled trial of lithium's effects on aggressive behavior, it was reported that of the six patients, three improved, two showed no change, and one worsened (Worrall, Moody, & Naylor, 1975). However, the positive effects may have been an artifact of the method of analysis used in this study (see Aman, 1983). Although the data are not conclusive, Tyrer, Walsh, Edwards, Berney, and Stephens (1984) have suggested that the following factors may be good predictors of a positive response to lithium by aggressive mentally retarded persons: female sex, overactivity, stereotypy, epilepsy, and a pretreatment rate of less than one aggressive episode per week. Furthermore, they suggest that lithium may not be effective with socially withdrawn males who have frequent aggressive outbursts.

Overall, there appears to be some indications for using lithium with mentally retarded persons, especially those with bipolar and recurrent unipolar depression. The data supporting its efficacy in controlling behavior problems are weak and need empirical verification. Given the adverse side effects of lithium (e.g., nephrotoxicity) and the absence of proven predictors of the drug's response in mentally retarded persons, one should be very cautious in its use.

SIDE EFFECTS

Antidepressants may have the following side effects: dry mouth, constipation, urinary retention, blurred vision, and mental confusion. Tricyclic antidepressants may also precipitate postural hypotension and tachycardia. The side effects of lithium include CNS confusional state, which occurs at serum levels around and above 1.5 mEq/l, and may include tremor, ataxia, sluggishness, and coma. Mild side effects may occur at therapeutic serum levels, the most common being gastrointestinal irritability. Finally, lithium may lead to renal and nephron toxicity (see Rapoport, Mikkelsen, & Werry, 1978 for further details).

Anxiolytics

Anxiolytics are used to treat a number of chronic conditions in nonretarded adults (e.g., insomnia, night terrors, mild anxiety) and sleep disorders and nonpsychotic anxiety in children. In the mentally retarded population, anxiolytics are often used to sedate patients with behavior problems.

PREVALENCE

Lipman's (1970) survey showed that anxiolytics (chlordiazepoxide and diazepam) were prescribed to about 8% of institutionalized mentally retarded residents, although more recent surveys report slightly higher figures: 9.4% (Intagliata & Rinck, 1985) and 12.7% (Hill et al., 1985). Prevalence in community settings ranges from about 2% to 12% (Aman et al., 1985; Fox & Westling, 1986; Hill et al., 1985; Intagliata & Rinck, 1985; Martin & Agran, 1985). Whether these drugs were employed as sedatives or antiepileptics (e.g., diazepam) or for behavioral control cannot be determined from the prevalence studies.

THERAPEUTIC EFFECTS

Only a handful of studies have investigated the effects of anxiolytics with mentally retarded patients. Of these, the best data are derived from studies of the benzodiazepines. Two uncontrolled studies (Krakowski, 1963; Pilkington, 1961) reported positive effects of chlordiazepoxide but these were based on clinical impressions. In a double-blind study that also utilized clinical impressions to measure behavior change (Zrull, Westman, Arthur, & Bell, 1963), no changes due to chlordiazepoxide were reported. In one of the better controlled studies (La Veck & Buckley, 1961), chlordiazepoxide actually increased undesirable behavior.

Two studies investigated the effects of diazepam on the behavior of mentally retarded persons, with one (Galambos, 1965) an uncontrolled study reporting positive results and the other (Zrull, Westman, Arthur, & Rice, 1964) a controlled study reporting no change. In a well-controlled study, Walters, Singh, and Beale (1977) found that mentally retarded children's hyperactive behavior worsened on lorazepam while inappropriate and inactive behaviors remained unchanged. In no controlled studies has any of the other anxiolytics shown much promise with mentally retarded persons.

In summary, it is clear that, while drugs of this class are used frequently in both institutional and community settings, there is a dearth of controlled studies on their efficacy with mentally retarded persons. The best controlled studies that are available (e.g., La Veck & Buckley, 1961; Walters et al., 1977; Zrull et al., 1964) indicate that at least the benzodiazepines (chlordiazepoxide, diazepam, and lorazepam) are contraindicated for this population. However, this conclusion is based on limited data, so further research is obviously warranted with this drug.

SIDE EFFECTS

Anxiolytics appear to produce few side effects in children other than sedative effects (i.e., drowsiness, disinhibition, and incoordination). However, there is some risk that psychological and physical dependence may develop with prolonged use (see Rapoport et al., 1978).

Stimulants

Stimulants are used primarily for the symptomatic management of children diagnosed as having attention deficit disorder with hyperactivity. Currently there are virtually no predictors of stimulant drug response in children, although there is a weak relationship between drug response and the degree of attention disorder (Barkley, 1976; Werry, 1982). Mentally retarded children often exhibit behaviors similar to those in children with attention deficit disorder with hyperactivity (e.g., short attention span, aggression directed at peers, impulsivity, and restlessness). It is likely that stimulants are prescribed for them on the basis of this similarity in behavior.

PREVALENCE

Stimulants are not widely used with mentally retarded persons. In Lipman's (1970) survey, less than 3% of institutionalized mentally retarded persons were prescribed drugs from this class. More recent surveys have reported even lower figures: 0.4% (Hill et al., 1985) and 1.2% (Intagliata & Rinck, 1985). Similar figures have been reported from community surveys: 0.3% (Intagliata & Rinck, 1985) and 1.0% (Hill et al., 1985). However, higher prevalence figures have been reported for mildly (5.5%) and moderately (3.4%) mentally retarded children attending public schools in Illinois (Gadow, 1985).

THERAPEUTIC EFFECTS

Aman (1983) has extensively reviewed studies published prior to 1982 where stimulant drugs were used with mentally retarded children. Most of these studies used double-blind, placebo-controlled designs and were methodologically adequate. With a few exceptions, they showed largely negative drug responses (but see Gadow, 1985 for another view). Aman concluded that "there is currently no compelling proof that the stimulants have a major role to play in the treatment of the mentally retarded" (pp. 485–486).

Two studies using stimulants have been published since Aman's (1983) review. Aman and Singh (1982) conducted a study with 28, 13- to 26-year-old severely retarded residents and reported no effects from using methylphenidate. Varley and Trupin (1982) conducted the other study with 10, 4- to 15-year-old mildly retarded hyperactive children from a public school and reported positive effects from the same drug. If this is a reliable and replicable finding, then it is likely that stimulants may be effective with young, mildly retarded children who do not have serious behavior problems (e.g., stereotypy). In addition, it may be that only hyperactive mentally retarded children and not the majority of the mentally retarded population are responsive to stimulant treatment.

SIDE EFFECTS

If the dosage does not exceed 1 mg/kg/day, then there are few, if any, long-term side effects. Larger doses may result in weight loss and growth retardation. Other side effects may be seen in the very early stages of treatment, but these are benign and quickly disappear. These are dose dependent and may include insomnia, toxic psychoses of the amphetamine type, choreiform-type movements, stomach-aches, and weepiness (Cantwell & Carlson, 1978).

Antiepileptics (Anticonvulsants)

Although antiepileptics are used primarily to control seizures, these drugs also have cognitive and behavioral effects (Stores, 1978). It has been estimated that the prevalence of epilepsy among mentally retarded persons is about 23% for the mildly/moderately retarded, 28% for the severely retarded, and almost 50% for the profoundly retarded (Corbett, Harris, & Robinson, 1975). Given these high rates, it is important that the effects of drugs used to control it are thoroughly investigated. An added reason is that antiepileptics are also used to control certain behavior problems of mentally retarded children, especially "those marked by episodic, violent outbursts of emotional, disruptive, or aggressive behavior" (Werry, 1982, p. 313).

PREVALENCE

Older surveys indicate that between 24% and 30% of institutionalized retarded persons were prescribed antiepileptics. In recent surveys, the rate has increased to between 36% and 42% (see Hill et al., 1985; Intagliata & Rinck, 1985). This is probably a result of there being an increasing proportion of profoundly retarded persons in institutions, since community integration is being initially undertaken with those who are less retarded. The prevalence figures in community samples vary over a wide range, and again it is likely that this range can be explained largely in terms of different levels of retardation. Two studies reported a figure of about 21% (Hill et al., 1985; Intagliata & Rinck, 1985), and another two between 45% and 48% (Fox & Westling, 1986; Martin & Agran, 1985).

THERAPEUTIC EFFECTS

The literature on the effects of antiepileptics has been reviewed extensively elsewhere (Aman, 1983; Gadow, 1986; Schain, 1983; Stores, 1978; Trimble, 1981) and, since no major advances have been made over the last few years, little time will be spent on it here. Briefly, the literature indicates that antiepileptics are used for both their seizure-controlling properties and for their psychotropic effects. Although there are data clearly showing their efficacy in controlling seizures, data showing direct psychotropic effects in terms of controlling behavior problems are meager and equivocal (Trimble & Reynolds, 1976). The whole area is in great need of further investigation.

SIDE EFFECTS

At high doses (blood levels), toxic effects such as tremor, blurring of vision, slurring of speech, drowsiness, mental confusion and uncoordination may result. Since a number of these side effects are very similar to the usual behavior of some severely and profoundly retarded persons, it is imperative that physicians and direct-care staff are vigilant about looking out for them. Periodic serum assays and neurological assessment are recommended for such cases.

Novel Psychoactive Agents

A number of novel psychoactive agents have been evaluated with mentally retarded and autistic patients. The rationale for their use has been the discovery of biochemical abnormalities associated with cognitive, behavioral, or motor problems in such patients that may be amenable to treatment through drugs.

FENFLURAMINE

It has been hypothesized that elevated levels of serotonin, a neurotransmitter, may be a causal factor in certain behavioral, cognitive, and motor problems in children (Campbell, Perry, Small, & Green, 1987). Since about 30% of autistic children have been found to have high serotonin levels (Ritvo et al., 1970), it has been suggested that a powerful antiserotonergic drug, like fenfluramine, may be useful in treating these problems by decreasing the child's serotonin levels to within the normal range. This hypothesis was tested in an open trial by Geller, Ritvo, Freeman, and Yuwiler (1982), who reported increased IQ and decreased blood serotonin levels in three autistic children. This study provided the impetus for an 18-center investigation of the effects of this drug with autistic children. The basic protocol for the studies involved double-blind, placebo-controlled conditions (2-week open placebo baseline, 1 month on placebo, 4 months on fenfluramine, and 2 months on placebo), with the dose of fenfluramine being 1.5 mg/kg/day for all subjects. Several measures were taken periodically including behavioral ratings, IQ, weight, and serotonin levels. Pooled data from 9 of the 18 centers, involving 81 autistic persons ranging in age from 2 to 24 years, have shown that about a third of them were strong drug responders (Ritvo et al., 1986). Positive results were also reported in an independent, open pilot study (Campbell et al., 1986), but this study had a number of methodological flaws.

Overall, the results of these studies are very encouraging but further work is required to establish the utility of this drug. Particularly important would be to find predictor variables of drug response other than just the level of blood serotonin. Readers interested in the general area of drug treatment of autism should consult the excellent overview by Campbell et al. (1987).

OPIATE ANTAGONISTS

Some recent studies suggest that opiate antagonists may provide an effective treatment for self-injury in developmentally disabled persons on the basis of the purported role of endogenous opioids in the regulation of pain (see Coid, Allolio, & Rees, 1983; Deutsch, 1986). Naloxone was reported to be effective in reducing self-injury in mentally retarded children in two studies (Richardson & Zaleski, 1983; Sandman et al., 1983), but not in two others (Beckwith, Couk, & Schumacher, 1986; Davidson, Kleene, Carrol, & Rockowitz, 1983). The efficacy of naltrexone for treating of self-injury has been investigated in only one study (Herman, Hammock, Arthur-Smith, Egan, Chatoor, Zelnick, & Boeckx, 1986), with two of three subjects showing a good response. Although current data on the efficacy of naloxone and naltrexone are mixed, there is enough theoretical interest in the pharmacological model of self-injury on which this treatment is based to warrant further investigation.

Several investigators have advanced the notion that abnormalities of the endogenous opioid system may be implicated in the behavioral and language problems often seen in autistic children (Panksepp & Sahley, 1987; Sandyk & Gillman, 1986). This means that opiate antagonists, such as naloxone and naltrexone, would be indicated to control such behaviors in this population. Two recent studies with autistic children (Campbell et al., 1988; Herman, Hammock, Arthur-Smith, Egan, Chatoor, Zelnick, Appelgate, & Boeckx, 1986) appear to support this suggestion. Decreases in stereotypies and increases in prosocial behaviors, including verbal behaviors, were reported. However, no clinically significant changes in their self-injurious behaviors were noted. Further controlled evaluations of the efficacy of opiate antagonists with this population are needed.

HYDROXYTRYPTOPHAN

There is equivocal evidence for the effectiveness of hydroxytryptophan (HTP) in certain childhood conditions. For example, 5-HTP has been used with trisomy-21 Down syndrome children in an effort to increase their platelet serotonin levels to normal levels (Pueschel, Reed, Cronk, & Goldstein, 1980; Weise, Koch, Shaw, & Rosenfeld, 1974). The usual finding has been that serotonin can be raised in some Down syndrome patients, but 5-HTP has little effect on their muscle tone, cognitive or adaptive functioning, developmental level, or social behavior.

A small number of investigators have used 5-HTP to treat self-injury in Lesch-Nyhan syndrome patients. In an uncontrolled study, Mizuno and Yugari (1975) administered L-5-HTP to four patients for 36 weeks and found that self-injury disappeared in all patients. Nyhan, Johnson, Kaufman, and Jones (1980) found that a combination of 5-HTP, carbidopa, and imipramine was effective in reducing self-injury in seven of nine Lesch-Nyhan patients, but tolerance developed within 3 months of initiating the drug regimen. The efficacy of 5-HTP in reducing self-injury in this population was not replicated in two other studies (Anderson, Hermann, & Dancis, 1976; Ciaranello, Anders, Barchas, Bergers, & Cann, 1976). As data on the efficacy of 5-HTP for treating self-injury in Lesch-Nyhan patients are limited further, systematic research appears to be in order.

PROPANOLOL

Propanolol, a β-adrenergic blocking agent, is usually prescribed for hypertension, angina pectoris, cardiac arrhythmias, and essential tremor, and is not really a drug for the treatment of psychiatric disorders. However, it has been found to effectively control violent and explosive behaviors in adult psychiatric patients (Ratey, Morrill, & Oxenkrug, 1983; Yudofsky, Williams, & Gorman, 1981). In the only study with mentally retarded patients, Ratey, et al. (1986) reported that, of 19 severely retarded patients given propanolol, 12 showed significant improvements in their aggressive and self-injurious behaviors, while another four showed moderate reductions in these behaviors. A low mean dose of 120 mg/day (range from 40 to 240 mg/day) was used, but seven patients exhibited side effects (hypotension and/or bradycardia) at 100 mg/day. The authors suggested that prolonged treatment on medication may have contributed to the therapeutic effects of propranolol at low doses. Although the findings of this study are encouraging, further research is needed to validate them.

Minerals, Diets, and Vitamins

The effect of minerals, diets, and vitamins on behavior has received considerable attention, both in the scientific and popular press. As several state-of-the-art papers summarizing what we currently know of this area with regard to the mentally retarded population have been published recently (e.g., Aman & Singh, 1988a; Singh, 1987; Waksman, 1983; Wender, 1986), only a general overview is presented here. Briefly, the literature indicates that a large number of different treatments have been used with this population at some time or other, including glutamic acid, celastrus paniculata, several vitamins, pituitary extract, sicca cell, and thyroid therapies. It can be stated with considerable confidence that controlled studies have generally reported negative outcomes with all of these substances (see Aman & Singh, 1988a).

Research data on glutamic acid (Astin & Ross, 1960), vitamin supplementation (Bronson GTC3 formula) (Harrell, Capp, Davis, Peerless, & Ravitz, 1981), and vitamin B_6 in autism (Rimland, 1973) provide, at best, equivocal support for their efficacy.

Although well-controlled studies have established that, at best, less than 5% of hyperactive children benefit from the Feingold diet (see Singh, 1987), the enthusiasm for it of some family physicians and parents has not diminished. At least two studies included mentally retarded children, but neither showed any effect of the diet (Harner & Foiles, 1980; Thorley, 1984). It is doubtful if the diet offers a viable alternative to other proven treatments for mentally retarded individuals.

Current Issues

At the recent NIMH-sponsored workshop on pharmacotherapy and mental retardation, Mouchka (1985) and Schroeder (1985) raised a number of issues regarding the pharmacological management of mentally retarded persons. The issue of people with dual diagnosis of mental illness (especially emotional disturbance) in addition to mental retardation (Reiss, Levitan, & Szyszko, 1982) received considerable attention. For a number of reasons that have been explored by both Mouchka (1985) and Schroeder (1985), these people appear to be not adequately served by either mental health or mental retardation facilities. This area is certainly in need of further study.

Schroeder (1985) also examined the need for better assessment instruments designed specifically for use with mentally retarded persons that would provide sensitive measures of change as a result of pharmacotherapy. He noted two instruments designed specifically for use with severely retarded individuals that had recently become available (see Aman & Singh, 1986; Matson, Kazdin, & Senatore, 1984). There appears to be a severe shortage of such instruments and it is imperative that this situation be rectified forthwith if we are to make real progress in assessing drug effects.

There are a number of other areas in need of research. Since some of them have been extensively reviewed or discussed elsewhere, they need not be repeated here. These include such important topics as withdrawal and tardive dyskinesias (Golden, 1988), measurement of drug blood levels in relation to behavioral outcome (Lewis & Mailman, 1988), and litigation and the use of drugs with persons with mental retardation (Beyer, 1988). In the remainder of this section, other areas are briefly reviewed.

Methodology

Since Sprague and Werry's (1971) seminal paper on the topic, the need for sound methodology has been a constant theme in the literature. The lack of methodological rigor in so many psychopharamacological studies with mentally retarded persons continues to be lamented even to the present day (see Aman & Singh, 1988). Certainly, some excellent experimental work has been done during the last 7 years, but far too many studies still do not meet the current requirements for well-controlled research. Also, a number of methodologically elegant studies published by Breuning and his colleagues in the early 1980s are, unfortunately, suspect (see Holden, 1987). While it is undoubtedly true that it can be difficult to achieve tight methodology in studies with mentally retarded persons, much more is possible than has hitherto been the case. Clearly, as researchers we have failed to heed the advice given 30 years ago by Greiner (1958), who said that if our aim is to help persons with mental retardation, we must "avoid the casual clinical trial of drugs. Make them good trials, or don't make them at all" (p. 347). There is simply no substitute for such good advice.

Effects on Learning

Given that the major problem of mentally retarded persons is one of learning, it is striking that there is precious little in the literature that indicates the effects drugs have on their learning, cognition, or work performance. Most drug studies with this population have focused on the effects on maladaptive behavior, and more recently, prosocial behavior. However, it is imperative that measures of other drug effects be incorporated in future studies. Several possibilities exist. One is for drug studies with mentally retarded school children to incorporate classroom measures, including observations of maladaptive and collateral behaviors and permanent product measures of academic performance. Drug studies with adults in workshops should include workshop performance measures (e.g., the number of work units completed in a given time). These measures should be included in studies in institutions as well. Experimental studies of drug effects should include a number of measures that have been found to discriminate between drug and no-drug conditions in other studies, both human and animal. These include operant paradigms, especially stimulus control paradigms (Heise, 1984; Heise & Milar, 1984), breadth of attention (Ullman, 1974), attention changes during discrimination learning (Singh & Beale, 1978), and incidental learning (Singh & Ahrens, 1978). As noted by Aman (1984), there is a paucity of studies on the effects of drugs on learning in this population and it behooves investigators to include at least some of these measures in all future studies.

Dosage Effects

Drugs may have differential effects on a given behavior or classes of behavior at different doses. Virtually all drug studies with mentally retarded persons have used a titrated dose, individualized for each subject, instead of a standardized dose based on body weight, blood level, or some other indicator. In the first dose-related study with mentally retarded persons, Singh and Aman (1981) reported that a low standardized dose of thioridazine was as effective as individualized doses given previously that had been determined by titration. Unfortunately, this remains one of the few dosage studies carried out with this population. Such studies are important if we are to prescribe the lowest dose to achieve a therapeutic effect for various behaviors.

Subject Sample

Gadow (1986) has astutely observed that "the study of psychopharmacotherapy in mentally retarded people is a science of institutions" (p. 144). Except for a handful of studies, all drug research has been carried out with institutionalized populations. When one considers that the overwhelming majority of mentally retarded persons reside in the community and not in institutions, it is apparent that the data from these studies must have limited generality. Various factors such as the institutional environment, philosophy of care, staffing ratios, and a host of other factors may affect the outcome of these drug studies. Hence it would be hazardous to infer from them that the results apply equally well to retarded people in the community. With the move toward community integration of retarded persons, the time is overdue for such studies to be carried out where the majority of our clients live.

A related issue is that we appear to have made little progress towards finding out what subject characteristics predict drug responses. As noted earlier, persons with high serotonin levels, such as some autistic children, may respond particularly well to drugs that normalize or reduce these levels. Also, recent developments of pharmacological models for treating self-injury have opened up a whole new area of research that will enable us to treat more appropriately subgroups of subjects with specific underlying neurochemical or psychiatric disorders (Gualtieri, Schroeder, Keppel, & Breese, 1986). It is only through such research that we will discover possible predictors of drug response for various subgroups of mentally retarded people.

Drugs and Alternative Treatments

In 1978, Sprague and Baxley argued that because of the potentially restrictive nature of pharmacotherapy, all drug treatments should be compared to some alternative treatment. With mentally retarded persons receiving medication for their behavior or psychiatric problems, the best alternative treatment is usually some form of behavior therapy, yet few investigators have directly compared these two therapies (Luiselli, 1986; Singh & Falconer, 1986). Recently, however, a number of studies have begun to investigate the combined effects of behavioral and pharmacological intervention for specific behavioral disorders. For example, the effects of combined treatment have been explored for such behaviors as self-injury (Durand, 1982; Luiselli, Evans, & Boyce, 1986), disruptive vocalizing (Luiselli & Evans, 1987), and stereotypic body rocking (Luiselli & Evans, 1987). This is an important area of research that should be explored more fully if we are to find the best possible interventions for mentally retarded persons with behavioral or psychiatric disorders. Readers interested in this area should consult Ackles (1986) and Schroeder, Lewis, and Lipton (1983) for a discussion of the rationale and methodology pertinent to pharmacological-behavioral treatment interactions and a comparison of the two treatments using either group or single-subject designs.

Conclusions

The experimental evidence attesting to the efficacy of pharmacological treatment of behavior disorders in the mentally retarded population is equivocal at best, with most studies lacking in methodological rigor. However, it is also clear that some patients do benefit from pharmacological treatment. What is needed is to search intensely for predictors of drug response that will assist clinicians in determining which patients will benefit the most from a particular treatment. It is only through systematic research that we will be able to advance our understanding of pharmacotherapy with mentally retarded persons to a point where clinicians will become comfortable in prescribing medication, knowing that the intervention will be effective.

Acknowledgments. Preparation of this chapter was supported by Grant G0068C3508 from the National Institute on Disability and Rehabilitation and Massey University (Psychology Department). We are grateful for the assistance provided by M. Winton Bell and the encouragement of Miki Winton and Judy Singh.

References

Ackles, P.A. (1986). Evaluating pharmacological-behavioral treatment interactions. In M. Hersen (Ed.), *Pharmacological and behavioral treatment interactions* (pp. 54–86). New York: Wiley.

Aman, M.G. (1983). Psychoactive drugs in mental retardation. In J.L. Matson & F. Andrasik (Eds.), *Treatment issues and innovations in mental retardation* (pp. 455–513). New York: Plenum Press.

Aman, M.G. (1984). Drugs and learning in mentally retarded persons. In G.D. Burrows & J.S. Werry (Eds.), *Advances in human psychopharmacology* (Vol. 3, pp. 121–163). Greenwich, CT: JAI Press.

Aman, M.G., Field, C.J., & Bridgman, G.D. (1985). City-wide survey of drug patterns among non-institutionalized retarded persons. *Applied Research in Mental Retardation*, 5, 159–171.

Aman, M.G., & Singh, N.N. (1980). The usefulness of thioridazine for treating childhood disorders: Fact or folklore? *American Journal of Mental Deficiency, 1980*, 331–338.

Aman, M.G., & Singh, N.N. (1982). Methylphenidate in severely retarded residents and the clinical significance of stereotypic behavior. *Applied Research in Mental Retardation*, 3, 345–358.

Aman, M.G., & Singh, N.N. (1983). Pharmacological intervention. In J.L. Matson, & J.A. Mulick (Eds.), *Handbook of mental retardation* (pp. 317–337). New York: Pergamon Press.

Aman, M.G., & Singh, N.N. (1986). A critical appraisal of recent drug research in mental retardation: The Coldwater studies. *Journal of Mental Deficiency Research, 30*, 331–338.

Aman, M.G., & Singh, N.N. (1988a). Introduction: Drug prevalence and patterns of drug use, programs to reduce medication use, measurement techniques, and future trends. In M.G. Aman & N.N. Singh (Eds.), *Psychopharmacology of the developmental disabilities* (pp. 1–28). New York: Springer-Verlag.

Aman, M.G., and Singh, N.N. (1988b). Vitamin, mineral, and dietary treatment. In M.G. Aman & N.N. Singh (Eds.). *Psychopharmacology of the developmental disabilities* (pp. 168–196). New York: Springer-Verlag.

Aman, M.G., Singh, N.N., & Fitzpatrick, J. (1987). The relationship between nurse characteristics and perceptions of psychotropic medications in residential facilities for the retarded. *Journal of Autism and Developmental Disorders, 17*, 511–523.

Aman, M.G., Singh, N.N., & White, A.J. (1987). Caregiver perceptions of psychotropic medication in residential facilities. *Research in Developmental Disabilities, 8*, 449–465.

Aman, M.G., Teehan, C.J., White, A.J., Turbott, S.H., & Vaithianathan, C. (in press). Haloperidol treatment with chronically medicated residents: Dose effects on clinical behavior and reinforcement contingencies. *American Journal of Mental Retardation.*

Aman, M.G., White, A.J., & Field, C.J. (1984). Chlorpromazine effects on stereotypic and conditioned behavior: A pilot study. *Journal of Mental Deficiency Research, 28*, 253–260.

Aman, M.G., White, A.J., Vaithianathan, C., & Teehan, C.J. (1986). Preliminary study of imipramine in profoundly retarded residents. *Journal of Autism and Developmental Disorders, 16*, 263–273.

Anderson, L.T., Hermann, L., & Dancis, J. (1976). The effects of L-5-hydroxytryptophan on self-mutilation in Lesch-Nyhan disease: A negative report. *Neuropaediatrie, 7*, 439–442.

Astin, A.W., & Ross, S. (1960). Glutamic acid and human intelligence. *Psychological Bulletin, 57*, 429–434.

Ayllon, T., Layman, D., & Kandel, H.J. (1975). A behavioral-educational alternative to drug control of hyperactive children. *Journal of Applied Behavior Analysis, 8*, 137–146.

Barkley, R.A. (1976). Predicting the response of hyperkinetic children to stimulant drugs: A review. *Journal of Abnormal Child Psychology, 4*, 327–348.

Barlow, D.H., & Hersen, M. (1984). *Single-case experimental designs* (2nd ed.). New York: Pergamon Press.

Bates, W.J., Smeltzer, D.J., & Arnoczky, S.M. (1986). Appropriate and inappropriate use of psychotherapeutic medications for institutionalized mentally retarded persons. *American Journal of Mental Deficiency, 90*, 363–370.

Beckwith, B.E., Couk, D.I., & Schumacher, K. (1986). Failure of naloxone to reduce self-injurious behavior in two developmentally disabled females. *Applied Research in Mental Retardation, 7*, 183–188.

Berchou, R.C. (1982). Effect of a consultant pharmacist on medication use in an institution for the mentally retarded. *American Journal of Hospital Pharmacy, 39*, 1671–1674.

Beyer, H.A. (1988). Litigation and the use of drugs in developmental disabilities. In M.G. Aman & N.N. Singh (Eds.), *Psychopharmacology of developmental disabilities.* New York: Springer-Verlag.

Blackwell, B., & Currah, J. (1973). The psychopharmacology of nocturnal enuresis. In I. Kolvin, R. McKeith, & S. Meadow (Eds.), *Bladder control and enuresis.* London: Heinemann.

Briggs, R., Hamad, C., Garrard, S., & Wills, F. (1985). A model for evaluating psychoactive medication use with mentally retarded persons. In J. Mulick & B. Mallany (Eds.), *Transitions in mental retardation: Advocacy, technology and science* (pp. 229–248). Norwood, NJ: Ablex.

Campbell, M., Perry, R., Polonsky, B.B., Deutsch, S.I., Palij, M., & Lukashok, D. (1986). An open study of fenfluramine in hospitalized young autistic children. *Journal of Autism and Developmental Disorders, 16*, 495–506.

Campbell, M., Perry, R., Small, A.M., & Green, W.H. (1987). Overview of drug treatment in autism. In E. Schopler & G.B. Mesibov (Eds.), *Neurobiological issues in autism* (pp. 341–356). New York: Plenum Press.

Campbell, M., Adams, P., Perry, R., Tesch, L., & Curren, E.L. (1988). Naltrexone in infantile autistim. *Psychopharmacology Bulletin, 24,* 135–139.

Cantwell, D.P., & Carlson, G.A. (1978). Stimulants. In J.S. Werry (Ed.), *Pediatric psychopharmacology* (pp. 171–207). New York: Brunner/Mazel.

Ciaranello, R.D., Anders, T.F., Barchas, J.D., Bergers, P.A., & Cann, H.M. (1976). The use of 5-hydroxytryptophan in a child with Lesch-Nyhan syndrome. *Child Psychiatry and Human Development, 7,* 127–133.

Coid, J., Allolio, B., & Rees, L.H. (1983). Raised plasma metenkephalin in patients who habitually mutilate themselves. *Lancet, 2,* 545–546.

Cooper, A.F., & Fowlie, H.C. (1973). Control of gross self-mutilation with lithium carbonate. *British Journal of Psychiatry, 22,* 370–371.

Corbett, J.A., Harris, R., & Robinson, R.G. (1975). Epilepsy. In J. Wortis (Ed.), *Mental retardation* (Vol. 3). New York: Brunner/Mazel.

Davidson, P.W., Kleene, B.M., Carrol, M., & Rockowitz, R.J. (1983). Effects of naloxone on self-injurious behavior: A case study. *Applied Research in Mental Retardation, 4,* 1–4.

Deutsch, S.I. (1986). Rationale for the administration of opiate antagonists in treating infantile autism. *American Journal of Mental Deficiency, 90,* 631–635.

Dostal, T., & Zvolsky, P. (1970). Antiaggressive effect of lithium salts in severe mentally retarded adolescents. *International Pharmacopsychiatry, 5,* 203–207.

Durand, V.M. (1982). A behavioral/pharmacological intervention for the treatment of self-injurious behavior. *Journal of Autism and Developmental Disorders, 12,* 243–251.

Ellenor, G.L., & Frisk, P.A. (1977). Pharmacist impact on drug use in an institution for the mentally retarded. *American Journal of Hospital Pharmacy, 34,* 604–608.

Ferguson, D.G., Cullari, S., & Gadow, K.D. (1987). Comment on the "Coldwater" studies. *Journal of Mental Deficiency Research, 31,* 219–222.

Field, D.J., Aman, M.G., White, A.J., & Vaithianathan, C. (1986). Single subject study of imipramine in a retarded woman with depressive symptoms. *Journal of Mental Deficiency Research, 30,* 191–198.

Fielding, L.T., Murphy, R.J., Reagan, M.W., & Peterson, T.L. (1980). An assessment program to reduce drug use with the mentally retarded. *Hospital and Community Psychiatry, 31,* 771–773.

Fox, L., & Westling, D.L. (1986). The prevalence of students who are profoundly mentally handicapped receiving medication in a school district. *Education and Training of the Mentally Retarded, 21,* 205–210.

Gadow, K.D. (1985). Prevalence and efficacy of stimulant drug use with mentally retarded children and youth. *Psychopharmacology Bulletin, 21,* 291–303.

Gadow, K.D. (1986). *Children on medication: Epilepsy, emotional disturbance, and adolescent disorders* (Vol. 2). San Diego: College-Hill Press.

Gadow, K.D. (1987). Comments on the community drug prevalence survey by Davis et al. (1982). *Journal of Mental Deficiency Research, 31,* 215–219.

Gadow, K.D., & Kalachnik, J. (1981). Prevalence and pattern of drug treatment for behavior and seizure disorder of TMR students. *American Journal of Mental Deficiency, 85,* 256–259.

Galambos, M. (1965). Long-term clinical trial with diazepam on adult mentally retarded persons. *Diseases of the Nervous System*, *26*, 305–309.

Geller, E., Ritvo, E.R., Freeman, B.J., & Yuwiler, A. (1982). Preliminary observations on the effects of fenfluramine on blood serotonin and symptoms in three autistic boys. *New England Journal of Medicine*, *307*, 165–169.

Goetze, U., Grunberg, R., & Berkowitz, B. (1977). Lithium carbonate in the management of hyperactive aggressive behavior of the mentally retarded. *Comprehensive Psychiatry*, *18*, 599–606.

Golden, G.S. (1988). Tardive dyskinesia and developmental disabilities. In M.G. Aman & N.N. Singh (Eds.), *Psychopharmacology of developmental disabilities*. New York: Springer-Verlag.

Greiner, T. (1958). Problems of methodology in research with drugs. *American Journal of Mental Deficiency*, *64*, 346–352.

Gualtieri, C.T. (1987). Letter to the editor. *Journal of Mental Deficiency Research*, *31*, 222–223.

Gualtieri, C.T., & Hawk, B. (1982). Antidepressant and antimanic drugs. In S.E. Breuning & A.D. Poling (Eds.), *Drugs and mental retardation* (pp. 215–234). Springfield, IL: Thomas.

Gualtieri, C.T., Schroeder, S.R., Keppel, J.M., & Breese, G.R. (1986). *Rational pharmacotherapy for self-injurious behavior: Testing the DI model*. Paper presented at the Gatlinburg Conference on Research and Theory in Mental Retardation and Developmental Disabilities.

Harner, I.C., & Foiles, R.A.L. (1980). Effect of Feingold's K-P diet on a residential mentally handicapped population. *Journal of the American Dietetic Association*, *76*, 575–580.

Harrell, R.F., Capp, R.H., Davis, D.R., Peerless, J., & Ravitz, L.R. (1981). Can nutritional supplements help mentally retarded children? An exploratory study. *Proceedings of the National Academy of Sciences*, *78*, 574–578.

Hartmann, D.P., Gottman, J.M., Jones, R.R., Gardner, W., Kazdin, A.E., & Vaught, R. (1980). Interrupted time-series analysis and its application to behavioral data. *Journal of Applied Behavior Analysis*, *13*, 543–559.

Hasan, M.K., & Mooney, R.P. (1979). Three cases of manic-depressive illness in mentally retarded adults. *American Journal of Psychiatry*, *36*, 1069–1071.

Heise, G.A. (1984). Behavioral methods for measuring effects of drugs on learning and memory in animals. *Medicinal Research Reviews*, *4*, 535–558.

Heise, G.A., & Milar, K.S. (1984). Drugs and stimulus control. In L.L. Iversen, S.D. Iversen, & S.H. Snyder (Eds.), *Handbook of psychopharmacology* (Vol. 18, pp. 129–190). New York: Plenum Press.

Heistad, G.T., Zimmerman, R.L., & Doebler, M.I. (1982). Long-term usefulness of thioridazine for institutionalized mentally retarded patients. *American Journal of Mental Deficiency*, *87*, 243–254.

Herman, B.H., Hammock, M.K., Arthur-Smith, A., Egan, J., Chatoor, I., Zelnick, N., & Boeckx, R.L. (1986). A biochemical role for opioid peptides in self-injurious behavior. *Scientific proceedings for the annual meeting of the American Academy of Child and Adolescent Psychiatry*, *2*, 29.

Herman, B.H., Hammock, M.K., Arthur-Smith, A., Egan, J., Chatoor, I., Zelnick, N., Appelgate, K., & Boeckx, R.L. (1986). Effects of naltrexone in autism: Correlation with plasma opioid concentrations. *Scientific proceedings for the annual meeting of the American Academy of Child and Adolescent Psychiatry*, *2*, 11–12.

Hill, B.K., Balow, E.A., & Bruininks, R.H. (1985). A national survey of prescribed drugs in institutions and community residential facilities for mentally retarded people. *Psychopharmacology Bulletin, 21*, 279–284.

Holden, C. (1987). NIMH finds a case of "serious misconduct." *Science, 235*, 1566–1567.

Inoue, F. (1982). A clinical pharmacy service to reduce psychotropic medication use in an institution for mentally handicapped persons. *Mental Retardation, 20*, 70–74.

Intagliata, J., & Rinck, C. (1985). Psychoactive drug use in public and community residential facilities for mentally retarded persons. *Psychopharmacology Bulletin, 21*, 268–278.

Jakab, I. (1984). Short-term effect of thioridazine tablets versus suspension on emotionally disturbed/retarded children. *Journal of Clinical Psychopharmacology, 4*, 210–215.

James, D.H. (1983). Monitoring drugs in hospitals for the mentally handicapped. *British Journal of Psychiatry, 142*, 163–165.

Kelly, J.T., Koch, M., & Buegel, D. (1976). Lithium carbonate in juvenile manic-depressive illness. *Diseases of the Nervous System, 37*, 90–92.

Krakowski, A.J. (1963). Chlordiazepoxide in the treatment of children with emotional disturbance. *New York State Journal of Medicine, 63*, 3388–3392.

Kratochwill, T.R., & Levin, J.R. (1980). On the applicability of various data analysis procedures to the simultaneous and alternating treatments designs in behavior therapy research. *Behavioral Assessment, 2*, 353–360.

LaMendola, W., Zaharia, E.S., & Carver, M. (1980). Reducing psychotropic drug use in an institution for the retarded. *Hospital and Community Psychiatry, 31*, 271–272.

La Veck, G.D., & Buckley, P. (1961). The use of psychopharmacological agents in retarded children with behavior disorders. *Journal of Chronic Disorders, 13*, 174–183.

Lewis, M.H., & Mailman, R.B. (1988). Drug blood levels: Measurement and relation to behavioral outcome in mentally retarded persons. In M.G. Aman & N.N. Singh (Eds.), *Psychopharmacology of developmental disabilities* (pp. 58–81). New York: Springer-Verlag.

Lion, J.R., Hill, J., & Madden, D.J. (1975). Lithium carbonate and aggression: A preliminary report. *Diseases of the Nervous System, 36*, 97–98.

Lipman, R.S. (1970). The use of psychopharmacological agents in residential facilities for the retarded. In F.J. Menolascino (Ed.), *Psychiatric approaches to mental retardation* (pp. 387–398). New York: Basic Books.

Luiselli, J.K. (1986). Behavior analysis of pharmacological and contingency management interventions for self-injury. *Journal of Behavior Therapy and Experimental Psychiatry, 17*, 275–284.

Luiselli, J.K., & Evans, T.P. (1987). Assessing pharmacological and contingency management interventions with mentally retarded adolescents in a residential treatment program. *Behavioral Residential Treatment, 2*, 139–152.

Luiselli, J.K., Evans, T.P., & Boyce, D.A. (1986). Pharmacological assessment and comprehensive behavioral intervention in a case of pediatric self-injury. *Journal of Clinical Child Psychology, 15*, 323–326.

Marholin, D. Jr., & Phillips, D. (1976). Methodological issues in psychopharmacological research. *American Journal of Orthopsychiatry, 46*, 477–495.

Martin, J.E., & Agran, M. (1985). Psychotropic and anticonvulsant drug use by mentally retarded adults across community residential and vocational placements. *Applied Research in Mental Retardation, 6*, 33–49.

Matson, J.L., & Barrett, R.P. (1982). *Psychopathology in the mentally retarded.* New York: Grune & Stratton.

Matson, J.L., Kazdin, A.E., & Senatore, V. (1984). Psychometric properties of the psychopathology instrument for mentally retarded adults. *Applied Research in Mental Retardation, 5,* 81–90.

Menolascino, F.J., Ruedrich, S.L., Golden, C.J., & Wilson, J.E. (1985). Diagnosis and pharmacotherapy of schizophrenia in the retarded. *Psychopharmacology Bulletin, 21,* 316–322.

Micev, V., & Lynch, D.M. (1974). Effect of lithium on disturbed severely mentally retarded patients. *British Journal of Psychiatry, 125,* 110.

Millichamp, C.J., & Singh, N.N. (1987). The effects of intermittent drug therapy on stereotypy and collateral behaviors of mentally retarded persons. *Research in Developmental Disabilities, 8,* 213–227.

Mizuno, T., & Yugari, Y. (1975). Prophylactic effects of L-5-hydroxytryptophan on self-mutilation in the Lesch-Nyhan syndrome. *Neuropaediatrie, 6,* 13–23.

Mouchka, S. (1985). Issues in psychopharmacology with the mentally retarded. *Psychopharmacology Bulletin, 21,* 262–267.

Mullerova, S., Novotna, J., Rehan, V., & Skula, E. (1974). Lithium treatment of behavioral disturbances in patients with defective intellect. *Activitas Nervosa Superior (Praha), 16,* 196.

Naylor, G.J., Donald, J.M., Le Poidevin, D., & Reid, A.H. (1974). A double-blind trial of long-term lithium therapy in mental defectives. *British Journal of Psychiatry, 124,* 52–57.

Nyhan, W.L., Johnson, H.G., Kaufman, I.A., & Jones, K.L. (1980). Serotonergic approaches to the modification of behavior in the Lesch-Nyhan syndrome. *Applied Research in Mental Retardation, 1,* 25–40.

Panksepp, J., & Sahley, T.L. (1987). Possible brain opioid involvement in disrupted social intent and language development in autism. In E. Schopler & G.B. Mesibov (Eds.), *Neurobiological issues in autism* (pp. 357–372). New York: Plenum Press.

Pilkington, T.L. (1961). Comparative effects of Librium and Taractan on behavior disorders of mentally retarded children. *Diseases of the Nervous System, 22,* 573–575.

Pueschel, S.M., Reed, R.B., Cronk, C.E., & Goldstein, B.I. (1980). 5-Hydroxytryptophan and pyridoxine: Their effects in young children with Down's syndrome. *American Journal of Diseases of Children, 134,* 838–844.

Rapoport, J.L., & Mikkelsen, E.J. (1978). Antidepressants. In J.S. Werry (Ed.), *Pediatric psychopharmacology: The use of behavior modifying drugs in children* (pp. 208–233). New York: Brunner/Mazel.

Rapoport, J.L., Mikkelsen, E.J., & Werry, J.S. (1978). Antimanic, antianxiety, hallucinogenic and miscellaneous drugs. In J.S. Werry (Ed.), *Pediatric psychopharmacology* (pp. 316–355). New York: Brunner/Mazel.

Rapport, M.D., Murphy, H.A., & Bailey, J.S. (1982). Ritalin vs response cost in the control of hyperactive children: A within subject comparison. *Journal of Applied Behavior Analysis, 15,* 205–216.

Ratey, J.J., Mikkelson, E.J., Smith, G.B., Upadhyaya, A., Zuckerman, H.S., Martell, D., Sorgi, P., Polakoff, S., & Bemporad, J. (1986). B-Blockers in the severely and profoundly mentally retarded. *Journal of Clinical Psychopharmacology, 6,* 103–107.

Ratey, J.J., Morrill, R., & Oxenkrug, G. (1983). Use of propranolol for provoked and unprovoked episodes of rage. *American Journal of Psychiatry, 140,* 1356–1357.

Reid, A.J., & Leonard, A. (1977). Lithium treatment of cyclical vomiting in a mentally defective patient. *British Journal of Psychiatry, 130,* 316.

Reiss, S., Levitan, G.W., & Szyszko, J. (1982). Emotional disturbance and mental retardation: Diagnostic overshadowing. *American Journal of Mental Deficiency, 86,* 567–574.

Revusky, S.H. (1967). Some statistical treatments compatible with individual organism methodology. *Journal of the Experimental Analysis of Behavior, 10,* 319–330.

Richardson, J.S., & Zaleski, W.A. (1983). Naloxone and self-mutilation. *Biological Psychiatry, 18,* 99–101.

Rimland, B. (1973). High-dosage levels of certain vitamins in the treatment of children with severe mental disorders. In D. Hawkins & L. Pauling (Eds.), *Orthomolecular psychiatry* (pp. 513–539). New York: W.H. Freeman.

Ritvo, E.R., Freeman, B.J., Yuwiler, A., Geller, E., Schroth, P., & Yokota, A. (1986). Fenfluramine treatment of autism: UCLA collaborative study of 81 patients at nine medical centers. *Psychopharmacology Bulletin, 22,* 133–147.

Ritvo, E.R., Yuwiler, A., Geller, E., Ornitz, E.M., Saeger, K., & Plotkin, S. (1970). Increased blood serotonin and platelets in infantile autism. *Archives of General Psychiatry, 23,* 566–572.

Rivinus, T.M., & Harmatz, J.S. (1979). Diagnosis and lithium treatment of affective disorder in the retarded: Five case studies. *American Journal of Psychiatry, 136,* 551–554.

Sandman, C.A., Datta, P.C., Barron, J., Hoehler, F.K., Williams, C., & Swanson, J.M. (1983). Naloxone attenuates self-abusive behavior in developmentally disabled clients. *Applied Research in Mental Retardation, 4,* 5–11.

Sandyk, R., & Gillman, M.A. (1986). Infantile autism. A dysfunction of the opioids. *Medical Hypotheses, 19,* 41–45.

Schain, R.J. (1983). Carbamazepine and cognitive functioning. In P.L. Morselli, C.E. Pippenger, & J.K. Perry (Eds.), *Antiepileptic drug therapy in pediatrics* (pp. 189–192). New York: Raven Press.

Schroeder, S.R. (1985). Issues and future research directions of pharmacotherapy in mental retardation. *Psychopharmacology Bulletin, 21,* 323–326.

Schroeder, S.R. (1988). Neuroleptic medications for persons with developmental disabilities. In M.G. Aman & N.N. Singh (Eds.), *Psychopharmacology of the developmental disabilities* (pp. 82–100). New York: Springer-Verlag.

Schroeder, S.R., & Gualtieri, C.T. (1985). Behavioral interactions induced by chronic neuroleptic therapy in persons with mental retardation. *Psychopharmacology Bulletin, 21,* 323–326.

Schroeder, S.R., Lewis, M.H., & Lipton, M.A. (1983). Interactions of pharmacotherapy and behavior therapy among children with learning and behavioral disorders. In K.D. Gadow (Ed.), *Advances in learning and behavioral disabilities* (Vol. 2, pp. 179–225). Greenwich, CT: JAI Press.

Shafto, F., & Sulzbacher, S. (1977). Comparing treatment tactics with a hyperactive preschool child: Stimulant medication and programmed teacher interventions. *Journal of Applied Behavior Analysis, 10,* 13–20.

Singh, N.N. (1987). Diet and childhood behavior disorders. In J. Birkbeck (Ed.), *Are we really what we eat?* (pp. 35–45). Auckland, New Zealand: Dairy Advisory Bureau.

Singh, N.N., & Ahrens, M.G. (1978). Incidental learning in the mentally retarded. *Exceptional Child, 35,* 53–63.

Singh, N.N., & Aman, M.G. (1981). Effects of thioridazine dosage on the behavior of severely mentally retarded persons. *American Journal of Mental Deficiency, 1981,* 580–587.

Singh, N.N., & Beale, I.L. (1978). Attentional changes during discrimination learning by retarded children. *Journal of the Experimental Analysis of Behavior, 29,* 527–533.

Singh, N.N., & Beale, I.L. (1986). Behavioral assessment of pharmacotherapy. *Behavior Change, 3,* 34–40.

Singh, N.N., & Falconer, K.M. (1986). *Effects of a drug alone and combined with a behavioral procedure on stereotypy and social behavior.* Paper presented at the Australian Behaviour Modification Association Conference, Sydney, Australia.

Singh, N.N., & Winton, A.S.W. (1984). Behavioral monitoring of pharmacological interventions for self-injury. *Applied Research in Mental Retardation, 5,* 161–170.

Sovner, R., & Hurley, A.D. (1983). Do the mentally retarded suffer from affective illness. *Archives of General Psychiatry, 40,* 61–67.

Sprague, R.L. (1987). Letter to the editor. *Journal of Mental Deficiency Research, 31,* 223–225.

Sprague, R.L., & Baxley, G.B. (1978). Drugs for behavior management, with comment on some legal aspects. In J. Wortis (Ed.), *Mental retardation and developmental disabilities* (Vol. 10, pp. 92–129). New York: Brunner/Mazel.

Sprague, R.L., & Werry, J.S. (1971). Methodology of psychopharmacological studies with the retarded. In N.R. Ellis (Ed.), *International review of research in mental retardation* (pp. 147–210). New York: Academic Press.

Stores, G. (1978). Antiepileptics (anticonvulsants). In J.S. Werry (Ed.), *Pediatric psychopharmacology* (pp. 274–315). New York: Brunner/Mazel.

Thorley, G. (1984). Pilot study to assess behavioural and cognitive effects of artificial food colours in a group of retarded children. *Developmental Medicine and Child Neurology, 26,* 56–61.

Trimble, M., & Reynolds, E.H. (1976). Anticonvulsant drugs and mental symptoms. *Psychological Medicine, 6,* 169–178.

Trimble, M.R. (1981). Anticonvulsant drugs, behavior, and cognitive abilities. In W.B. Essman & L. Valzelli (Eds.), *Current developments in psychopharmacology* (Vol. 6, pp. 65–91). New York: Spectrum.

Tryon, W.W. (1982). A simplified time-series analysis for evaluating treatment interventions. *Journal of Applied Behavior Analysis, 15,* 423–429.

Tu, J., & Smith, J.T. (1979). Factors associated with psychotropic medication in mental retardation facilities. *Comprehensive Psychiatry, 20,* 289–295.

Tu, J., & Smith, J.T. (1983). The Eastern Ontario survey: A study of drug-treated psychiatric problems in the mentally handicapped. *Canadian Journal of Psychiatry, 28,* 270–276.

Tyrer, S.P., Walsh, A., Edwards, D.E., Berney, T.P., & Stephens, D.A. (1984). Factors associated with a good response to lithium in aggressive mentally handicapped subjects. *Progress in Neuropsychopharmacology and Biological Psychiatry, 8,* 751–755.

Ullman, D.G. (1974). Breadth of attention and retention in mentally retarded and intellectually average children. *American Journal of Mental Deficiency, 78,* 640–648.

Varley, C.K., & Trupin, E.W. (1982). Double-blind administration of methylphenidate to mentally retarded children with attention deficit disorder: A preliminary study. *American Journal of Mental Deficiency, 86,* 560–566.

Waksman, S.A. (1983). Diet and children's behavior disorders: A review of the research. *Clinical Psychology Review, 3,* 201–213.

Walters, A., Singh, N.N., & Beale, I.L. (1977). Effects of lorazepam on hyperactivity in retarded children. *New Zealand Medical Journal*, *86*, 473–475.

Weise, P., Koch, R., Shaw, K.N.F., & Rosenfeld, M.J. (1974). The use of 5-HTP in the treatment of Down's syndrome. *Pediatrics*, *54*, 165–168.

Wells, K.C., Conners, C.K., Imber, L., & Delamater, A. (1981). Use of single-subject methodology in clinical decision-making with a hyperactive child in the psychiatric inpatient unit. *Behavioral Assessment*, *3*, 359–369.

Wender, E.H. (1986). The food additive-free diet in the treatment of behavior disorders: A review. *Developmental and Behavioral Pediatrics*, *7*, 35–42.

Werry, J.S. (1982). Pharmacotherapy. In B.B. Lahey & A.E. Kazdin (Eds.), *Advances in clinical child psychology* (Vol. 5, pp. 283–321). New York: Plenum Press.

Worrall, E.P., Moody, J.P., & Naylor, G.J. (1975). Lithium in nonmanic depressives: Antiaggressive effect and red blood cell lithium values. *British Journal of Psychiatry*, *126*, 464–468.

Wulbert, M., & Dries, R. (1977). The relative efficacy of methylphenidate (Ritalin) and behavior modification techniques in the treatment of a hyperactive child. *Journal of Applied Behavior Analysis*, *10*, 21–31.

Yudofsky, S., Williams, D., & Gorman, J. (1981). Propranolol in the treatment of rage and violent behavior in patients with chronic brain syndrome. *American Journal of Psychiatry*, *138*, 218–220.

Zimmerman, R.L., & Heistad, G.T. (1981). Correlates of psychotropic drug treatment at Cambridge State Hospital. In R. Young & J. Kroll (Eds.), *The use of medication in controlling the behavior of the mentally retarded* (pp. 123–132). Minneapolis: University of Minnesota.

Zrull, J.P., Westman, J.C., Arthur, B., & Bell, W.A. (1963). A comparison of chlordiazepoxide, d-amphetamine, and placebo in the treatment of the hyperkinetic syndrome in children. *American Journal of Psychiatry*, *120*, 590–591.

Zrull, J.P., Westman, J.C., Arthur, B., & Rice, D.L. (1964). A comparison of diazepam, d-amphetamine, and placebo in the treatment of the hyperkinetic syndrome in children. *American Journal of Psychiatry*, *121*, 388–389.

8
Professional Training

CAROL LEWIS AND RONALD S. DRABMAN

Behavioral medicine involves the application of learning-theory techniques (behavior therapy) to health-related problems. While the ultimate goal of behavioral medicine may be self-control of health-related behaviors by the child, it is often more practical to use some responsible other to bring about therapeutic change. This is particularly true with special populations such as developmentally disabled children. When children, parents, and/or significant others are taught behavioral techniques to control developmentally disabled children's problematic behavior related to health status, this subset of behavior therapy is referred to as behavioral medicine or behavioral pediatrics with developmentally disabled children.

The literature dealing with this application of behavioral medicine has generally used parents as the behavior-change agents. Parents have been taught to ensure adequate intake of nutrients and prevent physical problems such as muscle contractions and pressure sores in their developmentally disabled children (areas discussed in subsequent sections of this chapter). The literature is sparse, however, in the area of training nonpsychologist health care professionals to use behavioral medicine techniques with developmentally disabled children. It should be possible to teach most professional staff using procedures similar to those used with parents. A somewhat more sophisticated presentation could also be arranged for professional training. This training should cover at least a basic core curriculum and provide hands-on experience through practice.

Why should nonpsychologist health care providers learn behavioral medicine techniques and principles? The behavioral medicine practitioner needs to provide other professionals with a rationale that supports the use of these techniques with developmentally disabled children. She or he can point out that behavioral medicine techniques have been used to help developmentally disabled children reach their potential. For example, the physical mobility of these children has been increased by teaching them how to use a wheelchair, or ambulate with a walker, crutches, braces, or independently. Additionally, they have been taught to use various pieces of equipment as aids for communication, eating, bathing, and a number of other self-help skills. It is important for professionals to be aware that these and other problems within the developmentally disabled population have been addressed through the use of a number of different behavioral medicine techniques such as modeling, praise, feedback, and behavioral rehearsal. They also need to know that compliance with professional advice has been maintained through reinforcement and that inappropriate behaviors that might affect physical well-being have been eliminated through the use of extinction or punishment paradigms. In this way, a rationale can be developed so that professionals will be interested in learning to use behavioral medicine techniques to meet their patients' needs.

Just as the nonpsychologist health care provider needs training in the uses of behavioral medicine techniques, the behavioral medicine practitioner must be trained to work alongside the medical staff as part of the treatment team or as consultant to the team. The cooperation of the specialties is very important to the effectiveness of the behavioral medicine intervention. The medical staff can provide the behavioral medicine practitioner with extremely important information, such as medical contraindications for the use of certain reinforcers and punishers. The behavioral medicine practitioner must also be trained to work closely with other professionals, such as physical and occupational therapists. Cooperation among the specialties increases the likelihood of treatment success. It is particularly important for the developmentally disabled child's parents to be aware of the medical staff's support of the behavioral medicine intervention.

This chapter begins with an illustrative case that demonstrates the role that a behavioral medicine practitioner can serve as consultant to and teacher of other health-related professionals. Then general issues in training nonpsychologist health care providers are discussed. Next, the chapter reviews the literature on parent training with developmentally disabled children in the areas of developmental gain, physical therapy, occupational therapy, and pressure sores. The parent training literature is reviewed because it is important that nonpsychologist health care providers understand it and because there is little literature directly pertaining to training professional staff members in behavioral medicine. Each of the areas of parent training reviewed could easily be extended to the training of professional staff. The goals for training the following professionals are examined: physicians, nurses, physical therapists, occupational therapists, and teachers. The role of the psychologist as a behavioral medicine specialist is also discussed. Then, work aimed at discovering the effective components of packages designed to train parents is reviewed. Components found to be effective in parent training provide a starting point from which to develop effective professional training programs. The clinical significance and implications of this literature are then considered as they apply to professional training. Finally, important issues in developing behavioral medicine training programs for professionals who work with developmentally disabled children are discussed along with suggestions for future research.

Illustrative Case

Problem: Josh is a 5-year-old male with cerebral palsy. His physician and physical therapist (PT) judged him to be ready for ambulation training and initiated outpatient therapy. Josh and his mother attended physical therapy sessions several times a week. It became apparent early in treatment that Josh was afraid to walk outside of the safety of the stationary parallel bars. When placed in a walker, he would sit down when not supported by another person.

The PT consulted a behavioral medicine practitioner about Josh's failure to cooperate in ambulation training. The behavioral medicine practitioner did a functional analysis of the problem situation and determined several powerful reinforcers for Josh. Sweetened cereal, paired with social reinforcement, was selected to be used as the reinforcer in ambulation training.

The behavioral medicine practitioner developed a plan to shape Josh's ambulation using sweetened cereal. The practitioner observed the PT implementing the program with Josh over several therapy sessions. Problems were solved and adjustments made in the program. Thereafter, the PT implemented the program without direct supervision with occasional consultation provided by the behavioral medicine practitioner. In this way, Josh learned how to walk with a walker, and eventually learned to walk with no external supports. The sweetened cereal reinforcer was gradually faded out of the treatment so that social reinforcement alone maintained the desired behavior.

Training Nonpsychologist Health Care Providers: General Issues

In some ways, training professionals in the use of behavioral medicine techniques may be more difficult than training more naive individuals. This may be particularly true when considering health care providers and other professionals who work with special populations such as the developmentally disabled. The behavioral medicine practitioner who is designing a training program for professionals must take into account some of the attitudes of the professionals that may be encountered. For example, LeBow (1976) commented on the commonly accepted practice of and belief in "noncontingent caring" as a major obstacle to the adoption of behavioral techniques. These latter techniques require that reinforcement be delivered on a contingent basis (i.e. determined by behavior). Professionals working with developmentally disabled persons may feel that it is wrong to selectively withhold pleasurable events. The behavioral medicine practitioner must educate other professionals about the consequences of these various types of interaction.

Issues that arise when professionals are trained in the use of behavioral techniques were discussed by Mastria and Drabman (1979). First, there may be resistance to the use of these techniques on the part of the professionals. They may minimize the effects of behavior on health status. There may also be a lack of understanding and motivation to comply with the requirements of behavioral medicine techniques. Further, professionals sometimes question the ethics of behavior modification. Ethical issues should be addressed openly at the outset of training. Such issues may include the use of aversive techniques and the locus of decision making about behavior change. The cost/benefit ratio of professional training may also be of concern. Nonpsychologist health care providers may feel that it is not worth the time required to learn behavioral medicine techniques. The cost effectiveness of behavioral medicine treatments should be emphasized at the beginning of training. The professionals may need to be informed that they, as well as their patients, will benefit from the training. Lastly, behavioral medicine techniques should be presented to the professional as part of a comprehensive approach to patient care. Once again the impact of behavior on health status may need to be elucidated.

Several curricula for training professionals in the use of behavioral techniques are presented by Mastria and Drabman (1979). Their basic course consists of three main areas: learning theory, behavioral assessment, and treatment/research skills. They recommend the use of modeling as an instructional technique to teach the professionals behavioral procedures. The professional trainee should be provided with a rationale for the use of behavioral techniques. The content of the training course should be practical and aimed at providing more efficient and effective patient care.

In summary, nonpsychologist health care providers may hold attitudes that contribute to resistance to using behavioral medicine techniques. Training programs for these professionals should discuss such attitudes as well as ethical considerations, and the cost effectiveness of such treatment. A rationale for the use of behavioral medicine techniques should be provided early in training and the content of training should be practical and applied.

Research Findings That Illustrate Methods of Teaching and Material to Be Taught to Nonpsychologist Health Care Providers

Target: Developmental Gain

Parents have been trained to facilitate the developmental progress of their disabled children. General physical development is a very important target for behavioral medicine. Minor, Minor, and Williams (1983) used a participant modeling technique to teach 14 parents to be the primary developmental skill programmers for their developmentally disabled infants. Parents first watched an instructor perform the developmental tasks with infants, after which the parents themselves performed the tasks with their infants, receiving corrective feedback when necessary. Six months after pretest, the participant modeling group showed a mean developmental gain of 5.16 months. A comparison group of children (sample size of only five) who received more traditional clinic-based treatment showed a mean developmental gain of 2.03 months.

Developmental education of parents with developmentally disabled children was compared to child management education by Moxley-Haegert and Serbin (1983). Parents in the developmental education group conducted significantly more training sessions with their children and these children showed significantly more developmental gain than the child management group or a no-education control group.

SUMMARY

These two studies indicate that developmental progress can be facilitated by using modeling to train parents or professionals such as nurses and recreation therapists in developmental skill programming or educating them about appropriate development.

Target: Physical Therapy

Physical therapy is a very important component of the treatment of developmentally disabled children. These children often need to be stretched, taught particular physical skills that they have not developed spontaneously, taught to use wheelchairs, walk, or tolerate therapeutic seating arrangements. A small number of studies have looked at the use of behavioral medicine techniques to facilitate these tasks. A few of these have used parents as behavior-change agents. In the majority, however, the behavioral medicine practitioner carried out the treatment program directly. Effects of the behavioral medicine techniques are evaluated by looking at outcomes such as changes in the range of motion, number of steps able to walk with or without various aides, and length of time therapeutic seating is tolerated. Physical therapy evaluations generally provide the guidelines for developing the goals of treatment.

Body position is very important for most developmentally disabled children. A checklist has been developed for monitoring correct position in nonambulatory children who are not able to change position independently (Stephens & Lattimore, 1983). One investigation (Lattimore, Stephens, Favell, & Risley, 1984) showed that the use of this checklist by a supervisor in an institutional setting significantly increased the correct positioning of all target children. Another experimental condition in which information was provided for direct-care staff through a workshop did not significantly affect the positioning of the children.

In other investigations looking at body position, Grove and his associates (Grove, Dalke, Fredericks, & Crowley, 1975) established correct head position in mentally and physically handicapped children through the use of contingent reinforcement. Biofeedback was used by Woolridge and Russell (1976) to correct the head positioning of a child with cerebral palsy.

Use of adaptive seating devices has been shown to be associated with positive behavioral changes in multihandicapped, developmentally disabled children

(Hulme, Poor, Schulein, & Pezzino, 1983). Wheelchairs, travel chairs, or strollers with custom-made adaptations were used by the children for 1 or more years to produce greater postural stability. With the equipment the children went to significantly more new places in the community, spent less time lying down, sat more, became better able to sit upright rather than lean to one side, spent less time in the bedroom, became better able to visually track an object and to grasp objects independently, and improved in feeding.

A number of different behavior modification procedures were used by Gouvier and his colleagues (Gouvier et al., 1985) to reduce resistance to ambulation in physically disabled patients. Resistance to ambulation often arises due to fears, such as that of falling. Such fears are reality based in that falls sometimes result in injuries. Resistance can result in extremely slow progress in ambulation training. Some children are unwilling to proceed with ambulation training at all. Modeling and contingent music successfully increased the ambulation of both patients studied. Progressive desensitization has also been used to reduce the resistance to walking in a rehabilitation setting (Di Scipio & Feldman, 1971).

A 5-year-old mentally retarded child with spina bifida was taught to use crutches to walk to all of his classes through the use of contingent root beer and noise (noise was a reinforcer) (Horner, 1971). Contingent social reinforcement was used with a 4-year-old child with spina bifida to teach her to ambulate independently with braces and crutches both in physical therapy clinic and at home where parents served as therapists (Manella & Varni, 1981).

Two studies have looked at whether parents can carry out physical therapy exercises effectively at home with their physically handicapped children. Slight to marked changes in the movements of target joints were found after parents were taught simple physical therapy procedures (Rosenbaum, Keane, Drabman, & Robertson, 1981). In another study (Gross, Eudy, & Drabman, 1984), physical therapists taught parents of three developmentally disabled children procedures to elicit use of a target limb. Parental use of reinforcement (toys, Fruit Loops, praise) for desired behavior resulted in an improvement in extension of that limb.

There is some dispute about the frequency of therapy (physical and occupational) necessary to produce maximal benefit in the treatment of developmentally disabled children. This is important to consider because the amount of time a given professional will be able to conduct therapy may be limited. Jenkins and Sells (1984) found that children treated with motor therapies one and three times per week showed equivalent gain in gross motor skills. Conversely, Campbell, McInerney, and Cooper (1984) found that children who were provided with opportunities to perform target behaviors throughout the day showed faster motor improvement than when provided the opportunity only during therapy. It may be that differences in frequency of treatment are discernible only when daily and less than daily treatment are compared. Further research is indicated to elucidate the effects of this treatment variable.

The frequency of treatment needs to be determined on an individual basis with guidelines provided by the physical therapist. Practical issues need to be considered such as how much time the professional in question feels she has to devote to working with the child. Several arrangements may need to be tried. Assessment is a very important part of this process. The target skill should be monitored on a regular basis. The pattern change in this skill should be important in determining the frequency of treatment.

SUMMARY

Parents and professionals have been trained to use behavioral medicine techniques effectively to conduct physical therapy exercises with their developmentally disabled children. This literature should be used to help teach more professionals to work with developmentally disabled children on physical therapy exercises, adaptive seating, body positioning, and ambulation. Professionals may also be able to use these techniques to deal with other factors such as resistance to and fears of ambulation. The behavioral medicine practitioner should train the other professionals to conduct these treatment programs and deal with the issues that arise surrounding them.

Target: Occupational Therapy

Occupational therapy has much to offer developmentally disabled children in the areas of development of self-help skills, such as dressing and feeding, and in the training of gross and fine motor skills. The problem being addressed is sometimes a skills deficit and sometimes physical limitation. For instance, a child may not have developed the motor skills necessary to feed himself or herself or he or she may not have sufficient motor control to use eating utensils independently. In the former case, therapeutic eating may be used to enhance development of the appropriate muscles. In the latter case, aides may be used to maximize the independent eating of the child. Behavioral medicine utilizes functional assessment of the particular problem in order to determine the nature of the problem. A variety of different causes can result in similar presenting problems. Functional assessment allows the therapist to determine if the presenting problem is due to a skills deficit, noncompliance, fear, physical limitations, or other etiologies. In terms of parent training, occupational therapists have traditionally given parents activities to perform with their children at home (Anderson & Hinojosa, 1984). These activities, in a behavioral framework, could also be used with the children by other health care professionals.

An interesting application of self-help skills in occupational therapy is bathing independence. Shillam, Beeman, and Loshin (1983) worked on this skill area with 19 wheelchair-bound or bedridden patients in a rehabilitation center. All 19 received some bathing equipment such as tub benches, bathtub chairs, shower chairs, or wheelchair shower-commodes. Flexible hoses, long-handled sponges, and grab bars were also used. All patients showed increases in bathing independence post-therapy. This was statistically significant for the group as a whole. The decrease in bathing assistance required was beneficial for the patient's self-esteem and also reduced family or paid-aide time needed for this activity.

SUMMARY

There is only a small amount of literature on methods of successfully training parents or professionals in occupational therapy skills within a behavioral medicine framework. This is in spite of parents traditionally being given occupational therapy exercises to use with their children at home. As with the other areas, these professionals should be taught to increase the effectiveness of occupational therapy exercises with developmentally disabled children by the use of behavioral medicine techniques. They need to be taught how to conduct a functional assessment to determine the characteristics of a particular problem and what type of intervention would best address it. They also need to learn how to collect data throughout assessment and treatment phases so that changes can be detected.

Target: Pressure Sores

A very serious potential problem for wheelchair-bound developmentally disabled children or those wearing splints or braces is pressure sores (also called bedsores, decubitus ulcers, and ischemic ulcers). They result from skin and underlying tissue being traumatized by pressure, shear, or friction (DeLisa & Mikulic, 1985). Healing may be a lengthy process, particularly if the ulcers become infected. Infection may be difficult to diagnose if deep tissue is involved (Sugarman, 1985).

Pressure sores can be prevented through proper care. Once they have developed, treatment may be expensive in terms of time, money, and pain. For example, pressure sore development may result in a wheelchair-bound child having to lay flat on his or her stomach until the sore has healed. Behavioral treatments that address this problem show clearly how behavior change can prevent medical problems. In practice, however, professionals often do not take the time to use programs with susceptible individuals to avoid the problem before it occurs.

A number of devices have been suggested to help prevent pressure sores. At least 12 different kinds of beds and mattresses and eight kinds of wheelchair cushions have been developed (DeLisa & Mikulic, 1985). Once the sores are present, at least 14 physical agents and 38 topical applications have been reported as appropriate treatments (DeLisa & Mikulic, 1985).

Obviously, prevention is preferable to treatment. In addition to the special cushions mentioned above, a behavioral program has been developed to prevent development of pressure sores in wheelchair-bound individuals. This program involves the patient doing push-ups in the wheelchair at regular intervals (at least one every 10 to 20 minutes) in order to relieve the pressure (Malament, Dunn, & Davis, 1975). In one study (Malament, Dunn, & Davis, 1975), providing the patient with information about what he or she should do did not result in a sufficient number of push-ups to prevent pressure sores. Several devices have been developed to facilitate the execution of these wheelchair push-ups at an effective rate. One such device sounds a 30-second alarm at the end of any 10-minute interval in which a push-up is not done (Malament, Dunn, & Davis, 1975). The patient may avoid the alarm by doing a push-up, which then starts the next interval. The alarm can also be terminated by doing a push-up. Push-ups must be of at least 4 seconds duration. This device also records push-up frequency. It has proven effective in producing an adequate number of push-ups in at least one study (Malament, Dunn, & Davis, 1975).

A more recent study (Merbitz, King, Bleiberg, & Grip, 1985) has shown that simply electronically recording frequency of lift-offs yields wide variability in frequency. The relationship between lift-off frequency and pressure sore development also appears to be somewhat variable between individuals (Merbitz et al., 1985). Future research with developmentally disabled persons should extend this literature to look at characteristics of the health care provider and his or her interactions with the patient as they are related to pressure sore prevention and treatment.

SUMMARY

Pressure sore development can be avoided through the application of appropriate behavioral medicine techniques. Therefore, it is extremely important that professionals working with children likely to develop pressure sores have knowledge of preventive behavioral medicine techniques.

Analysis of Treatment Components

Several investigations have begun to look at what variables produce the most effective treatment package for training parents of developmentally disabled children. It might be assumed that components that lead to effective use of the treatments by parents would also effectively train professionals. Even where the problems in question are not health related, the findings about parent training in general are relevant to this aspect of behavioral medicine. Hudson (1982) used four parent training conditions in his investigation of factors that facilitate gain in developmentally disabled children. The groups were: 1) verbal instruction, 2) verbal instruction plus teaching of behavioral principles, 3) verbal instruction plus the use of modeling and role playing, and 4) a wait-control group. Results indicated that parents needed to be taught with techniques that directly shaped their responding (modeling and role playing) in order to affect their children's behavior.

Baker and his group at the UCLA Project for Developmental Disabilities also looked at the effectiveness of various formats for parent training (Brightman, Baker, Clark, & Ambrose, 1982). Parents of 66 moderately to severely retarded children (aged 3 to 13 years) participated in either group or individual training to reduce behavior problems and teach self-help skills or were assigned to a delayed training control group. After 3 months of training, trained parents knew more about behavior modification and were better at using these principles than control parents. Children of trained parents tended to have reduced behavior problems but showed no differences on self-help skills. Further, there were no differences between parents trained using an individual versus a group format.

The UCLA group has also looked at other important aspects of parent training of developmentally disabled children, such as the effect of nonspecific factors on treatment gains and the prediction of treatment outcome. Baker and Brightman (1984) taught one group of parents behavior modification knowledge and skills and another group advocacy knowledge and skills. After approximately 10 weeks of treatment each group of parents showed gains, but primarily on instruments particular to their training program. This demonstrates the specificity of the effects on treatment gains.

Discriminant analysis has been used to classify parental proficiency at conducting a behavioral program with their developmentally disabled children (Clark & Baker, 1983). Parents of 103 moderately to severely retarded children were classified as either high or low proficient after participating in a 10-week group treatment aimed at increasing their children's self-help skills and reducing their behavior problems. The model correctly classified 76% of the parents. Low-proficient parents were of lower socioeconomic status, had expected greater problems in teaching their children, and had less previous experience with behavior modification. At a 6-month follow-up, factors predictive of low rate of follow-through were marital status (unmarried), low proficiency at the end of training, and low likelihood of teaching their children prior to the program. Several questions arise when these findings are extended to professional training. Will professionals who expect greater problems in training children, have less previous experience with behavior modification, and show a lower proficiency at the end of training be less likely to use the behavioral medicine skills they are taught?

Remediation for parents showing low proficiency at the end of training was conducted by Baker and McCurry (1984). These parents were taught skills in a school-based group format supplemented by live modeling, observation of teaching, individual supervised teaching, and videotaped feedback (Brightman, Ambrose, & Baker, 1980). There were significant treatment gains, but maintenance of these gains over 6 months varied according to teaching proficiency at the end of treatment. Skill levels were low at all points, however, compared to the sample used to develop the classification formula (Clark & Baker, 1983). Therefore, as might be expected, those who learned the skills well actually used them more. This indicates the need for assessment of learning after professionals have been trained in behavioral medicine.

Clinical Significance of Parent Training Research

The parent training literature has a number of implications for professional training of behavioral medicine with developmentally disabled children. The research has shown that many parents trained in behavioral techniques can effectively provide care and treatment for their developmentally disabled children at home with professional supervision. This care includes not only shaping appropriate and acceptable behaviors, but also facilitating developmental progress, skill acquisition, and preventing physical problems. If parents can learn how to use these skills with their children, professionals should be able to do the same.

The time required by the behavioral medicine practitioner to provide these services for developmentally disabled children can be quite extensive and costly. Training parents and other professional staff members to provide some of these services can reduce their costs. It also may allow the child to receive needed therapy on a more frequent basis, an arrangement that might not otherwise be feasible.

Within the traditional, professional treatment model wherein each member works only in one area, developmentally disabled children receive only limited services. They may also require periodic hospitalization in order to have extensive services provided directly by each professional staff member. Effective professional training provides the opportunity for developmentally disabled children to receive more frequent and intensive treatment under the supervision of a smaller number of professionals. Therefore, it has the potential of reducing the number or duration of those costly, extensive hospitalizations.

Professionals who are trained in behavioral medicine can often provide developmentally disabled children with more cost-effective treatment. They can prevent health problems that might arise due to problematic behavior and reduce problems that adversely affect health status. The behavioral medicine practitioner should train the other professionals to use the behavioral techniques with developmentally disabled children so that the behavioral medicine practitioner serves only as a consultant, not as a direct-care provider.

The parent training literature indicated that certain characteristics of parents are associated with lower skills in conducting behavioral programs with their developmentally disabled children after receiving training (Clark & Baker, 1983). Some of these characteristics may be associated with lower proficiency of professionals who have been trained in behavioral medicine to use with developmentally disabled children. These characteristics include expectations of great problems in teaching the children and little prior experience with behavior modification. Future research should investigate the relationship of these factors and proficiency of skills in professionals after behavioral medicine training in order to develop treatment components that would counteract these effects.

Implications of Behavioral Medicine Interventions on Medical Components of Chronic Care

Behavioral medicine interventions for developmentally disabled children should affect a number of the medical aspects of chronic care. First, child behavior problems may reduce the effectiveness of medical interventions. Behavioral medicine programs could decrease the problem behaviors, thereby increasing efficacy of the medical intervention. For example, a child cannot obtain the maximum benefit from an arm splint if he or she constantly removes it. A behavioral medicine treatment program that decreases the child's frequency of removing the splint would be of obvious clinical benefit. Behavioral techniques can also facilitate cooperation of the developmentally disabled child in therapeutic activities. It is difficult to make therapeutic progress with a child who is fighting, screaming, or involved in constant self-stimulatory behavior.

Physical and occupational therapy exercises conducted within a behavioral medicine framework may facilitate ambulation, use of arms and legs, and development of both gross and fine motor skills. Therapist-prescribed exercises used within that framework might also reduce contractions of muscle groups due to the inactivity of those groups. This could facilitate the availability of the muscles for use in such activities as transferring from bed to wheelchair. As noted previously, behavioral medicine programs implemented by professionals can help prevent other problems common to developmentally disabled children, such as pressure sores from misuse of adaptive equipment. Therefore, it is strongly recommended that training programs for nonpsychologist health care providers include a behavior medicine specialist on the teaching faculty. Students need to be exposed to both didactic and practicum experience in this area.

Goals of Training

There are several critical training issues relevant to many professionals being trained in behavioral medicine with developmentally disabled children. Each of these issues should be addressed within a program designed for the particular group of professionals being trained.

Recognizing Disabilities and Syndromes

Professionals who have not previously worked with developmentally delayed children may not be familiar with the presenting characteristics of developmental disabilities. The first goal of a training program is to teach professionals how to recognize features associated with developmental disabilities. The professional must be able to identify the developmentally disabled child before services can be offered to the child. Additionally, early identification of such children by professionals will lead to early intervention and improved programs for the children.

Identifying Problem Behaviors

Certain types of problem behaviors are found more commonly than others in developmentally disabled children. Professionals should be familiar with what these problem behaviors are, so that they will inquire about them, and if they are present, interventions will be designed and implemented. Early identification of problem behaviors may result in easier treatment of the problem, as well as reduced stress on the family.

Coursework

Training programs should include coursework dealing with the conceptual framework and practical application of behavioral medicine principles. Learning principles should be taught. Discussions should also include the advantages and disadvantages of behavioral medicine intervention and problems commonly addressed with behavioral medicine techniques.

Practicum/Supervision

All professionals being trained in behavioral medicine should have practicum experience with behavioral medicine applications in developmental disabilities supervised by an experienced behavioral medicine practitioner. The importance of this "hands-on" experience should not be underestimated. It allows the professional trainee to have firsthand "success" experiences with behavioral medicine applications with the benefit of expert supervision.

Knowledge of Consultants/Resources

By the end of training, professionals should be aware of what types of problems are best addressed by behavioral medicine techniques and where to find behavioral medicine practitioners to either consult or refer the patient when necessary. Lists of such resources should be provided to the "graduate."

Issues Relevant to Specific Professional Fields

Physicians

While the nonpsychiatrist physician generally will not directly implement behavioral medicine programs with developmentally disabled children, physician training should nevertheless address all of the issues discussed above. Information about referral sources is particularly important to provide to physicians.

Nurses

Nurses generally spend greater amounts of time with patients than do physicians. Therefore, they are more likely to actually implement behavioral medicine programs with developmentally disabled children. Since nurses are often the "gatekeepers" to patient care, they will need to learn firsthand that behavioral medicine can prove cost effective if used appropriately. Specifically, nurses can use behavioral medicine techniques to address compliance behaviors, help teach patients how to reduce both pre- and postoperative fears, and train self-care skills.

Physical and Occupational Therapists

Therapists should be taught which of the types of problems they often see can be addressed by behavioral medicine techniques and why these techniques are often the treatment of choice. Therapists can be taught how to apply behavioral medicine principles to such problems as teaching an uncooperative developmentally disabled child how to walk, use a previously neglected limb, eat foods of different textures, and stop tantrum behavior that interferes with treatment.

Teachers

Although teachers generally work in a nonmedical setting, those who work with developmentally disabled children often have situations where use of behavioral medicine techniques would be appropriate. Developmentally delayed children often receive education in coordination with other services such as physical and occupational therapy. Their teachers can be trained in behavioral medicine techniques so that problems can be addressed in a comprehensive fashion.

Programs aimed at training teachers in the use of behavioral medicine methods should address all of the issues outlined above. Because teachers work with children for many hours in the course of a day, they would likely be implementing behavioral medicine programs themselves. Training for them should emphasize practicum experience and information about consultants. Behavioral medicine techniques can be used by teachers to increase the likelihood of children participating in the classroom by identifying the most effective means of instruction for a particular developmentally disabled child or decrease interfering behaviors such as self-stimulation and throwing a tantrum.

Psychologist as Behavioral Medicine Specialist

Training for psychologists who are behavioral medicine specialists is quite extensive. A number of shortcomings in graduate training for clinical psychologists have been identified, however (Drabman, 1985), and should be duly addressed. Psychologists who identify themselves as behavioral medicine specialists should have received extensive supervised experience with real clinical populations. Graduate programs should strive to make experience with medical patients available to their students. Experience with pediatric patients would be especially important to clinical psychology graduate students who want to later identify themselves as behavioral pediatrics specialists. Hands-on research experience with these medical populations should also be provided during graduate training since research in medical settings often presents difficulties unique to the setting. These research skills should be taught so practitioners can continue to increase their knowledge of behavioral medicine. Psychologists who do not have research skills cannot effectively "read between the lines" of publications so they cannot adequately gain knowledge of newly developing techniques and therefore are doomed to obsolescence.

Important Issues to Consider in Developing Behavioral Medicine Teaching Programs

The motivation of the professional to carry out behavioral medicine programs should be carefully evaluated. The professional should be assisted in realistically determining the amount of time he or she has to devote to behavioral medicine programs. This would then indicate the role that he or she should assume as the program consultant or hands-on implementor. If the professional reserves for him- or herself the task of direct implementation of the program and yet is not able to be there to conduct it as needed, the program is unlikely to succeed. It may be necessary to delegate responsibility for direct implementation to others.

Professionals other than the behavioral medicine practitioner may feel themselves incompetent to carry out treatment programs. Alternately, they may believe that developmentally disabled children, especially those who also have a chronic illness, should not be forced to change their behavior regardless of the positive or negative consequences. These issues must be resolved in training if behavioral medicine techniques are to be successful. The task of the behavioral medicine practitioner may be to work to alter the professional's attitudes prior to attempting programming. Appropriate expectations should also be fostered about the course of treatment and its interaction with the developmental status of a disabled child. Where needed, education should be provided about the course of development and its implications for behavioral treatment.

Reinforcers and punishing agents for use in behavioral medicine interventions with developmentally disabled children should be chosen carefully. It is very important that professionals be taught how to arrive at appropriate selections using careful methods to avoid choices that might be dangerous to the child. Sometimes there are medical contraindications that dictate against use of particular agents as reinforcers or punishers. The behavioral medicine practitioner must be very careful not to recommend use of any such agents. Potential disasters can be averted by checking out possible reinforcers or punishers with medical staff before program implementation. For example, the feeding status of the child should be considered when selecting food items for reinforcers. It is important to know whether the child enjoys eating, can chew, and what texture of food he or she can currently manipulate.

Professionals should also be taught to consider the particular disabilities of a child when developing a behavioral medicine program. To illustrate, visually impaired children should always be told what is being done and should be touched as much as possible. Textured toys may be very effective reinforcers for them.

Other children may be engaging in so much self-stimulatory behavior that external reinforcers are ineffective. The type and extent of disability of each individual child should be considered in order to develop the most effective program.

Future Research Directions for Training Nonpsychologist Health Care Providers

Continued research is necessary to further elucidate which methods most effectively train professionals to provide care and treatment for developmentally disabled children. Research should look at the treatment components used (e.g., in vivo modeling, viewing videotapes, reading a manual) and whether or not the professionals actually use the behavior medicine techniques and for how long. The attitudes of professionals undergoing training in behavioral medicine techniques should also be assessed pre-and posttraining. In addition, the relationship between skill acquisition and attitudes would be a worthwhile topic for future research.

After training, research should assess the amount of time various types of professionals actually implement behavioral programs and the amount of time they act as consultants to direct-care staff. The transfer of training between trained professional and other staff members should be investigated. If the trained professional adopts the role of consultant or supervisor he or she needs to be able to accurately convey the principles of behavioral medicine to whomever directly implements the programs.

The amount of contact after training between the behavioral medicine practitioner and the trained professional should be looked at as related to treatment effectiveness. Once trained, the professional may or may not seek out the behavioral medicine practitioner for additional information, classification, or assistance. That is assuming the professional is indeed using the behavioral medicine techniques.

Aspects of interventions that professionals are better able and more likely to carry out should be determined. If these can be found, then the behavioral medicine practitioner's time and effort would best be spent teaching professionals these aspects of behavioral medicine. It would also be interesting to look at the types of developmentally disabled children with which professionals are most effective in conducting behavioral medicine interventions. Particular emphasis could be given in training for types of disabilities and problems that are particularly problematic to treat using behavioral medicine techniques. It is in the best interest of the behavioral medicine practitioner to provide the professional trainee with as much assistance as possible so that success experiences are more likely (positive reinforcement!).

Quality of professional-developmentally disabled child interactions should also be evaluated posttraining. The interaction itself may be affected as well as the attitudes of the professional toward the child and the child's family toward the professional as more attention is shown to the child. It should be noted that these attitudes may affect treatment effectiveness.

Conclusion

Nonpsychologist health care providers can be trained in the effective use of behavioral medicine techniques with developmentally disabled children. Research has shown that parents have been trained to effectively reduce their developmentally disabled children's behavior problems and facilitate acquisition of self-help skills and language, cognitive, and physical development. Research has yet to elucidate the most effective treatment package for professional training.

The attitudes of professionals toward behavioral medicine techniques should be evaluated and discussed prior to training. The content of training should be practical and include both coursework and clinical experience. Professionals should be assisted in developing a role in the use of behavioral medicine techniques with developmentally disabled children that they will realistically be able to fulfill.

References

Anderson, J., & Hinojosa, J. (1984). Parents and therapists in a professional partnership. *American Journal of Occupational Therapy, 38*(7), 452–461.

Baker, B.L., & Brightman, R.P. (1984). Training parents of retarded children: Program-specific outcomes. *Behavior Therapy & Experimental Psychiatry, 15*(3), 255–260.

Baker, B.L., & McCurry, M.C. (1984). School-based parent training: An alternative for parents predicted to demonstrate low teaching proficiency following group training. *Education and Training of the Mentally Retarded, 19*(4), 261–267.

Brightman, R.P., Ambrose, S.A., & Baker, B.L. (1980). Parent training: A school-based model for enhancing parent performance. *Child Behavior Therapy, 2*, 35–47.

Brightman, R.P., Baker, B.L., Clark, D.B., & Ambrose, S.A. (1982). Effectiveness of alternative parent training formats. *Behavior Therapy & Experimental Psychiatry, 13*(2), 113–117.

Campbell, P.H., McInerney, W.F., & Cooper, M.A. (1984). Therapeutic programming for students with severe handicaps. *American Journal of Occupational Therapy, 38*(9), 594–602.

Clark, D.B., & Baker, B.L. (1983). Predicting outcome in parent training. *Journal of Consulting and Clinical Psychology, 51*(2), 309–311.

DeLisa, J.A., & Mikulic, M.A. (1985). Pressure ulcers: What to do if preventive management fails. *Postgraduate Medicine, 77*, 209–220.

Di Scipio, W.J., & Feldman, M.C. (1971). Combined behavior therapy and physical therapy in the treatment of a fear of walking. *Behavior Therapy & Experimental Psychiatry, 2*, 151–152.

Drabman, R.S. (1985). Graduate training of scientist-practitioner-oriented clinical psychologists: Where we can improve. *Professional Psychology: Research and Practice, 16*, 623–633.

Gouvier, W.D., Richards, J.S., Blanton, P.D., Janert, K., Rosen, L.A., & Drabman, R.S. (1985). Behavior modification in physical therapy. *Archives of Physical Medicine and Rehabilitation*, *66*, 113–116.

Gross, A.M., Eudy, S., & Drabman, R.S. (1984). Training parents to be physical therapists with their physically handicapped child. *Journal of Behavioral Medicine*, *5*, 321–327.

Grove, D.N., Dalke, B.A., Fredericks, H.D., & Crowley, R.F. (1975). Establishing appropriate head positioning with mentally retarded and physically handicapped children. *Behavioral Engineering*, *3*, 53–59.

Horner, R.D. (1971). Establishing use of crutches by a mentally retarded spina bifida child. *Journal of Applied Behavior Analysis*, *4*, 183–189.

Hudson, A.M. (1982). Training parents of developmentally handicapped children: A component analysis. *Behavior Therapy*, *13*, 325–333.

Hulme, J.B., Poor, R., Schulein, M., & Pezzino, J. (1983). Perceived behavioral changes observed with adaptive seating devices and training programs for multihandicapped, developmentally disabled individuals. *Physical Therapy*, *63*, 204–208.

Jenkins, J.R., & Sells, C.J. (1984). Physical and occupational therapy: Effects related to treatment, frequency, and motor delay. *Journal of Learning Disabilities*, *17*(2), 89–95.

Lattimore, J., Stephens, T.E., Favell, J.E., & Risley, T.R. (1984). Increasing direct care staff compliance to individualized physical therapy body positioning prescriptions: Prescriptive checklists. *Mental Retardation*, *22*(2), 79–84.

LeBow, M.D. (1976). Applications of behavior modification in nursing practice. In M. Hersen, R. Ester, & P. Miller (Eds.), *Progress in behavior modification* (Vol. 2, pp. 137–177). New York: Academic Press.

Malament, I.B., Dunn, M.E., & Davis, R. (1975). Pressure sores: An operant conditioning approach to prevention. *Archives of Physical Medicine and Rehabilitation*, *56*, 161–165.

Manella, K.J., & Varni, J.W. (1981). Behavior therapy in a gait-training program for a child with myelomeningocele. *Physical Therapy*, *61*(9), 1284–1287.

Mastria, M., & Drabman, R. (1979). Development of behavioral competence in medical settings. In J. Regis McNamara (Ed.), *Behavioral approaches to medicine: Application & analysis*. New York: Plenum Press.

Merbitz, C.T., King, R.B., Bleiberg, J., & Grip, J.C. (1985). Wheelchair push-ups: Measuring pressure relief frequency. *Archives of Physical Medicine and Rehabilitation*, *66*, 433–438.

Minor, S.W., Minor, J.W., & Williams, P.P. (1983). A participant modeling procedure to train parents of developmentally disabled infants. *Journal of Psychology*, *115*, 107–111.

Moxley-Haegert, L., & Serbin, L.A. (1983). Developmental education for parents of delayed infants: Effects on parental motivation and children's development. *Child Development*, *54*, 1324–1331.

Rosenbaum, M.S., Keane, T.M., Drabman, R.S., & Robertson, S.J. (1981). Goniometry in assessing a program to establish appropriate responses in physically handicapped children. *Behavioral Assessment*, *3*, 325–334.

Shillam, L.L., Beeman, C., & Loshin, P.M. (1983). Effect of occupational therapy intervention on bathing independence of disabled persons. *American Journal of Occupational Therapy*, *37*(11), 744–748.

Stephens, T.E., & Lattimore, J. (1983). Prescriptive check list for positioning residential clients. *Physical Therapy*, *63*, 1113–1115.

Sugarman, B. (1985). Infection and pressure sores. *Archives of Physical Medicine and Rehabilitation*, *66*, 117.
Woolridge, C.P. & Russell, G. (1976). Head positioning training with a cerebral palsied child: An application of biofeedback techniques. *Archives of Physical Medicine and Rehabilitation*, *57*, 407–414.

9
Behavioral Medicine Consultation

DON P. SUGAI AND JAMES K. LUISELLI

Preceding chapters in this volume examine a variety of behavioral medicine assessment and treatment methodologies. As advances in prevention, risk reduction, and therapeutic management continue to evolve, it is likely that psychologists and practitioners with specialized training in behavioral medicine will encounter greater opportunities for clinical practice. Many clinicians, for example, will receive requests to provide program-wide and individual case consultation. Conducting professional consultation is a multifaceted endeavor that encompasses many skill areas. In addition to the obvious prerequisite of clinical competency, effective consultation demands strong interpersonal skills, a knowledge of service delivery systems, efficient time management, and a broad-based understanding of multiple disciplines. Unfortunately, very little has been written concerning the process of behavioral consultation. The majority of publications on this topic have focused on the *academic training* of consultants, primarily within the discipline of school psychology (Bergan, 1977; Kratochwill & Bergan, 1978). Other discussions have consisted of brief overviews of consultation in such areas as geriatrics (MacDonald, 1983), psychiatry (Hersen & Bellack, 1978), and behavior therapy in private practice (Kaplan, 1987).

This chapter discusses the psychologist's role as a behavioral medicine consultant with developmentally disabled persons. The authors' intent is to analyze the goals of consultation, present a conceptual framework for implementing consultative services, and review methods to enhance therapeutic success. Also included are illustrative case examples within applied and medical settings. In setting forth this material, the authors have attempted to synthesize the small body of written information currently available with their own clinical experiences and working methodologies. Although written primarily for psychologists and behavioral clinicians, the content of the chapter should be applicable to other professional disciplines. The ultimate objective is to provide practitioners with a better understanding of how to plan, implement, and evaluate behavioral medicine consultation with developmentally disabled persons.

Overview

The behavioral medicine psychologist can serve as a consultant in several capacities. Some individuals may be employed full time within a variety of clinical settings and may be requested to provide consultation as a function of this position. For example, a psychologist who is a member of a pediatrics or psychiatry department at a university-affiliated medical center may be asked to consult on different cases referred from other departments. Many psychologists in these settings also serve on in-house evaluation and treatment teams (e.g., pediatric developmental evaluation teams and feeding clinics) and/or supervise parent training groups. Activities of this type frequently generate requests for consultation. Consultation is also a common enterprise for psychologists who are employed in residential treatment programs such as psychiatric hospitals, private schools, and extended-care facilities.

Psychologists in private practice also encounter many opportunities for behavioral medicine consultation. Many psychology group practices, as an example, receive frequent referrals from pediatricians, neurologists, and general practitioners. Clinicians involved in family therapy also may make referrals to the behavioral medicine specialist. Other referral sources include public school programs, special education collaboratives, and day rehabilitation settings. Usually, requests from these agencies entail the assessment of individual clients and recommendations for designing and implementing a systematic treatment plan. Consultation of this type can be particularly productive since a successful outcome with one client oftentimes leads to additional referrals.

Behavioral consultation generally serves one of three functions: staff consultation, case consultation, and consultation-liaison work. Because of the increased effort to integrate behavioral psychology into care-providing institutions and facilities, a number of authors and researchers have described strategies and goals for staff consultation (Ayllon & Michael, 1959; Graziano, 1971; Poser, 1967; Tharp & Wetzel, 1969; Thoresen, 1971). Bellack and Franks (1975) have outlined four components for consideration in the development of a staff consultation program. Essentially, these four components include: 1) the development of reasonable goals of consultation with regard to the establishment of skills and expertise in staff members, 2) the development of a format by which to provide integrated instruction and training to facilitate staff compliance and performance, 3) specific strategies by which the consultant can successfully interact with staff to convey information and to serve as a model, and 4) specific means by which to meet the needs of the individual staff members and facilitate learning of material in a stimulating and interesting fashion.

Generally, the principal focus of behavioral consultation involves either case consultation or consultation-liaison work, the primary difference between these being that case consultation tends to have a specific problem focus or patient-related issue, while consultation-liaison work involves not only specific case material but also case coordination and/or staff issues relative to a particular patient. Although consultation-liaison services tend to be specific to the hospital or institutional environment, their primary emphasis is consultation regarding specific case management. Kratochwill and Bergan (1978) define behavioral consultation as "a problem-solving model designed to assist consultees in defining problems and evaluating the attainment of consultation goals and the effectiveness of plans implemented to achieve these goals." (p. 377) They termed the strategies of this model as problem identification, problem analysis, plan implementation, and program evaluation. Certainly, in behavioral medicine consultation these strategies serve as a foundation for the development of both treatment and assessment programs. It is important to consider that the empirical framework and methodology that enhances such consultative endeavors (typically not found in other disciplines or treatment programs) is the specific forte of the behavioral consultant. This empirical framework provides for the operational definition of problem areas, the means by which to quantify these target problems, and methods by which to measure the changes brought forth by programming as well as strategies for treatment follow-up and maintenance.

To conduct effective behavioral consultation, four requirements become salient and require consideration. First, it is essential that the consultant develop a knowledge and understanding of the clinical-medical system in which he or she will be working as well as an understanding of the structure of administration within that system. Hersen and Bellack (1978), in referring to this as the "politics" of the consultation setting, note the importance of recognizing the "interpersonal forces, undercurrents, and informal networks that determine much of the day-to-day hospital operation" (p. 77). Although their specific reference is to the hospital environment, it is suggested that the same considerations be applied to other consultation settings. Certainly, an understanding of the system and the workings of the administration in the consultation environment provides the consultant with useful guidelines and resources from which to draw.

A second requirement is that the consultant have strong interpersonal skills, as the consulting environment can often prove to be both socially challenging and hostile. It is not unusual in the daily endeavors of the behavioral consultant to encounter those who might be skeptical, suspicious, or even overtly hostile. These feelings and sentiments arise not only because of a sense of professional intimidation but more often because of the staff's lack of familiarity with or strong personal bias against the orientation or philosophy espoused by the consultant. In these situations, it is important that the consultant draw upon his or her interpersonal skills of assertiveness in carrying out consultation duties, while remaining sensitive to issues posed by the consultee staff or, even, a general sense of apprehension and skepticism regarding new ideas and interventions that they might have.

A third requirement of the behavioral consultant is that he or she be able to function in an interdisciplinary setting. Generally, consultation, such as in behavioral medicine, often takes place in a hospital or similar setting, thus necessitating cooperative efforts of individuals from different clinical professions.

Successful consultation within such systems requires an understanding of the role of each of these individuals and an understanding of each of their areas of expertise in addition to the limits of the consultant's own role in working with them.

Finally, once these preliminary requirements of understanding the political and work environment are met, the expertise of the consultant and substantive issues of the consultation can now become the focus. Having addressed the politics, the personalities, and the professional interests involved in the consultation environment, the behavioral consultant can then draw upon his or her specific expertise in the assessment, formulation and implementation of treatment, staff training, and research regarding the specific case problem.

Nature and Demands of Consultation

Although behavioral consultation can take place in a variety of settings, the consultation environments common to developmentally disabled persons include hospitals, schools, residential facilities, and homes. Though specific demands and considerations of behavioral consultation vary depending on the settings, there are several critical features that are consistent across these diverse environments.

Interdisciplinary Focus

One of the more common issues to be addressed in many consultation environments is the need to recognize the interdisciplinary nature of the staff as well as their differing levels of professional training and expertise. In addressing this issue the consultant must be able to work cooperatively with individuals while maintaining a positive and productive interaction style. Mesibov and Johnson (1982) describe the role of the pediatric psychologist in the consultation process. Specifically, they focus on three consultation environments (i.e., the medical, school, and residential settings), and note that in each of these the ability to recognize the interworkings of an interdisciplinary staff as well as the politics and hierarchies within each of these settings is necessary for successful performance.

The behavioral consultant's success in being able to perform in the interdisciplinary environment hinges largely on his or her ability and willingness to learn about the roles of the other contributors and care providers and to understand how these roles interface with the role of the consultant. Typically, this can be accomplished by meeting with these individuals formally or within the framework of case coordination with discussion regarding each person's role, perspectives on the case, and what their own expectations of the behavioral consultant might be. Usually, each individual and discipline represented will have some particular expectation of the consultant related to how the intervention might impact directly on his or her own involvement with the case. Furthermore, each discipline representative will expect some recognition of his or her own expertise and potential contributions to the treatment and management of a particular case.

This "give-and-take" process is one of information sharing and facilitates the development of guidelines and a data base by which the behavioral consultant can begin his or her work.

In most consultation environments, it is often the case that staffs as a whole tend to be unfamiliar with behavioral theory, applied behavioral analysis, and the empirically based methodology upon which behavioral consultation is founded. Furthermore, it is not unusual for some individuals to be wary of or even resistant to understanding or learning the theory, application, and practice of behavior modification. Bellack and Franks (1975) noted that open resistance is common when staffs are presented with the theory and intervention styles of behavior modification. They also point out that these attitudes are generally the result of misconceptions or pervasive myths regarding specific behavioral interventions such as aversive therapies or similar treatment strategies. Hersen and Bellack (1978) note that resistance can also be the result of individuals' concerns regarding "the behavior therapist's interest in quantifying human behavior" (p. 63). They explain that while it is necessary to approach empirically the targeted problem for both programmatic and research purposes, such quantification is sometimes interpreted and used as a way of assessing the competence of staff members. That is, that the "objective evaluation of patient progress necessarily implies some evaluation of staff performance" (p. 63). The implications of such negative interpretations by some staff members of the role of the behavioral consultant together with the possibility of program changes that these same individuals might not be prepared for or willing to accept can pose serious problems for the behavioral consultant. Certainly, the ability of the behavioral consultant to convey information and provide training in the implementation of behavioral techniques while being sensitive to these concerns requires deft social skills and a strong commitment to behavioral principles.

Administrative Concerns

Another important issue for consideration by the behavioral consultant is that often he or she enters the consultation environment with little or no administrative authority. As these are environments in which high expectations are often placed on the consultant, even amidst poor staff support and overt resistance, it is generally necessary to determine the source and seek out some level of administrative authority and support. The absence of authority can become an issue when the consultant is involved in the implementation of programming in which it is necessary to outline and direct staff functioning or in assigning specific duties to staff members. Resistance from consultee staff resulting from uncertainty, intimidation, or hostility is not unusual and requires that the consultant be both considerate and informed in the designation of duties, selection of staff, and development of programming, while having the overt support of the authority figure(s). Also, because most staff will generally be unfamiliar with behavioral intervention strategies, concrete direction and instruction will be necessary. Furthermore, in an effort to facilitate the implementation of programming and to help motivate a wary staff, it is often necessary for the consultant to function as a role model in the performance of duties. While these are all useful strategies for working with a cautious, unsupportive, or hostile staff, it is most useful for the consultant to contract with the institutional authorities such that some degree of power or directed support is assigned to the consultant and conveyed to the staff. This, together with careful planning and familiarity with the institution and its staff, will help to prevent conflicts that could undermine or compromise the consultant's work.

Role Definition

In a related area of concern, it is not unusual for the behavioral consultant to experience difficulties with staff personnel regarding the definition of his or her role and function. Generally, when a consultant is hired, it is for the purpose of addressing issues or problems that have posed particular concerns and obstacles to the institution and to the staff. As such, there often develops an unrealistic expectation that the behavioral consultant is the expert who can provide a "quick fix" for these problems. These exaggerated expectations often are the result of misconceptions regarding the work and the limitations of what the behavioral consultant can do as well as the limitations and constraints imposed by the institution. It is necessary that the consultant work within the framework and guidelines of the consultee institution with the expectation that staff members or selected personnel can carry out this work and maintain programming. For this reason, the work of the behavioral consultant must be carefully tailored to meet the specific needs of the consultee staff, with interventions carefully designed so that they can be realistically implemented and sustained by them. Again, most issues resulting from misconceptions regarding what the consultant can and is expected to do can be addressed through careful contracting and discussions with staff. Attention should be focused on the specific pattern at hand and realistic expectations established regarding what can be done given the limitations and constraints of the consultation environment. To further clarify and emphasize this point, it is often necessary to restate at periodic intervals during consultation the parameters of the consultant's ability in addressing the specific problems for which he or she has been contracted.

Staff training that concretely and realistically describes the potential contributions and limitations of the consultant's approach, as well as the responsibilities of the staff, can also serve to clarify the role and expectations of the behavioral consultant. This type of staff training involves presentation and instruction in the use of protocols and strategies of behavior modification interventions and their application in the consulting environment. As such, appropriate and reasonable target goals and objectives can be identified, a methodology outlined, and a quantifiable means of assessing outcome established. Such efforts clarify for the staff what is to be expected regarding behavior change and how this is to be effected. It is this type of approach and reliance on an empirical methodology that has fostered the integration of behavioral consultation into medicine, education, rehabilitation, and other disciplines.

Bellack and Franks (1975) note that consultees often tend to view the role of the consultant and the consultation contract in a circumscribed fashion. They explain that the expectation of the consultee staff is for the consultant to "tell me what to do with a client without necessarily teaching or changing me" or to "teach me a technique" (p. 389). Thus, Bellack and Franks suggest that the behavioral consultant contract specifically to address a designated problem and to work with the staff on how to implement the appropriate intervention program to address this problem. They further note that " more in-depth or more extensive presentation" concerning theoretical issues or more staff training should be a separate contracted goal. Bellack and Franks also suggest that when staff members are able to experience some immediate clinical success as a result of consultation and are reasonably comfortable with the means by which this was achieved, issues of resistance and poor compliance are reduced. Thus, the authors suggest that treatment program planning incorporate some early success experience, where possible, to facilitate staff support, cooperation, and motivation.

Staff Integration

One of the more general issues confronting the behavioral consultant is the simple fact that he or she is not a member of the "on-line" staff. Among staff members, the notion often evolves that the consultant is some sort of "big shot" who is "going to tell us what to do" and "change the way we like to do things." Although such sentiments are not necessarily pervasive, they can turn the efforts of the behavioral consultant into a frustrating experience punctuated by occasional encounters with both overt and passive hostilities from staff members that can serve to isolate the consultant from the staff. Others who have studied this process of consultation concur that the most successful means by which to address this problem is to shed "the outsider" role and to literally become part of the "on-line" staff. Petrillo and Sanger (1980), Geist (1977), and Mesibov and Johnson (1982) all stress the importance of direct participation by the consultant in the clinical intervention and management of a case, thus serving as a role model while demonstrating a willingness to work cooperatively with the staff members. Geist (1977) describes this process as the consultant becoming a part of the milieu and, as such, becoming part of the working staff. In doing so, the behavioral consultant must be both empathic and sensitive to staff issues while providing them with direction and instruction. Despite the efforts of the consultant and the benefits of the strategies suggested by him or her, some resistance can remain for which more direct discussion might be necessary. In this event, appropriate assertiveness in addition to a restatement of the contractual agreement describing the role and the expectations of the consultant can be useful in assuaging such concerns.

It is essential that the behavioral consultant always consider that he or she is, in fact, "an outsider" whose responsibility it is to be sensitive to the issues and the concerns of the staff while meeting the objective of the consultation contract. Oftentimes it is a useful strategy to plan a meeting with staff members simply for the sake of listening to the ideas, concerns, and anxieties of the staff with which one will be working. This gesture is one that is generally recognized and appreciated by staff, although the ultimate benefit is realized in increased understanding of some of the staff and environmental variables that could impact on program development and implementation.

Time-Limited Function

Another issue that should be considered both in consultation contracting and in the development of relationships with the consultee staff is that the behavioral consultant's work is generally time limited. This tends to result in some degree of limited visibility. That is, it is generally not possible or reasonable for the behavioral consultant to be "on line" with the consultee staff on a day-to-day basis. Because of this, it is the responsibility of the behavioral consultant to develop a model of intervention that is easily understood and implementable by staff members that will facilitate some degree of autonomous functioning in program implementation. In the initial phases of the consultation process, it is important that the behavioral consultant be represented at each step of programming, including goal and objective formation, development of treatment strategies, and implementation of assessment procedures and outcome studies. Furthermore, it is important that the consultant provide a reliable schedule by which staff members can access the consultant for his or her expertise as they proceed with the day-to-day implementation of programming. This accessibility of the behavioral consultant, together with a carefully designed and implemented treatment program, will help to reduce concerns that can develop from decreased visibility.

Throughout the consultation process, it is important for the behavioral consultant to acknowledge and encourage the independent functioning of staff members in their successful implementation of the intervention program. It is also important to consider that open communication and mutual efforts in maintaining communication provides access to the consultant for information purposes and to provide a means by which staff members can express their concerns or questions regarding programming. Mechanisms for establishing and maintaining effective mutual communication should be formally integrated into the consultation contract.

Stages of Consultation

Since specific models of consultation generally offer idiosyncratic consultation formats, it is generally true that behaviorally based consultation engenders a consistent treatment and assessment format that relies heavily on its empirical foundation. Four stages of consultation become evident in examining the behavioral consultation format (Kratochwill & Bergan, 1978). These are: 1) problem identification, 2) problem analysis, 3) intervention, and 4) program evaluation. Each of these stages incorporates into its format a quantifiable means by which to measure and track behavior change so that reasonable assessments can be made regarding treatment outcome and program effectiveness. Bergan (1977) and Hersen and Bellack (1978) have systematically identified similar methodologies for each of these stages that are based upon measurable behavior change and calculated manipulations of the consultation environment.

Problem Identification

Before behavioral consultation can be clinically implemented, a specific problem or issue must be identified and some agreement reached within the consulting environment that behavioral consultation would be useful and necessary. Typically, problems or issues that are identified by staff personnel and targeted for consultation are the more difficult cases or can be clinical concerns that go beyond the work capacity or even the skill level of the consultee staff. In these situations, a contact person, preferable one who is familiar with the case, initiates the consultation process by presenting the identified problem to the behavioral consultant. Conversations and meetings between the behavioral consultant and staff members serve as a formal process for the identification and analysis of the issues, with some consideration given to the subjective and objective data available. Furthermore, these initial information-sharing sessions can help to determine the impact of the identified problem on the consultee environment and ways in which the problem has been sustained. Because referring staffs typically lack behavioral expertise and sophistication, the data they have to offer tend to be crude and vague, frequently more narrative than empirical. Also, the data and information initially collected by the consultee staff can often be clouded and biased by the extent of frustration and helplessness that they have experienced. It is often useful if the consultant can relieve some of these initial anxieties and concerns by providing a more empirically based context in which to view the identified problem that is objective and constructive.

One of the early goals in the problem identification stage of consultation is to provide staff members with a more formal means by which to collect information and data that will help to further define and delineate the referral problem. Behaviorally oriented clinicians and researchers have produced many instruments and strategies for the identification of target behaviors and the collection of early or preintervention data. One instrument, the Behavior Management, Planning, and Programming Form (BMPPF), described by Luiselli (1981), provides for an accumulation of in-depth information to help in both problem identification and treatment program development. The BMPPF generates useful and specific information regarding the presenting problem such as its estimated frequency of occurrence, the approximate duration of the occurrence of the behavior, the relative effectiveness of previous interventions, and specific case characteristics. This particular format, as suggested by Luiselli, has been found to be extremely useful in consultation regarding developmentally disabled populations, as information and characteristics regarding an individual's physical, sensory, intellectual, language, and social functioning are collected.

It is important during this initial phase of consultation that a working understanding of the politics, day-to-day operations, and general resources within the consulting environment is developed. As noted earlier, effective consultation almost always requires close cooperation with the consultee staff, especially those individuals who have had extensive contact with the identified target population. This type of cooperative relationship not only helps to facilitate the processes of information gathering and problem identification, but also contributes to the smooth implementation of intervention programming. Efforts made during this stage of consultation to become familiar with the consulting environment, to develop a working relationship with staff members, and to gain the confidence of the staff will help to lay a foundation for effective consultation. Furthermore, consideration given to maintaining consultant visibility, accessibility as a resource person, and sensitivity to staff issues will serve to assuage concerns or anxieties that might develop regarding staff roles and responsibilities in implementing the consultant's program.

The last phase of problem identification involves establishing agreement between the consultant and staff members on an operational definition of the target problem. Such a definition must be specific, concrete, and provide a clear and quantifiable target behavior. At the same time, such specificity must not prove to be overwhelming to the consultee staff in their efforts to observe and quantify these behaviors. It is important to strike a balance between determining an operation definition of the target behavior that will allow for the collection of valid data, while also being functional in terms of the ease of program implementation so as to encourage staff support and cooperation.

Having developed an operational definition of the target behavior, the establishment of a methodology for the collection of data and strategies for measuring treatment outcome now become the focus of consultation. By breaking down the target behavior to increments that are simple and observable, strategies such as frequency measures, interval measures, or checklists can be easily implemented. It is important to carefully consider the methodology to be used in data collection and how it can be adapted to the consulting environment. Because data collection often proves to be the most difficult and time-consuming aspect of a behavioral intervention for the consultee staff, involving staff members in designing this process is often both efficacious and politically savvy. Furthermore, because the more empirical and scientifically sound strategies for data collection are often difficult to implement in the consulting environment and are subject to the constraints of staff limitations, meticulous contracting and discussions with these staff members can help to formulate a workable strategy. Thus, having developed an operational definition of the target behavior and a plan for the collection of data, the next phase of behavioral consultation is data collection.

Problem Analysis and Assessment

Problem analysis and assessment is very much dependent on the careful identification and definition of the referral problem. In developing strategies to address the problem, it is necessary to establish measures that can determine the extent of the problem, assess the rate of occurrence of the problem, and provide some means by which to evaluate the outcome of the intervention. The initial phase of assessment involves the collection of data to provide a baseline measure of the target behavior. It is during this baseline phase of data collection that the consultant and staff must work closely to ensure that the assessment techniques are reasonable and realistic given environmental and staff constraints. It is important that the consultant be actively involved in this phase of data collection to ascertain that the procedures being implemented by the consultee staff are in line with the recommended empirical format. This early cooperative effort between the consultant and staff can help to address miscommunications or misunderstandings that might arise with the implementation of programming.

The amount of time needed for collecting baseline data is often determined by the degree of difficulty encountered in establishing a reliable method of response recording and achieving some consistent measure of the target behavior. Because the reliability of the data being collected is important to maintain throughout the consultation process, two considerations are noteworthy. First, since nonprofessional staff are often involved in the data collection process, it is important to determine the reliability of reports between the different observers and correct problems as they occur. Correcting such problems usually involves either a revision of the operational and concrete definition of the target behavior or the provision of additional instruction and training to staff members in accurately measuring these behaviors. Second, because more of the responsibility for program implementation will be gradually transitioned to the consultee staff over the course of consultation, it is essential that the staff be both comfortable with and skilled in method of data collection. Once the accurate and reliable collection of data has been established, consultation can proceed to the design and implementation of clinical programming.

Intervention

Having defined and collected baseline data about the target behavior, the consultant is now prepared to design and implement a treatment program. Certainly, a strength of the behavioral consultant's approach is the variety of techniques and strategies that have been developed, researched, and adapted for a diversity of specialized populations. These techniques and strategies comprise the consultant's clinical repertoire and are the essence of what the consultee staff has requested. Typically, it is the behavioral technique rather than the theoretical orientation of the consultant that he or she has been hired to produce. This consideration is important with regard to staff training and preparation. Bellack and Franks (1975) and Hersen and Bellack (1978) note that the application of the technique should initially be stressed before the theoretical framework upon which it is based. These authors suggest that an early goal of consultation should be to allow the consultee to participate in the implementation of behavioral programs and to experience the success that this often brings. Hersen and Bellack (1978) point out that with this success, the consultee tends to be "more amenable to an in-depth evaluation of the basis for the technology being used" (p. 83). It is the consultant's responsibility to be active and visible in the demonstration of treatment procedures, in modeling the staff role in the clinical interventions, and in explaining how treatment has been adapted for the consultee environment. Thus, as a visible clinical resource and with some early success experience built into the behavioral intervention, the consultant can often expect a greater degree of enthusiasm and support from the consultee staff.

In designing a clinical intervention there are a number of considerations that must be acknowledged and addressed by the behavioral consultant and the consultee staff. Perhaps most important in these considerations is the identification of the independent variables or environmental variables that affect the target problem. As part of the preintervention observation and definition of the target behavior, it is important to identify those environmentally based stimuli that interact with the target behavior. Often, these variables serve to stimulate the occurrence of the target problem behavior and contribute to its maintenance. By identifying these environmental variables and, in a systematic and concrete fashion, establishing the relationship between these and the target behavior, the behavioral consultant can help the consultee staff to develop an understanding of the rationale regarding the design of the intervention and how it is to be implemented.

Another important consideration regarding treatment design involves identifying possible secondary gains resulting from a problem behavior, as well as how these tend to further reinforce it. In such cases, the intervention should also focus on these secondary gains and reinforcements and attempt to systematically alter them. Consideration should also be given to understanding the limitations of the consultation environment and staff so as to offer programming that can be realistically implemented. Often, this tends to be more of a logistical issue and requires that the consultant assess whether staffing and resources are sufficient to carry out the intervention and that the demands placed on the staff do not overly distract from their regular duties.

As part of treatment development it is important to monitor the effectiveness of the intervention throughout the consultation and to modify the treatment or methodology as deemed necessary. Modification of programming is necessary when: 1) the intervention has failed to effect the desired change in the target problem, 2) the assessment procedures being used do not yield reliable or valid data, or 3) the staff encounters problems that interfere with the implementation of programming. While these issues generally tend to be case specific, they do require attention from the consultant so that a more effective program can be designed. Once these program "bugs" have been identified and corrected, the revised intervention program is implemented, data are recorded, and a new assessment is made regarding treatment effectiveness. Again, it is important to stress that the consultant closely monitor and supervise the implementation of the modified treatment program to ascertain that a consistent approach is followed by the staff and that reliability is maintained in the collection of data. Many of these considerations and concerns can be addressed directly with the staff who probably are best able to advise the consultant on issues of compliance, motivation, and how the intervention can be better adapted to the consultee environment. As the intervention proceeds, and the desired changes occur in the target behavior, additional evaluation of the intervention and its effectiveness in addressing the target behavior becomes necessary. It is at this time that consideration also be given to the gradual withdrawal of formal intervention procedures and the formulation of maintenance programming.

Evaluation and Follow-Up

As part of consultation contracting regarding the formulation and implementation of treatment procedures, it is also necessary to include strategies for treatment and follow-up evaluations. Treatment evaluation is an integral feature of any behavioral intervention and, as such, has frequently been described and discussed in the behavior modification literature. Hersen and Barlow (1976), Kratochwill (1978), and others have extensively reviewed single-case design and time-series research formats that provide for the evaluation of treatment procedures by measuring the impact of the manipulation of independent variables on dependent variables, or the target behaviors. Operationally, this allows for the identification and examination of different environmental stimuli that contribute to the development and maintenance of the target behavior. Finally, with regard to the consultation contract, treatment evaluation provides data upon which the termination of the intervention program can be effected once the agreed-upon criteria or goals have been met.

It is important to stress that treatment evaluation methods can easily be integrated into program designs and provide evidence regarding the effectiveness and benefit of the intervention. Furthermore, this type of outcome data can be used to encourage the consultee staff in their efforts and to further facilitate their cooperation and motivation. By having staff members participate in the process of determining reasonable criteria for the assessment of treatment outcome, they are better able to monitor the results and impact of their work. In the event that treatment outcome does not meet expectations, staff members reviewing these data can have some input regarding the need and rationale for modification of the intervention.

As part of any intervention program, it is expected that the programmed environmental changes that have served to reduce or eliminate the target behavior will be maintained and eventually integrated into the consultation environment. However, researchers have reported that the termination of formal intervention programming has often resulted in the deterioration of the recently implemented environmental change, thus allowing the recurrence of the target behavior (Marholin & Siegel, 1978). For this reason, it is essential to have a maintenance program in place at the time of formal termination of consultation services that can be implemented by the staff without the direct input of the behavioral consultant.

Maintenance programming not only contributes to the long-term impact of the consultant's work, but also facilitates the transitioning of the administration of programming to the consultee staff. Maintenance programming involves the continuation of existing intervention procedures with the elimination or reduction of the more burdensome features of the consultant's program, such as the comprehensive collection of data, which can be achieved by implementing fewer and shorter observation periods by staff members. Another strategy for maintenance programming would include the gradual withdrawal of tangible reinforcement systems and transitioning to more "naturally occurring" reinforcing stimuli such as social attention. The implementation of social reinforcement strategies contingent upon the performance of appropriate behaviors that are incompatible with the target behavior is another useful technique that can be used in program maintenance.

Follow-up evaluations are important in determining the long-term success of the consultant's program and the degree to which treatment effect has been successfully maintained in the consultation environment. Follow-up evaluation typically involves implementing formal data collection, using procedures identical to those used during the initial phase of treatment evaluation. These data yield information regarding whether there has been a symptom or problem regression or if there has been an increase in the frequency of the target behavior. The timing of the follow-up evaluation is often a subjective decision, although in contracting for behavioral consultation, a follow-up period of 2 to 6 months is generally sufficient. Hersen and Barlow (1976) have described a number of follow-up assessment procedures and how these yield specific data regarding treatment outcome as determined by the status of the independent and dependent variables.

Behavioral Consultation Within Clinical Settings

The various phases and stages of behavioral consultation outlined previously describe a process of service delivery that is applicable to most clinical settings. However, it has also been noted that various settings differ with regards to the goals, objectives, and demands of consultation. Therefore, to be maximally effective, the methodology of consultation must be adapted to the particular setting. In this section, the authors discuss setting-specific concerns for behavioral medicine consultation within medical, residential, and school environments, including several illustrative case examples.

Medical Settings

Roberts, Maddux, Wurtele, and Wright (1982) suggest three models of consultation that occur within the medical setting. Although the four elements of behavioral consultation (i.e., problem identification, problem analysis and assessment, intervention, and evaluation and follow-up) apply to each of these models, the format with which the consultant operates does vary somewhat.

In the independent functions model, Roberts et al. (1982) describe the consultant as a "specialist" who, independent of the consultee staff, implements the diagnostic evaluation and treatment of a patient. This model does not promote a collaborative endeavor between the consultant and the consultee, except for the exchange of referral and outcome information. The authors note that this model of consultation is prevalent in medical settings because of the traditional arrangement of the subspecialty consultant and the primary care practitioner. As such, throughout this consultation model the referring physician continues to manage the "medical aspects" of the presenting problem and defers to the behavioral consultant on matters related to the biobehavioral and psychosocial issues.

Another consultation format, the indirect psychological consultation model, establishes direct consultation to the referring physician but with little direct contact with the patient. While more collaboration regarding patient diagnosis and treatment exists between professionals in this model, it is typically limited to a specific problem focus. Christophersen and Rapoff (1980) describe a similar consultation model in which they taught medical staff specific treatment procedures for the management of encopresis and enuresis being used by a pediatric psychologist. In this format, the consultant's input can take the form of staff supervision, the didactic presentation of assessment treatment strategies through lectures, grand-round presentations or in-service training. This consultation format has become increasingly more common in medical settings and especially so with the addition of behavioral medicine subspecialists to hospital staffs and medical school faculties.

The third model of behavioral consultation in medical settings described by Roberts et al. (1982) is the collaborative team model. In this consultation format, the behavioral clinician becomes a member of a collaborative, interdisciplinary evaluation and treatment team that can also include physicians, psychologists, physical therapists, occupational therapists, social workers, audiologists, speech and language pathologists, and education specialists. This interdisciplinary team model has become more popular in recent years and has been incorporated into a variety of hospital departments including Oncology-Hematology (Koocher, Sourkes, & Keane, 1979; Sugai 1982), Neurology (Sugai 1983a), Surgery (Geist, 1977), Child Development and Pediatrics (Russo & Varni, 1982), Gastroenterology (Schaefer, 1979; Sugai & Benedetto, 1985), and Neonatal Intensive Care Units (Magrab & Davitt, 1975). In the collaborative team model, the behavioral consultant often participates in case coordination responsibilities as well as the more traditional endeavors of behavioral assessment and treatment. Furthermore, the role of the consultant often includes teaching and training responsibilities with regard to the other team members as well as to medical, psychology, and social work interns and residents.

An example of the behavioral psychologist's role in an interdisciplinary team model was described by Suagi (1983b). In this case, a 28-month-old girl with diagnoses of failure-to-thrive and physical and cognitive developmental delays was referred for pediatric inpatient hospitalization with the goal of treating food refusal and emesis during meals. Behavioral consultation was provided as part of a comprehensive "feeding team" comprised of a pediatrician, pediatric dietary specialist, and occupational therapist specializing in oral-motor functioning. Each of these disciplines, in addition to the consulting pediatric psychologist, completed individual diagnostic assessments to determine the etiology of the

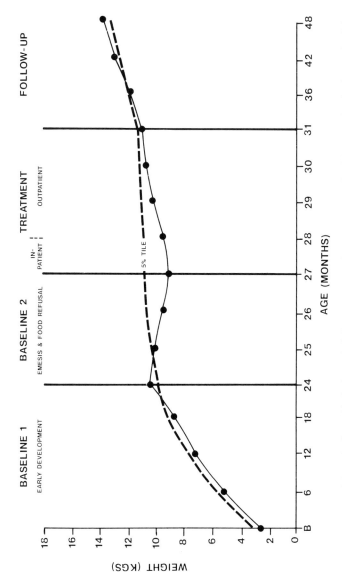

FIGURE 9.1. Weight gain from birth through follow-up evaluation as compared with normal velocity at the 5th percentile. The child was a 28-month-old girl receiving behavioral consultation within an inpatient hospital setting.

child's feeding problems. These assessments failed to identify a specific organic etiology and, therefore, a behaviorally based, contingency management treatment program was designed by the consultant. Procedures included a standardized method of food presentation, social reinforcement of food acceptance, withdrawal of attention (time-out) contingent upon food-refusal behaviors, and cue-contingent distraction following preemetic responses. Training was conducted with nursing staff and the child's foster mother. Treatment was implemented and evaluated during inpatient feeding sessions and meals scheduled during outpatient and follow-up home visits. Figure 9.1 shows that with the introduction of treatment, an increase in weight was established and sustained throughout the inpatient and outpatient phases of programming. Furthermore, with the termination of formal treatment, weight increase was maintained at the 5th percentile. Figure 9.2 presents the frequency of emesis during inpatient feeding sessions and documents the reduction and eventual elimination of vomiting behavior associated with application of the treatment program.

Mesibov and Johnson (1982) in describing medical consultation by pediatric psychologists identify several points that require some consideration. First, they emphasize that the role of the consulting psychologist in a medical setting tends to be different from that of the traditional role of the psychologist. While acknowledging that the consulting psychologist often participates in some "traditional consultative activities," they explain that the function of the consultant tends to interface with the more medically oriented issues such as use of and compliance in taking medications, preparation for medical procedures, and pain management. These issues often impact on when and how intervention programs are designed and implemented, thus necessitating that communications be maintained with the other professionals who are involved in the care of the patient. Depending on the nature of the presenting medical problem, the role of the consultant regarding patient care or his or her interactions with other health care professionals can vary greatly as can the consultants' actual contact time with the patient. As noted earlier, behavioral consultation services, whether direct or indirect, always require maintaining close communication with the primary care physician or other involved in the coordination of health care services. Mesibov and Johnson (1982) note that this issue focuses specifically on the relationship between the consulting psychologist and interdisciplinary medical treatment and evaluation team members. A third consideration concerns the behavioral consultant's extensive repertoire of intervention and assessment strategies and techniques and how these can be implemented within the medical setting or in addressing problems that have a medical component. As previously noted, behavioral specialists have contributed their treatment and assessment skills to address a variety of medical problems while maintaining a staunch adherence to a format that stresses empirically based assessment and treatment. Certainly, the recent development and recognition of autonomous departments of behavioral medicine in hospital settings underscores the contribution and value of this approach.

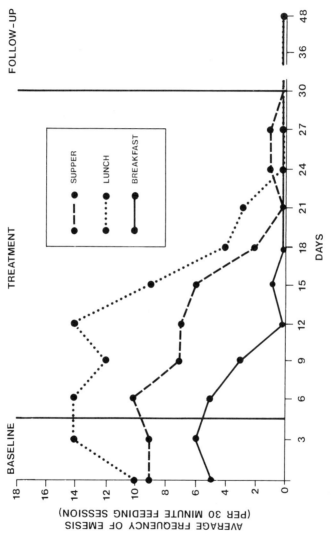

FIGURE 9.2. Reduction of emesis during inpatient hospitalization.

Another important contribution of the consulting psychologist in the medical environment is in the area of teaching and training. In teaching hospitals and other clinical settings, the consultant can play an important role in the education of medical, psychology, and social work interns and residents. Consulting psychologists sometimes participate in clinical patient rounds and are called upon to present both case-specific and more general clinical information regarding behavioral assessment and intervention with these patients. Such consultation activities not only provide training and supervision for residents, students, and interns, but also help to further define the role and clinical breadth of the behavioral specialist. In discussing consultation-liaison psychiatry, Enelow (1980) emphasizes the importance of teaching as a function of consultation. Although this reference is specific to the role of psychiatric consultation in medical settings, it is certainly applicable to behavioral consultation and its function in educating hospital staff while providing both direct and indirect clinical service. Teaching and training responsibilities through seminars, didactic presentations, and formal lectures as part of medical school curricula further help to establish the behavioral clinician and consultant as an integrated member of the health care community.

Finally, another focus for the behavioral consultant is the integration of research as part of clinical treatment design and program implementation. Because much of the behavioral consultant's clinical repertoire relies on quantification skills, the utility of his or her contribution is immediately recognized in such areas as treatment evaluation, program assessment, and research design. Inasmuch as treatment design and evaluation are a strength of the behavioral consultant and are typically not part of basic medical training, and given the increasing emphasis on medical utilization review and the need for the assessment of treatment outcome, the value of behavioral consultation in medical settings becomes even more evident. This integration of empirically based behavioral medicine with traditional clinical medicine has served to create an important role for behavioral consultation in medicine.

Residential Settings

Behavioral consultation, especially with the developmentally disabled population, commonly takes place in residential settings. Treatment strategies and important issues involved in providing behavioral consultation for developmentally disabled persons in residential settings have been addressed by a number of researchers. Mesibov and Johnson (1982) describe issues and methodologies involved in the residence-based treatment of special-needs populations such as the mentally retarded. Creer and Christian (1976) have written extensively about the behavioral treatment and management of chronically ill and handicapped children in their residential settings. Kazdin (1973) and Schinke and Wong (1977) describe consultation issues related to residential-staff training pertaining to management of developmentally disabled individuals. As with behavioral consultation in a medical setting, a general protocol exists for the behaviorally based assessment of target problems, treatment formulation, and the assessment of treatment outcome and effectiveness in residential settings. However, in consulting in a residential setting, there are additional important considerations regarding staff participation and in the development of an understanding of the operations and functions of the "system" within the residential environment.

Unlike behavioral consultation in medical or educational settings, a residential population tends to have a more chronic and dependent need for services from the staff personnel. Furthermore, the resources within the residential setting or of its staff tend to be more limited than in other consultation environments. As such, in performing residential-based behavioral consultation it is generally true that staff training is an important goal of any intervention program. Kazdin (1973) and Nay (1978) emphasize the importance of working with the staff members of a residential setting, not only in program implementation and the instruction of behavior modification techniques, but also in areas such as staff communication and motivation. Luiselli (1981) also stresses the importance of developing a comfortable working relationship between the behavioral consultant and staff members of the residential setting. Luiselli suggests that this can be accomplished by emphasizing an objective and empirically based approach typical of behavioral treatment, while avoiding the use of overly technical information and terminology in communication with the staff. Considerations such as these help to facilitate staff support and their confidence in behavioral treatment programming and the competence of the consultant.

Staff involvement is an important component of the behavioral consultant's program both in data collection and treatment implementation. McInnis (1976) notes that staff training is crucial for successful program outcome and that careful and precise program development and the cooperative implementation of these programs facilitates attaining the consultation objectives while also providing some success experience for staff members. It is not unusual, however, for some resistance to exist on the part of staff members to learn or develop new skills for the purpose of implementing the consultant's programming. Hersen and Bellack (1978) make a distinction between staff training and staff consultation, in that the former often implies an institutional commitment to staff training and program changes while the latter tends to be more case specific. They do note, though, that for both approaches it is important to attend to staff issues and concerns, not only regarding the learning of new skills, but also staff and consultant relations and issues of motivation. Such efforts enhance sustained staff cooperation and facilitate the eventual transitioning of programming responsibilities for the consultant to the residential placement staff.

Sugai and Benedetto (1985) provided behavioral consultation to a residential group-home to manage emesis of a 4-year-old mildly retarded, developmentally disabled girl. Data on the frequency of emesis were recorded during breakfast and supper meals by members of the group-home staff. In addition, the teaching staff at the child's classroom collected data within the lunch meal. Both residential and classroom staffs were trained to implement a treatment program that combined social reinforcement for appropriate feeding and contingent auditory

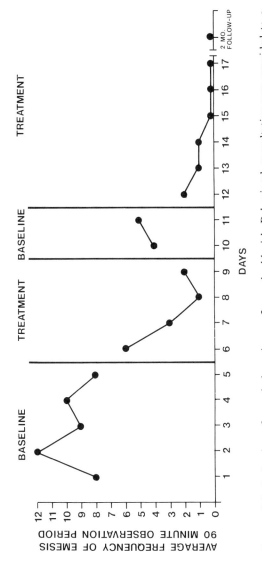

FIGURE 9.3. Reduction of emesis in a 4-year, 2-month-old girl. Behavioral consultation was provided to a residential group-home setting.

distraction to direct the child's attention away from initiating or completing emetic behavior. Procedures were evaluated using an ABAB reversal design. The results, presented in Figure 9.3, indicated that the treatment program was very successful in eliminating emesis and that the effects were maintained at a 2-month follow-up assessment.

School Settings

In recent years the role of behavioral psychologists working with developmentally disabled, learning disabled, and medically compromised children has expanded to include consultation services in the classroom. One problem area in which this has become particularly true is with attention deficit disordered, hyperactive youngsters. Traditionally, behavioral and pediatric psychologists have been involved in the evaluation and development of behavioral programs for these youngsters. More recently, however, they have been called upon to provide consultation to school personnel on issues including behavior management, academic performance, social skills, and stress management. Studies by Ross and Ross (1976) and Safer and Allen (1976) have emphasized the need to integrate behavioral management techniques that control the behavior of hyperactive youngsters and teach them behavioral self-management, while also developing programs that adequately address their educational needs in light of specific learning problems, such as short attention span, poor focal attention, and distractibility. Recent studies by Rosenthal and Allen (1978), Barkley (1985), and others clearly note the interrelationship between educational problems and behavioral problems with this population, and stress the importance of coordinating programming and interventions to address both problems.

Other areas in which school-based behavioral consultation has become more evident is in the management of youngsters who have medical disorders such as cancer (Katz, Kellerman, Rigler, Williams, & Siegel, 1977), chronic or serious illness such as asthma or epilepsy (Kaplan, Smith, & Grobstein, 1974; Holdsworth & Whitmore, 1974; Gershwin & Klingelhofer, 1986), and developmental disabilities (Cyphert, 1973; Molnar & Taft, 1975; Zigler & Muenchow, 1979). Recent research has also reviewed the role of behavioral consultation in addressing school-based management of dietary programs, feeding problems, and eating disorders (Coates, Jeffrey, & Slinkard, 1981; Sugai & Benedetto, 1985; Williams, Carter, Arnold, & Wynder, 1979), the management of anxiety disorders and stress in the classroom (Russell & Carter, 1978), and the development and enrichment of children's social-interactional skills (Michelson, Sugai, Wood, & Kazdin, 1983; Sheppard, Shank, & Wilson, 1973). Given the variety of problem behaviors and issues addressed by the behavioral consultant, it is again important to note that the format and guidelines for consultation are based on a scientific and empirically based methodology while addressing the health and psychological needs of this population.

Luiselli (in press) described the school-based treatment of a health-threatening behavior displayed by a 6-year-old deaf, mentally retarded boy with a medical diagnosis of cytomegalovirus (CMV). This child engaged in high-rate spitting

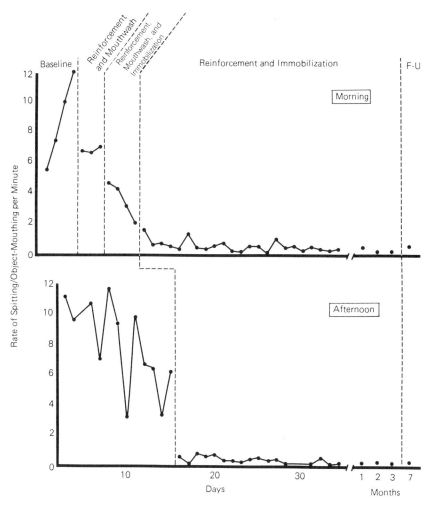

FIGURE 9.4. Frequency of spitting and object mouthing by a 6-year-old boy with cytomegalovirus. Behavioral consultation was provided to a special-education classroom.

and object mouthing and, as a result, projected and drooled saliva onto himself, other persons, and materials. The presence of saliva was unhygienic and problematic in that it represents one medium for transmission of the virus. Through consultation with the classroom teachers, two play periods during the day were selected as the settings for data collection. Staff recorded the frequency of spitting and object mouthing during these periods within the context of a multiple-baseline design. The initial treatment phase consisted of reinforcement of non-expectorating behaviors plus contingent application of diluted mouthwash as a mildly aversive consequence. This program did not establish clinical control until a response-contingent immobilization procedure (gently holding hands down for

3 seconds) was added to the treatment package. Subsequently, the mouthwash procedure was discontinued while the reinforcement plus immobilization strategy was maintained. As shown in Figure 9.4, this combination of procedures was responsible for rapid response suppression. Results of a 7-month follow-up assessment revealed therapeutic maintenance in the absence of continued treatment.

Summary

This chapter discusses several issues relating to the process of behavioral medicine consultation to developmentally disabled persons. Effective consultation is dependent, in part, on an understanding of the demands and operating procedures of the clinical setting. Critical features of most consultation environments include an interdisciplinary focus, the nature of the administrative hierarchy, clear role definition, integration with on-line staff, and a time-limited function. In accordance with other behavioral consultation models, specific stages of consultation are reviewed with regards to goals, objectives, and methods to promote therapeutic success. Consultation practices within medical, residential, and school settings are discussed to highlight some of the idiosyncratic concerns that apply to specific clinical environments. The case examples that are presented demonstrate how the behavioral medicine consultant can serve as an empirical clinician and, in that role, deliver effective therapeutic services while conducting meaningful applied research.

Although this chapter discusses many facets of behavioral medicine consultation, it is worth noting that most consultant behaviors have been generated by individual "learning histories" without the benefit of systematic research. Thus, we need to evaluate various consultative protocols with regards to cost efficiency, durability, and clinical outcome. Data are also lacking on the most effective format for delivering consultation services (e.g., case review, interdisciplinary team). It would be informative to have consultees rate their acceptability of and satisfaction with the methods and results of consultation through social validity assessment. Furthermore, what are the best approaches to train behavioral medicine consultants? Research on these and similar topics would provide essential information on how to improve the methodology of clinical consultation and service to clients.

References

Ayllon, T., & Michael, J. (1959). The psychiatric nurse as a behavioral engineer. *Journal of Experimental Analysis of Behavior, 2*, 323–334.

Barkley, R.A. (1985). Attention deficit disorders. In P.H. Bornstein & A.E. Kazdin (Eds.), *Handbook of clinical behavior therapy with children* (pp. 158–215). Homewood, IL: Dorsey Press.

Bellack, A.S., & Franks, C.M. (1975). Behavioral consultation in the community mental health center. *Behavioral Therapy, 6*, 388–391.

Bergan, J.R. (1977). *Behavioral consultation*. Columbus, OH: Merrill.

Christophersen, E.R., & Rapoff, M.A. (1980). Pediatric psychology: An appraisal. In B.B. Lahey & A.E. Kazdin (Eds.), *Advances in clinical child psychology* (Vol. 3) (185–221). New York: Plenum Press.

Coates, T.J., Jeffrey, R.W., & Slinkard, L.A. (1981). Heart, healthy eating and exercise: Introducing and maintaining changes in health behaviors. *American Journal of Public Health, 71*, 15–23.

Creer, T.L., & Christian, W.P. (1976). *Chronically ill and handicapped children: Their management and rehabilitation*. Champaign, IL: Research Press.

Cyphert, F.R. (1973). Back to school for the child with cancer. *Journal of School Health, 43*, 215–217.

Enelow, A.J. (1980). Consultation-liaison psychiatry. In H.I. Kaplan, A.M. Freedman, & B.J. Sadock (Eds.), *Comprehensive textbook of psychiatry* (Vol. 2, pp. 1980–1985). Baltimore: Williams & Wilkins.

Geist, R. (1977). Consultation on a pediatric surgical ward: Creating an empathic climate. *American Journal of Orthopsychiatry, 47*, 432–444.

Gershwin, M.E., & Klingelhofer, E.L. (1986). *Asthma: Stop suffering, start living*. Reading, MA: Addison-Wesley.

Graziano, A.M. (1971). *Behavior therapy with children*. Chicago: Aldine.

Hersen, M., & Barlow, D.H. (1976). *Single case experimental designs: Strategies for studying behavior change*. New York: Pergamon Press.

Hersen, M., & Bellack, A.S. (1978). Staff training and consultation. In M. Hersen & A.S. Bellack (Eds.), *Behavior therapy in the psychiatric setting* (pp. 58–87). Baltimore: Williams & Wilkins.

Holdsworth, L., & Whitmore, K. (1974). A study of children with epilepsy attending ordinary schools. *Developmental Medicine in Child Neurology, 16*, 746–758.

Kaplan, D.M., Smith, A., & Grobstein, R. (1974). School management of the seriously ill child. *Journal of School Health, 44*, 250–254.

Kaplan, S.J. (1987). *The private practice to behavior therapy*. New York: Plenum Press.

Katz E.R., Kellerman, J., Rigler, D., Williams, K.O., & Siegel, S.E. (1977). School intervention with pediatric cancer patients. *Journal of Pediatric Psychology, 2*, 72–76.

Kazdin, A.E. (1973). Issues in behavior modification with mentally retarded persons. *American Journal of Mental Deficiency, 78*, 134–140.

Koocher, G.P., Sourkes, B.M., & Keane, W.M. (1979). Pediatric oncology consultations: A generalizable model for medical settings. *Professional Psychology, 10*, 467–274.

Kratochwill, T. (Ed.). (1978). *Single subject research: Strategies for evaluating change*. New York: Academic Press.

Kratochwill, T.R., & Bergan, J.R. (1978). Evaluating programs in applied settings through behavioral consultation. *Journal of School Psychology, 16*, 375–386.

Luiselli, J.K. (1981). Consultation in the residential treatment of visually impaired children. *Journal of Visual Impairment and Blindness, 75*, 353–357.

Luiselli, J.K. (in press). *Multicomponent behavioral treatment of high-rate spitting and object-mouthing in a child with cytomegalovirus. Journal of the Multihandicapped Person*.

MacDonald, M.L. (1983). Behavioral consultation in geriatric settings. *The Behavior Therapist, 6*, 172–174.

Magrab, P.R., & Davitt M.K. (1975). The pediatric psychologist and the developmental follow-up of intensive care nursery infants. *Journal of Clinical Child Psychology, 4*, 16–18.

Marholin, D., II, & Siegel, L.J. (1978). Beyond the law of effect: Programming for the maintenance of behavioral change. In D. Marholin, II (Ed.), *Child behavior therapy.* New York: Gardner Press.

McInnis, T. (1976). Training and maintaining staff behaviors in residential treatment programs. In R.L. Patterson (Ed.), *Maintaining effective token economies.* Springfield, IL: Thomas. (pp. 95–166).

Mesibov, G.B., & Johnson, M.R. (1982). Intervention techniques in pediatric psychology. In J. Tuma (Ed.), *Handbook for the practice of pediatric psychology* (pp. 110–164). New York: Wiley.

Michelson, L., Sugai, D.P., Wood, R.P., & Kazdin, A.E. (1983). *Social skills assessment and training with children: An empirically based handbook.* New York: Plenum Press.

Molnar, G.A., & Taft, L.T. (1975). Cerebral Palsy. In J. Wartis (Ed.), *Mental retardation and developmental disabilities: An annual review* (pp. 121–134). New York: Brunner-Mazel.

Nay, W.R. (1978). Intra-institutional "roadblocks" to behavior modification programming. In D. Marholin II (Ed.), *Child behavior therapy* (pp. 446–459). New York: Gardner Press.

Petrillo, M., & Sanger, S. (1980). *Emotional care of hospitalized children.* Philadelphia: Lippincott.

Poser, E.G. (1967). Training behavior therapists. *Behavior Research and Therapy, 5,* 37–41.

Roberts, M.C., Maddux, J.E., Wurtele, S.K., & Wright, L. (1982). Pediatric care: Health care psychology for children. In T. Millon, C. Green, & R. Meagher (Eds.), *Handbook of clinical health psychology* (pp. 191–226). New York: Plenum Press.

Rosenthal, R.H., & Allen, T.W. (1978). An examination of attention arousal and learning dysfunctions of hyperkinetic children. *Psychological Bulletin, 85,* 689–715.

Ross, D.M., & Ross, S.A. (1976). *Hyperactivity: Research, theory, and action.* New York: Wiley.

Russell, H.L., & Carter, J.L. (1978). Biofeedback training with children: Consultation, questions, applications, and alternatives. *Journal of Clinical Child Psychology, 7,* 23–25.

Russo, D.C., & Varni, J.W. (1982). Behavioral pediatrics. In D. Russo & J. Varni (Eds.), *Behavioral pediatrics: Research and practice* (pp. 3–24). New York: Plenum Press.

Safer, D.J., & Allen, R.P. (1976). *Hyperactive children: Diagnosis and management.* Baltimore: University Park Press.

Schaefer, C.E. (1979). *Childhood encopresis: Causes and therapy.* New York: Van Nostrand Reinhold.

Schinke, S.P., & Wong, S.E. (1977). Evaluation of staff training in group homes for retarded persons. *American Journal of Mental Deficiency, 82,* 130–136.

Sheppard, W.C., Shank, S.B., & Wilson, D. (1973). *Teaching social behavior to young children.* Champaign, IL: Research Press.

Sugai, D.P. (1982). *Covert rehearsal and cue-controlled relaxation: Three case studies.* Paper presented at the meeting of the Association for the Advancement of Behavior Therapy, Los Angeles, CA.

Sugai, D.P. (1983a). *The treatment of the disorder in children using covert rehearsal and cue-contingent relaxation.* Paper presented at the meeting of the Association for the Advancement of Behavior Therapy, Washington, DC.

Suagi, D.P. (1983b). *Behavioral assessment and treatment of psychogenic failure-to-thrive: Three case studies.* Paper presented at the meeting of the Association for the Advancement of Behavior Therapy, Washington, DC.

Sugai, D.P., & Benedetto, L. (1985). *Treatment of encopresis related to chronic constipation and emesis in young children using cue-contingent distraction techniques.* Paper presented at the meeting of the Association for the Advancement of Behavior Therapy, Houston, TX.

Tharp, R.G., & Wetzel, R.J. (1969). *Behavior modification in the natural environment.* New York: Academic Press.

Thoresen, C.E. (1971). *Training behavioral counselors.* Paper presented at Third Banff International Conference on Behavior Modification.

Williams, C.L., Carter, B.J., Arnold, C.B., & Wynder, E.L. (1979). Chronic disease risk factors among children: The "Know Your Body" study. *Journal of Chronic Diseases, 32,* 505–513.

Zigler, E., & Muenchow, S. (1979). Mainstreaming: The proof is in the implementation. *American Psychologist, 34,* 993–996.

Author Index

Subject Index